ADVANCES IN NEUROLOGY
VOLUME 17

Advances in Neurology

INTERNATIONAL ADVISORY BOARD

Advances in Neurology
Volume 17

Treatment of Neuromuscular Diseases

Edited by

Robert C. Griggs, M.D.
Departments of Neurology,
Medicine, Pathology, and Pediatrics
University of Rochester
Rochester, New York

Richard T. Moxley, III, M.D.
Departments of Neurology and
Pediatrics
University of Rochester
Rochester, New York

Raven Press ▪ New York

Raven Press, 1140 Avenue of the Americas, New York, New York 10036

Made in the United States of America

International Standard Book Number 0-89004-113-x
Library of Congress Catalog Card Number 75-43197

Library of Congress Cataloging in Publication Data
Main entry under title:

Treatment of neuromuscular diseases.

    (Advances in neurology; v. 17)
    Bibliography
    Includes index.
    1. Neuromuscular diseases — Congresses. I. Griggs,
Robert C. II. Moxley, Richard T. III. Series.
[DNLM: 1. Neuromuscular diseases — Therapy — Congresses.
2. Neuromuscular diseases — Diagnosis — Congresses. W1
AD684H v. 17 / WE550 T784 1976]
RC321.A276   vol. 17   [RC925] 616.8'08s [616.7'4]   75-43197
ISBN 0-89004-113-X

Foreword

This volume on the Treatment of Neuromuscular Diseases coincides with the fiftieth anniversary of the University of Rochester School of Medicine, the twenty-fifth anniversary of the founding of the Muscular Dystrophy Association Clinic at Rochester, and the tenth anniversary of the establishment of the Department of Neurology at the medical school.

Fifty years ago, there was almost nothing known about muscle disease except for the clinical descriptions and some broad classifications of the muscle dystrophies. Twenty-five years ago, steroid therapy was becoming popular, and it was found effective in the then-named menopausal muscular dystrophy which proved to be inflammatory. Ten years ago, more specific mechanisms for the muscle disorders were being found with the fructifying union of biochemistry, physiology, immunology, and neurology.

A few years ago, it would have been an impertinence to discuss treatment of these disorders. It will become obvious that great strides have taken place, but it will be equally obvious that we have a way to go. New treatments will come only as we come to understand the basic mechanisms of normal and abnormal neuromuscular function. The arrangement of this symposium emphasizes the logical move from disordered structure and function to efforts to correct these abnormalities.

Robert J. Joynt, M.D., Ph.D.
Professor and Chairman
Department of Neurology
University of Rochester School of
Medicine and Dentistry

Preface

This volume commemorates the 50th anniversary of the University of Rochester School of Medicine and Dentistry.

It presents information on the evaluation and management of patients with neuromuscular diseases, as well as a review of areas of research likely to lead to advances in the treatment and understanding of these conditions. Introductory chapters focus on the approach to the neuromuscular diseases and the evaluation of the weak patient. Subsequent chapters review the management of those neuromuscular diseases for which treatment is available including myasthenia gravis, polymyositis, dermatomyositis, periodic paralysis, myotonia, and neuropathies. Genetic counseling is discussed and the management of pulmonary, cardiac, and orthopedic complications of the progressive neuromuscular diseases is reviewed. Additional sections present an overview of areas of investigation likely to lead to new therapy for neuromuscular diseases including discussions of immunologic, histologic, electrophysiologic, biochemical, and metabolic studies.

The volume is not intended to be a comprehensive text on either clinical or investigative aspects of neuromuscular disease but to serve as a "state of the art" discussion of current and future therapy. The volume is written by clinicians and investigators experienced in all aspects of the treatment of neuromuscular disease and is aimed at the physician who sees patients with neuromuscular disease as either a major or occasional portion of his practice. It is also pertinent for those with a special investigative interest in neuromuscular disease since much of the work is either previously unpublished or unavailable in a single source.

The Editors

Advances in Neurology Series

Contents

Contributors

Michael H. Brooke
Department of Neurology and Jerry Lewis Neuromuscular Research Center
Washington University School of Medicine
St. Louis, Missouri 63110

Mark J. Brown
Department of Neurology
Hospital of the University of Pennsylvania
Philadelphia, Pennsylvania 19104

Christopher Clark
H. Houston Merritt Clinical Research Center for Muscular Dystrophy and Related Diseases
Department of Neurology
College of Physicians and Surgeons
Columbia University
and
Neurological Institute of the Presbyterian Hospital
New York, New York 10032

Jules Cohen
Cardiology Unit
Department of Medicine
University of Rochester School of Medicine and Dentistry
Rochester, New York 14642

Salvatore DiMauro
H. Houston Merritt Clinical Research Center for Muscular Dystrophy and Related Diseases
College of Physicians and Surgeons
Columbia University
and
Neurological Institute
Presbyterian Hospital
New York, New York 10032

Peter James Dyck
Department of Neurology
Mayo Clinic and Mayo Foundation
Rochester, Minnesota 55901

Abraham B. Eastwood
H. Houston Merritt Clinical Research Center for Muscular Dystrophy and Related Diseases
College of Physicians and Surgeons
Columbia University
and
Neurological Institute
Presbyterian Hospital
New York, New York 10032

W. King Engel
National Institutes of Neurological and Communicate Disorders and Stroke
National Institutes of Health
Bethesda, Maryland 20014

David Goldblatt
Department of Neurology
University of Rochester School of Medicine and Dentistry
Rochester, New York 14642

Robert C. Griggs
Departments of Neurology, Medicine, Pathology, and Pediatrics
University of Rochester School of Medicine and Dentistry
Rochester, New York 14642

William J. Hall
Departments of Medicine and Pediatrics
University of Rochester School of Medicine and Dentistry
Rochester, New York 14642

T. R. Johns
Department of Neurology
University of Virginia Jerry Lewis
*   Neuromuscular Center*
University of Virginia
Charlottesville, Virginia 22904

William R. Markesbery
Departments of Neurology and Pathol-
*   ogy*
University of Kentucky College of
*   Medicine*
Lexington, Kentucky 40506

Michael P. McQuillen
Department of Neurology
The Medical College of Wisconsin
Milwaukee, Wisconsin 53226

Richard T. Moxley, III
Departments of Neurology and Pedi-
*   atrics*
University of Rochester School of
*   Medicine and Dentistry*
Rochester, New York 14642

Gary J. Myers
Departments of Pediatrics, Neurology,
*   and Obstetrics and Gynecology*
University of Rochester School of
*   Medicine and Dentistry*
Rochester, New York 14620

Marcelo Olarte
H. Houston Merritt Clinical Research
*   Center for Muscular Dystrophy and*
*   Related Diseases*
Department of Neurology
College of Physicians and Surgeons
Columbia University
and
Neurological Institute of the Presby-
*   terian Hospital*
New York, New York 10032

Audrey S. Penn
H. Houston Merritt Clinical Research
*   Center for Muscular Dystrophy and*
*   Related Diseases*
Department of Neurology
College of Physicians and Surgeons
Columbia University
and
Neurological Institute of the Presby-
*   terian Hospital*
New York, New York 10032

Lewis P. Rowland
H. Houston Merritt Clinical Research
*   Center for Muscular Dystrophy and*
*   Related Diseases*
Department of Neurology
College of Physicians and Surgeons
Columbia University
and
Neurological Institute of the Presby-
*   terian Hospital*
New York, New York 10032

Peter T. Rowley
Departments of Medicine, Pediatrics,
*   and Microbiology*
University of Rochester Medical Cen-
*   ter*
Rochester, New York 14642

Irwin M. Siegel
Department of Orthopaedic Surgery
*   and Muscle Disease Clinic*
Strauss Surgical Group Associates
L. A. Weiss Memorial Hospital
and
Department of Orthopaedic Surgery
Abraham Lincoln School of Medicine
and
Muscle Disease Clinic
University of Illinois
Chicago, Illinois 60612

Advances in Neurology, Vol. 17, edited by
R. C. Griggs and R. T. Moxley, III. Raven Press,
New York © 1977.

Perspectives on the Treatment of Neuromuscular Disease

Robert C. Griggs

*Departments of Neurology, Medicine, and Pediatrics, University of Rochester
School of Medicine and Dentistry, Rochester, New York 14642*

INTRODUCTION

The contributors to this volume consider recent major advances in the treatment of the neuromuscular diseases. This chapter presents a brief overview of the classification of neuromuscular disease and summarizes the approach to the patient suspected of having neuromuscular disease in the light of current therapy. A number of considerations in the management of neuromuscular disease not discussed elsewhere in the volume are reviewed briefly. The following chapter by Moxley highlights those research areas in which significant therapeutic advances may be looked for in the near future.

CLASSIFICATION OF THE NEUROMUSCULAR DISEASES

The traditional subdivision of the motor unit into four parts, although oversimplified and perhaps naive in the light of current speculation as to etiology of a number of so-called myopathies, has merit in providing an approach to the diagnosis and evaluation of patients with neuromuscular disease. Table 1 summarizes the clinical features of characteristic examples of (a) anterior horn cell disease, (b) peripheral neuropathy, (c) neuromuscular junction disease, and (d) myopathy. It should be noted that the anterior horn cell, the peripheral nerve, and the proximal portion of the neuromuscular junction are, in fact, all part of one cell—the anterior horn cell and its peripheral extension. The subdivision into the four traditional categories of neuromuscular disease is, therefore, somewhat arbitrary, and it has been increasingly recognized that a defect apparently limited to the distal portion of the anterior horn cell may, in fact, reflect more proximal pathology in the neuron.

The classification of neuromuscular diseases into these categories has been based on specific electromyographic and muscle biopsy patterns. This has in large part been due to a meager basic understanding of the etiology of these conditions. Nonetheless, because disease nosology has been drawn

1

TABLE 1. *Classification of the neuromuscular diseases*

Site of involvement	Anterior horn cell	Peripheral nerve	Neuromuscular junction	Muscle
Example	Amyotrophic lateral sclerosis	Nutritional neuropathy	Myasthenia gravis	Polymyositis
Distribution of weakness	Asymmetric limb or bulbar	Symmetrical distal	Extraocular, bulbar, proximal limb	Symmetrical proximal limb, bulbar
Atrophy	Marked early	Moderate	Usually slight	Slight early, severe late
Sensory symptoms	Cramps	Paresthesias, hypoesthesia	None	Aching
Characteristic features	Fasciculations	Tremor	Diurnal fluctuation	
Reflexes	Variable (depends on degree of upper motor neuron involvement)	Decreased out of proportion to strength	Normal	Parallel strength

along these lines, it is reasonable to maintain this subdivision if only as a framework for discussion of evaluation and management.

RECOGNITION OF NEUROMUSCULAR DISEASE

Physicians experienced in the diagnosis of neuromuscular diseases have come to realize that the most difficult part of the management of neuromuscular disease is recognizing the appropriate diagnostic category for a given patient. Thus, a large number of patients are seen with complaints of "weakness," "cramps," or "stiffness," which defy specific diagnosis. On the other hand, a smaller but impressive number of patients endure true cramps, myoglobinuria, fatigue, myotonia, or other symptoms and are subjected to the hazards of general anesthesia, contraindicated medications, or severe exercise during athletic or military training without diagnosis being established.

Symptoms Suggesting Neuromuscular Disease

"Weakness," the finding common to the majority of neuromuscular diseases, is surprisingly uncommon as a chief complaint. Patients more characteristically complain of an inability to perform a specific activity at home or work, such as lifting an object of specific weight that previously was easily managed, rising from a chair, or climbing a flight of stairs. In children, parents may note that a child does not achieve specific motor skills at an age comparable to his peers or older siblings. Although a complaint of "weakness" or "fatigue" can occur in myasthenia gravis and occasionally in other neuromuscular diseases, such complaints more commonly reflect a cause outside the motor unit such as anemia, congestive heart failure, or depression. Limb weakness is often of insidious onset whereas ocular and bulbar weakness is more often abrupt in presentation since a deficit such as diplopia, dysphonia, dysphagia, or ptosis is difficult to ignore for more than a brief time.

If the history supports a loss of muscle function, a number of complaints are important including (a) diurnal fluctuation in strength, (b) pain, (c) cramps, (d) stiffness, (e) fasciculations, and (f) paresthesias. Fluctuation in strength is characteristic of disorders of neuromuscular transmission in which strength is usually worse later in the day. Muscle pain, cramps, or stiffness are surprisingly uncommon in diseases of muscle, although they may occur in a minority of patients with dermatomyositis or polymyositis and characteristically in disorders of glycogen and lipid metabolism. Pain and cramps are more often seen in patients with anterior horn cell or peripheral nerve disease. Fasciculations in a weak patient are usually indicative of anterior horn cell or less commonly peripheral neuropathic disease. Paresthesias point to peripheral neuropathy but may also occur in the Eaton-Lambert syndrome. As isolated presenting complaints, however, symptoms such as fatigue, pain, cramps, and fasciculations do not usually indicate neuromuscular disease. Thus, although patients with diseases of the neuromuscular junction such as myasthenia gravis or the Eaton-Lambert syndrome characteristically have fatigue, this complaint in isolation also indicates disease remote from the neuromuscular system. Muscle pain, cramps, or stiffness are often without clear diagnostic significance, and fasciculations are often benign in the patient without weakness.

Inability to establish diagnosis in patients with these complaints may not necessarily indicate that no disease is present. In fact, patients with the recently characterized disorders such as the glycogen and lipid storage disease discussed by DiMauro and Eastwood (*this volume*) defied diagnosis until quite recently and were often felt to have complaints on a psychogenic basis. The existence of forme frustes of a number of neuromuscular diseases such as myotonic dystrophy, facioscapulohumeral dystrophy, and Fabry's disease should also raise concern that patients with undiagnosed complaints could represent such a situation. Similarly, the recent recognition that occasional carriers of neuromuscular disease such as Duchenne and Becker dystrophy may manifest moderately severe features of the illness (22,24) raises the possibility that heterozygotes of other recessive conditions could have moderate and undiagnosable symptoms.

In addition to those complaints clearly referable to the neuromuscular system, a number of other clinical findings should raise the possibility of neuromuscular disease, including (a) skeletal deformity, such as scoliosis, club foot, or pes cavus; (b) unexplained dyspnea owing to respiratory insufficiency; and (c) cardiac disease suspected to be related to myopathy. Neuromuscular diseases with multisystem involvement, such as myotonic dystrophy or the collagen diseases, may also present with complaints outside the peripheral neuromuscular system. Often the symptoms point to pathology in the central nervous system, joints, eyes, or elsewhere.

Examination of the Patient with Neuromuscular Disease

Patient examination is considered in detail by Brooke (*this volume*). He emphasizes the activities that normal individuals can perform and stresses functional testing of patients in these activities. "Formal testing" using the Medical Research Council 0 to 5 scale is often difficult to interpret in terms of the question, "Is weakness present?" Formal testing is notoriously unreliable in sequential follow-up of a patient, and although sometimes helpful, it should never substitute for functional testing. Functional testing permits (a) reproducible evaluation by more than one examiner; (b) assessment of strength by history (for example, by telephone); (c) allowance for differences because of age, size, gender, and to some extent, physical conditioning; and (d) sequential follow-up during therapeutic trial. A system of sequential functional testing such as that described by Brooke is essential for the evaluation of any patient with neuromuscular disease undergoing treatment.

Laboratory Evaluation

As summarized in Table 2, evaluation of patients with neuromuscular disease is directed toward determining: (a) which of the four categories of neuromuscular diseases best describes the patient; and (b) what specific condition in this category he resembles. To answer these questions, one must perform certain laboratory evaluations. All patients should have serum "muscle enzyme" determinations (serum glutamic oxaloacetic transaminase, lactate dehydrogenase, and creatine phosphokinase), electrocardiogram, and a screening pulmonary function test. Most should have electrophysiological studies as discussed by McQuillen (*this volume*). Muscle biopsy (see Chapter 10) and nerve biopsy (see Chapter 14) are indicated in selected patients. Taken together, these tests usually permit determination of whether an illness is due to muscle or nerve disease. A number of other specific tests may be indicated in selected cases such as immunologic studies, endocrine evaluation, or metabolic studies.

In the patient with a potentially treatable neuromuscular disease, laboratory criteria to permit sequential follow-up are of obvious importance. Although most of the diagnostic techniques summarized in Table 2 permit some degree of reliability for sequential follow-up during the treatment, several have marked limitations. Muscle biopsy, for example, represents only a relatively small number of fibers, and marked variation can occur because of sampling error (1). Even within muscles sampled from the same patient at the same time, muscle pathology can vary from normal to severely abnormal in adjacent sites or in identical muscles from different limbs. Nerve conductions (10) and creatine phosphokinase (16) similarly have a considerable degree of spontaneous variation that has not been well characterized for many conditions. Thus, there remains a need for additional criteria for the sequential follow-up of the course of neuromuscular disease in terms of both following therapy and documenting the natural history of illness.

SUMMARY OF THE MANAGEMENT OF THE NEUROMUSCULAR DISEASES

Anterior Horn Cell

Although none of the anterior horn cell diseases is amenable to specific therapy, much can be done to help patients with these diseases.

TABLE 2. *Laboratory evaluation of patients with neuromuscular disease — characteristic findings*

Site of involvement	Anterior horn cell	Peripheral neuropathy	Neuromuscular junction	Myopathies
Example	Amyotrophic lateral sclerosis	Nutritional neuropathy	Myasthenia gravis	Polymyositis
Creatine phosphokinase	Normal or slightly elevated	Normal	Normal	Elevated
Electromyography	Recruited motor units, number decreased; size and duration increased; spontaneous activity marked	Recruited motor units, number normal or decreased; size and duration often increased; spontaneous activity usually abnormal	Recruited motor units, normal number initially; size and duration normal; spontaneous activity normal	Motor units recruited more rapidly than normal, size of potential decreased; spontaneous activity occasionally abnormal
Motor nerve conduction velocity	Early — normal	Usually normal or slightly slowed in axonal neuropathy — usually slowed in demyelinating neuropathy	Normal	Normal
Repetitive nerve stimulation	Usually normal	Usually normal	Decremental response	Normal
Muscle biopsy	Early — single-fiber atrophy; late — grouped atrophy, fiber type grouping	Same as anterior horn cell although grouped atrophy less striking	Variable — slight or moderate atrophy frequent	Muscle necrosis, phagocytosis; inflammatory reaction

AMYOTROPHIC LATERAL SCLEROSIS

As indicated by Goldblatt (*this volume*), there is no specific therapy for this disorder, which is the commonest of the anterior horn cell diseases. Although supportive treatment can prolong life and minimize complications, the major role of the physician, at least in initial management, is to exclude possible treatable diseases. Advanced amyotrophic lateral sclerosis is distinctive and precludes any differential diagnosis. However, early in its course, it may resemble cervical spinal cord disease, conditions with increased parathormone, or recurrent hypoglycemia. Diseases of anterior horn cell mimicking amyotrophic lateral sclerosis have been observed in association with previous poliomyelitis, lead poisoning, and irreversible anticholinesterase poisoning. These entities have not proved to be much more treatable than amyotrophic lateral sclerosis itself, but their prognosis is less dire. Occasional patients with amyotrophic lateral sclerosis may have myasthenic features (15), but neither anticholinesterase medication nor guanidine has been associated with prolonged benefit. A trial of these agents has been recommended by some (11).

Infantile Spinal Muscular Atrophy (Werdnig-Hoffmann Disease)

As discussed by Myers (*this volume*), neuromuscular disease in the infant presents as a hypotonic, floppy baby. Since Werdnig-Hoffmann disease is untreatable and progresses to death in the majority of cases within several years, the most important point in management of the patient is establishing the diagnosis. This condition is usually autosomal recessive and is likely to recur in subsequent pregnancies. As with amyotrophic lateral sclerosis, it is also important to exclude the large number of disorders such as the congenital myopathies (6) and congenital fiber type dysproportion (5), which can simulate Werdnig-Hoffmann disease but have a much more benign prognosis.

Juvenile Spinal Muscular Atrophy (Kugelberg-Welander Disease)

Juvenile spinal muscular atrophy can simulate slowly progressive muscular dystrophy and is without specific treatment. It is, however, amenable to orthopedic and pulmonary management of complications as discussed for the muscular dystrophies. It is of particular importance to identify patients with this condition to avoid the error of mistakenly calling this condition Duchenne dystrophy. Not only is the prognosis for Kugelberg-Welander disease more benign, but the hereditary pattern is usually autosomal recessive or occasionally autosomal dominant. Genetic counseling of females and others within the family is vastly different than for Duchenne dystrophy.

Peripheral Neuropathy

Brown (*this volume*) presents an overview of the neuropathies, emphasizing those in which specific therapy is available. Even in those without specific therapy, bracing and reconstructive surgery (25) may be helpful for distal weakness and deformity. Patients with sensory deficit require careful attention to the potential for perforating ulcers and subsequent infection. Neurotrophic (Charcot) joints must be sought since they also carry a risk of skin ulceration and infection (23).

Neuromuscular Junction Disease

MYASTHENIA GRAVIS

As discussed by Johns (*this volume*), corticosteroid therapy has revolutionized the treatment of myasthenia gravis. Although anticholinesterase agents and thymectomy remain of major importance in the treatment of myasthenia gravis, corticosteroids have proved beneficial in a majority of patients unresponsive to other forms of therapy. Immunosuppressive therapy has been widely used in Europe with some success (13) but has received only limited trial in this country.

EATON-LAMBERT SYNDROME

Another form of myoneural junction disease, the Eaton-Lambert or myasthenic syndrome, is noteworthy for its dramatic therapeutic response to guanidine hydrochloride (20). The toxicity of guanidine is being increasingly well characterized in view of the large experience in therapeutic trials with amyotrophic lateral sclerosis (17) and includes weakness and liver, marrow, and nervous system toxicity (18). It should be noted that guanidine therapy, although occasionally successful in myasthenia gravis, usually has a deleterious effect and indicates the need for careful distinction between this disease and the Eaton-Lambert syndrome (2).

Myopathies

The major treatable myopathies are considered in detail in this volume. They include Rowland and co-workers' discussion of dermatomyositis and polymyositis, Griggs's commentary on myotonic disorders and periodic paralysis, and DiMauro and Eastwood's description of lipid storage myopathies. Moxley considers endocrine aspects of muscle disease, and it bears emphasis that proximal weakness can complicate virtually any endocrine gland hypo- or hyperfunction. The treatment of these disorders is that of the underlying endocrinopathy. Whether these conditions represent myopathy or neuropathy is open to considerable question since usual biochemical and histologic changes of myopathy are absent (21). Similarly, each of the collagen vascular diseases can be associated with proximal weakness. In some patients, this weakness is caused by an inflammatory myopathy typical of polymyositis. In others, the basis for the weakness is unclear. As with endocrine-related neuromuscular disease, the treatment of these "myopathies" is usually that of the underlying collagen disease. The treatment of polymyalgia rheumatica and associated giant cell arteritis is well detailed elsewhere (8). There is increasing evidence that this condition is, in fact, an inflammatory disease of joints. Signs of joint effusion in symptomatic joints by isotopic scanning are seen in virtually all patients (19). Usual laboratory criteria for muscle disease are absent in this condition, and it appears that the disorder involves the joints rather than muscle.

Undiagnosed Proximal Weakness

A substantial number of patients with proximal weakness defy specific diagnosis. In the absence of a positive family history, a diagnosis of chronic polymyositis is always difficult to exclude since although the criteria for the classic case are quite good (1) diagnostic criteria remain hazy in atypical patients. In the treatment of chronic disabling proximal weakness of adulthood or childhood, the question usually comes down to a decision about whether or not to use a trial of corticosteroids. As Rowland et al. (*this volume*) discussed, even the treatment of classic dermatomyositis or polymyositis is fraught with difficulty because of complications of corticosteroids. Treatment of less easily characterized patients is even more challenging.

THE MUSCULAR DYSTROPHIES

Despite advances in understanding the etiology of muscular dystrophies as described by Moxley, the four major muscular dystrophies—Duchenne dystrophy, myotonic dystrophy, facioscapulohumeral dystrophy, and limb-girdle dystrophy—remain without specific treatment. As discussed in the chapter on the myotonic disorders, certain features of myotonic dystrophy are treatable, but the progressive weakness of this, as for the other dystrophies, is not amenable to therapy. As Rowley (*this volume*) discussed, the incidence of the X-linked disease Duchenne dystrophy can be reduced by carrier detection or antenatal sexing of the fetus. Similarly, a proportion of cases of myotonic dystrophy can be diagnosed antenatally using genetic linkage studies (9).

OCULOPHARYNGEAL MUSCULAR DYSTROPHY

The relatively rare condition oculopharyngeal dystrophy is treatable in terms of its major manifestations. This condition is characterized by ptosis, ophthalmoparesis, dysphagia, and slight extremity weakness. Typically starting after age 40, it is particularly prevalent in French-Canadians and in Spanish-Americans in the southwestern United States. The ptosis can be corrected by operative procedures (3). A Silastic suspension sling of the upper eyelid appears to be the most satisfactory approach since (a) operative procedure is minimal, (b) ptosis less commonly recurs than after plastic procedures involving resection of lid, and (c) the lid elevation can be reversed by simple removal of the suspending Silastic loop (thus permitting lowering of the lid if exposure keratitis occurs).

Dysphagia, the other major manifestation of oculopharyngeal dystrophy, is also amenable to surgical correction. Dysphagia is usually associated with a cricopharyngeus muscular functional constriction of the hypopharynx, which impedes the progress of the bolus of food from mouth to esophagus. Section of the cricopharyngeus muscle is often totally curative of the dysphagia (14). A similar surgically correctable "constriction" can occur in other neuromuscular diseases including dermatomyositis and the bulbar palsy associated with motor neuron disease.

Management of Complications of Myopathies

Treatment of pulmonary, cardiac, and orthopedic manifestations of the muscular dystrophies, in particular Duchenne dystrophy, is discussed in this volume by Hall, Cohen, and Siegel, respectively, and much can be done to prolong mobility and maintain health in these patients.

CORTICOSTEROID THERAPY

Side effects of corticosteroids reviewed in detail elsewhere (12) present a major limitation for their use in any chronic disease. Although one cannot withhold corticosteroid treatment from a bed- or respiratory-dependent patient with myasthenia gravis, the treatment of ocular or other relatively restricted forms of myasthenia gravis must be undertaken with caution. The most disabling side effects of corticosteroids include osteoporosis, myopathy, glucose intolerance, and decreased resistance to infection. Cosmetic problems such as striae, obesity, and hirsutism may have profound psychological implications. Cataracts are less of a problem since they can be removed. The relationship of ulcer disease to corticosteroids is presently unclear (4). Virtually all side effects of corticosteroids continue to occur, although with reduced frequency and severity, in patients on alternate-day therapy (12). The possibility that the osteopenia and likelihood of bony collapse related to corticosteroids can be reduced by the concomitant administration of calcium and vitamin D may represent a major advance in the treatment of patients with neuromuscular disease (7).

The paradox of having to treat proximal weakness with an agent that causes proximal weakness remains a clinical dilemma. It seems likely that even in patients improving rapidly on corticosteroid therapy, some degree of steroid atrophy may develop. In chronically treated patients, such atrophy is virtually assured. Avoidance of the particular troublesome 9-alpha fluorinated agents such as triamcinolone may lessen the severity of this atrophy.

Because of the toxicity of corticosteroids, the decision to introduce these agents must always be balanced against the possible benefit to be derived. The modest weakness of even a proven polymyositis may not warrant the large doses of corticosteroids necessary to alter the course of the illness.

REFERENCES

1. Bohan, A., and Peter, J. B. (1975): Polymyositis and dermatomyositis. *N. Engl. J. Med.,* 292:344–347, 403–407.
2. Brown, J. C., and Johns, R. J. (1969): Clinical and physiological studies of the effect of guanidine on patients with myasthenia gravis. *Johns Hopkins Med. J.,* 124:1.
3. Callahan, A. (1966): *Reconstructive Surgery of the Eyelids and Ocular Adnexa,* pp. 98–99. Aesculapius Publishing Co., Birmingham, Alabama.
4. Conn, H. O., and Blitzer, B. L. (1976): Nonassociation of adrenocorticosteroid therapy and peptic ulcers. *N. Engl. J. Med.,* 294:473–479.
5. Dubowitz, V., and Brooke, M. H. (1973): Muscle biopsy: A modern approach. In: *Major Problems in Neurology, Vol. 2,* pp. 280–283. W. B. Saunders Co., Philadelphia.
6. Greenfield, J. G., Cornman, T., and Shy, G. M. (1958): The prognostic value of the muscle biopsy in the "floppy infant." *Brain,* 81:461–484.
7. Hahn, B., and Hahn, T. (1976): Reduction of steroid osteopenia by treatment with 25 OH vitamin D and calcium. *Arthritis Rheum.,* 19:800.
8. Hunder, G. G., Sheps, S. G., Allen, G. L., and Joyce, J. W. (1975): Daily and alternate-day corticosteroid regimens in treatment of giant cell arteritis. *Ann. Intern. Med.,* 82:613–618.
9. Insley, J., Bird, G. W. G., Harper, P. S., and Pearce, G. W. (1976): Prenatal prediction of myotonic dystrophy. *Lancet,* 1:806.
10. Kominami, N., Tyler, H. R., Hampers, C. L., and Merrill, J. P. (1971): Variations in motor nerve conduction velocity in normal and uremic patients. *Arch. Intern. Med.,* 128:235–239.
11. Liversedge, L. A., and Campbell, M. J. (1974): Motor neurone diseases. In: *Disorders of Voluntary Muscle, 3rd Ed.,* edited by J. N. Walton, pp. 790–791. Churchill Livingstone, London.
12. Melby, J. C. (1974): Systemic corticosteroid therapy: pharmacologic and endocrinologic considerations. *Ann. Intern. Med.,* 81:505–512.
13. Mertens, H. G., Balzereit, M., and Leipert, M. (1969): The treatment of severe myasthenia gravis with immunosuppressive agents. *Eur. Neurol.,* 2:321.
14. Mills, C. P. (1973): Dysphagia in pharyngeal paralysis treated by cricopharyngeal sphincterotomy. *Lancet,* 1:455.
15. Mulder, D. W., Lambert, E. H., and Eaton, L. M. (1959): Myasthenic syndrome in patients with amyotrophic lateral sclerosis. *Neurology (Minneap.),* 9:627.
16. Munsat, T. L., Baloh, R., Pearson, C. M., and Fowler, W. (1973): Serum enzyme alterations in neuromuscular disorders. *J.A.M.A.,* 226:1536–1543.

17. Norris, F. H. (1973): Guanidine in amyotrophic lateral sclerosis. *N. Engl. J. Med.,* 288:690.
18. Norris, F. H., Eaton, J. M., and Mielke, C. H. (1974): Depression of bone marrow by guanidine. *Arch. Neurol.,* 30:184–185.
19. O'Duffy, J. D., Wahner, H. W., and Hunder, G. G. (1976): Joint imaging in polymyalgia rheumatica. *Mayo Clin. Proc.,* 51:519–524.
20. Oh, S. J., and Kim, K. W. (1973): Guanidine hydrochloride in the Lambert-Eaton syndrome. *Neurology (Minneap.),* 23:1084–1090.
21. Patten, B. M., Bilezikian, J. P., Mallette, L. E., Prince, A., Engel, W. K., and Aurbach, G. D. (1974): Neuromuscular disease in primary hyperparathyroidism. *Ann. Intern. Med.,* 80:182–193.
22. Roses, A. D., Roses, M. J., Miller, S. E., Hull, K. L., and Appel, S. H. (1976): Carrier detection in Duchenne muscular dystrophy. *N. Engl. J. Med.,* 294:193–198.
23. Sinha, S., Munichoodappa, C. S., and Kozak, G. P. (1972): Neuroarthropathy (Charcot joints) in diabetes mellitus. *Medicine (Baltimore),* 51:191–210.
24. Skinner, R. (1974): Becker muscular dystrophy—clinical and genetic studies. *Excerpta Medica,* 334:89.
25. Stillwell, G. K. (1975): Rehabilitation procedures. In: *Peripheral Neuropathy, Vol. II,* edited by P. J. Dyck, P. K. Thomas, and E. H. Lambert. W. B. Saunders Co., Philadelphia.

Advances in Neurology, Vol. 17, edited by
R. C. Griggs and R. T. Moxley, III. Raven Press,
New York © 1977.

Research Trends Pertinent to the Management of Neuromuscular Diseases

Richard T. Moxley, III

Departments of Neurology and Pediatrics, University of Rochester School of Medicine and Dentistry, Rochester, New York 14642

INTRODUCTION

This chapter reviews recent research trends in the study of neuromuscular diseases. Other chapters in this volume discuss specific research approaches and they are referenced in the text. This review highlights the recent experimental work that may lead to advances in the prevention and treatment of neuromuscular diseases.

The pathophysiology of most diseases affecting muscles is unclear. Numerous investigative approaches are being pursued, but most fall within one of the categories of: (a) nerve-muscle interaction, (b) cell membrane and intracellular regulation, (c) vascular supply to nerve and muscle, or (d) axonal transport. This chapter discusses each of these four categories including the specific disease states in each category. Experimental findings have been selected for each specific disease state within a given category to indicate the recent research progress that is being made in the study of that disease. At the same time, speculation has been included to suggest a connection between the research observations and their therapeutic implications. Many of the studies mentioned in the discussion of these four areas provide information very likely to influence the management of patients, whereas other investigations give a new vantage point from which to view disease pathophysiology.

NERVE-MUSCLE CELL INTERACTION

Muscular Dystrophies

An important trophic nerve-muscle interaction has been well known for years (17,24). Recently research interest in this relationship has been stimulated by the neurogenic theory of the etiology of muscular dystrophy (36,37). Electrophysiologic studies by McComas and co-workers have suggested a neural etiology for several muscular dystrophies. These researchers have reported a loss of functioning motor units in Duchenne dystrophy and in limb-girdle, facioscapulohumeral, and myotonic muscular dystrophy, which they have attributed to "sick" nerve supply (38). This neural etiology hypothesis has received support from animal experiments, which have indicated the vital role of the motor nerve supply in determining the characteristics of the skeletal muscle it supplies. Buller and colleagues (8) as well as other researchers (44), have demonstrated in cross-innervation studies using normal rats that whether a muscle fiber is red or white is determined by the nerve supply. Salafsky (46) and more recently Dubowitz and Neerunjun (40) have shown that when normal or dystrophic muscle is transplanted into a normal mouse, it will regenerate with the dystrophic muscle retaining its dystrophic characteristics. However, when normal or dystrophic muscle is implanted into a dystrophic host, there is no regeneration. These results have suggested that neurons are by themselves capable of producing the myopathic state in muscle.

Despite the interesting experimental observations just noted, there are conflicting data. For example, Cosmos and Douglas (12) have evaluated the response of normal and dystrophic mouse muscle to cross-innervation from mouse sciatic nerve. Preliminary observations have demonstrated no significant difference in muscle weight or histochemical appearance in normal versus dystrophic muscle, regardless of whether the sciatic nerve came from a normal or dystrophic litter mate. Based on their experimental findings, Cosmos and Douglas have offered two alternative hypotheses to the neurogenic etiology theory. They suggest that dystrophic muscle itself may be unable to receive neural input in a normal manner or that dystrophic muscle fails to transmit a trophic substance centripetally to attract properly the peripherally growing terminals of motor neurons. Caution is necessary when considering the animal experiments mentioned in this and the preceding paragraph. No exactly analogous animal model for any of the human muscular dystrophies is available. Any conclusions about the etiology of a particular muscular dystrophy that come from animal studies require careful validation in patients.

Two separate recent investigations of myoneural junction appearance in human muscular dystrophies (14) and (**W. R. Markesbery,** *this volume*) have also questioned the nerve cell etiology of these disorders. The chapter by Markesbery describes the light and electron microscopic findings in the common muscular dystrophies, and emphasizes that the changes are nonspecific and do not point clearly to a neural etiology.

A report by Drachman and Fambrough (14) raises further questions about the neural etiology. Their results indicate that in denervating states such as amyotrophic lateral sclerosis, the skeletal muscle outside the myoneural junction area develops a marked increase in the number of receptor sites for acetylcholine. This increase in extrajunctional acetycholine receptors has been generally accepted as an indication of denervation (4,32,48). None of the nine myotonic dystrophy patients they have studied showed an increase in extrajunctional acetylcholine receptor sites. Their observations do not support the hypothesis of a neurogenic etiology to myopathic muscle changes.

As these selected articles indicate, the role of nerve supply to muscle in the causation of various muscular dystrophies is unclear. If a specific neural etiology for any of the muscular dystrophies can be determined, therapeutic agents directed toward correcting abnormal nerve metabolism or restoring proper nerve cell structure will become an obvious area for pharmacologic research.

Lower Motor Neuron Disorders

Motor denervating diseases (anterior horn cell and peripheral neuropathy) represent another area in which research on nerve-muscle interaction continues to be of paramount importance. McQuillen (*this volume*) has reviewed the most recent electrodiagnostic techniques that are used in studying the pathophysiology of neuromuscular diseases.

Stalberg and co-workers (47) in the past few years have been using a technique that records the electrical activity in individual muscle fibers (47). One application of this technique has been to evaluate the pattern of firing of individual muscle fibers by the terminal nerve branches of a single motor neuron. This allows an estimation of the variability in time required for the contraction of the individual muscle fibers that compose a motor unit. This variability has been called "jitter" (47). This technique can be used to study any disease that affects the size or pattern of firing of a motor unit. Stalberg et al. have demonstrated in their work that there is a great variation in the time necessary to fire each muscle of a myasthenic motor unit. This single-fiber recording technique may prove valuable in following the reinnervation that occurs during the recovery phase of many neuropathic disorders (49).

The nature of the trophic influence of nerve on muscle continues to be studied by research on the denervation of muscle in animal models. Investigations by Thesleff (48) have described specific changes in rat skeletal muscle that occur within the first several days after denervation. Before any obvious sign of atrophy in the muscle, there are striking changes in its electrophysiologic characteristics. There is a fall in the resting membrane potential and a spread of acetylcholine receptor sites outside the myoneural junction area. Also, a change in the physicochemical properties of the motor neuron membrane is indicated by a decrease in the number of sodium sites responsible for propagation of the nerve action potential. Other animal research has shown that after nerve transmission has been blocked by surgical incision of the nerve, botulinus toxin, or diphtheria toxin, acetylcholine receptors spread to the extrajunctional areas (13,29,34). Stimulation of the nerve distal to the diphtheria toxin block prevents the spread of acetylcholine receptors to the extrajunctional areas (34). Other investigations have demonstrated that direct and continuous electrical stimulation of denervated limb muscles or diaphragm prevents the appearance of extrajunctional acetylcholine receptors (15,34). Experiments have demonstrated that the spread of these receptors beyond the myoneural junction can be prevented by the addition of inhibitors of protein synthesis, such as actinomycin D (22).

In summary, the research findings noted above emphasize the important role that the motor nerve supply has on the electrophysiologic and biochemical characteristics of muscle distal to it. They indicate that muscle inactivity appears to be an important factor in the establishment of the denervation changes observed. Direct electrical stimulation of weakened skeletal muscles of patients may become an adjunctive treatment for lower motor neuron disorders. Exercise therapy, which leads to increased physiological nerve firing, for weakened muscles in peripheral neuropathy may also become a serious therapeutic consideration. Both direct stimulation of muscle and exercise have been used as anecdotal therapy in the past. However, these approaches may need a more thorough evaluation in the near future.

Myasthenia Gravis

Myasthenia gravis is another disease whose understanding has been broadened by recent research on nerve-muscle cell interactions. Present and past neurophysiologic research has shown that neuromuscular transmission is abnormal in myasthenia (7,23). Decreased amplitude of miniature end-plate potentials in resting myasthenic muscle and declining amplitude of the compound muscle action potential after repetitive nerve stimulation are two of the more characteristic findings that have demonstrated abnormal neuromuscular transmission (11,19). As better animal models for myasthenia gravis have been developed, the immunologic aspects of myasthenia gravis have come to be viewed as a very important factor in the causation of this disease and in particular in the production of neuromuscular transmission defects (27,42). Audrey Penn has reviewed much of this research in her chapter in this volume, and T. R. Johns has referred to this investigative approach in his discussion on the treatment of myasthenia gravis.

The development of techniques to measure antibodies to skeletal muscle end-plate acetylcholine receptors has led to the determination of circulating antibody levels in patients (3). It now appears that the abnormalities in nerve-muscle interaction in myasthenia gravis may be caused by a diminished number of muscle end-plate acetylcholine receptors because of antibody binding at these sites. This decreased number of receptors correlates with high titers of circulating antibodies in both animal and human myasthenia studies (1). Antibody detection techniques may provide an important means in the immediate future whereby clinicians can monitor the clinical course of a myasthenic patient.

In addition to these immunologic studies, tissue culture techniques have been applied to the investigation of lymphocyte interactions. Penn (*this volume*) discussed tissue culture studies in patients with polymyositis and dermatomyositis. These studies have shown that a selected population of lymphocytes obtained from patients with either of these two diseases are toxic to normal muscle cells in the culture. This observation has been confirmed in several other systems (25,30,36) and has prompted the hypothesis that immunologic injury to muscle in the inflammatory myopathies may be mediated through selective lymphocytes that attach to the muscle membrane. These lymphocyte studies may provide a laboratory method for assessing the activity of polymyositis or dermatomyositis, and serial evaluations of a patient's lymphocyte toxicity to muscle cells may prove useful in tailoring a patient's therapeutic regimen (9).

The animal disease model studies and tissue culture techniques that have been mentioned may provide an opportunity to test *in vitro* certain medications that are suspected of being pharmacologically useful in patients. An example of such an application has been presented by Engel (*this volume*). In their laboratory, they have grown muscle cells in tissue culture from patients with acid maltase deficiency. Various agents have been added to these cultures to evaluate their effectiveness in reversing the metabolic defect that characterizes this disease. After an effective agent is found, it can then be tried in animal disease models and patients. Future research using these investigative approaches will help to clarify pathophysiology and aid in developing potential therapeutic agents.

CELL MEMBRANE AND INTRACELLULAR METABOLIC REGULATION

Duchenne Dystrophy

The field of biochemical genetics has prompted research investigation of the physical and biochemical regulatory properties of the membranes of different tissues, such as red blood cells, white cells, fibroblasts, fat cells, liver cells, and skeletal muscle membrane. Duchenne dystrophy is a disease with a clear sex-linked recessive history in the majority of patients, and detailed biochemical *in vitro* studies of muscle from affected individuals have failed to demonstrate an enzyme deficiency or any intracellular accumulation of a toxic metabolite (43). Since there is no obvious metabolic defect inside the muscle cell, researchers have recently asked if Duchenne dystrophy might be a disease that primarily affects muscle membrane. Roses, Appel, and co-workers (39,45) have demonstrated increased membrane phosphorylation in red blood cells and skeletal muscle from patients with Duchenne muscular dystrophy. Although no clear correlation between these abnormalities of membrane phosphorylation and a specific intracellular metabolic malregulation has been uncovered, these data certainly suggest that some membrane abnormality is present. Additional investigation by Appel's group has demonstrated with *in vitro* studies that the calcium-stimulated potassium efflux in intact red blood cells of patients with Duchenne muscular dystrophy is increased (2). The pathophysiologic significance of this abnormality remains to be clarified. However, it is another piece of evidence to support the hypothesis that an abnormal membrane may be the causative factor in this type of muscular dystrophy.

The abnormality of calcium-stimulated red blood cell potassium efflux in Duchenne dystrophy may provide an important detection technique for the carrier state. At present, the use of creatine phosphokinase assays at best detects no more than 70 to 80% of known carriers of the disease (52). If the potassium efflux (or membrane phosphorylation) method approaches 100% sensitivity in the study of known carriers, it may provide a significant assistance to the genetic counseling and the preventive medical approach to the treatment of Duchenne dystrophy. It may also allow antenatal diagnosis of affected fetuses. Rowley (*this volume*) discussed our present genetic counseling approach to Duchenne dystrophy and pointed out the limitation that exists with carrier identification using the creatine phosphokinase technique.

Myotonic Dystrophy

Myotonic dystrophy is an autosomal dominant disorder affecting many different tissues with the major pathologic impact being on skeletal muscle (see Griggs, "The Myotonic Disorders and the Periodic Paralyses," *this volume*). Because many geneticists have suspected that autosomal dominant disorders are likely to be the result of an abnormal cell membrane, investigations of red blood cell and skeletal muscle membrane in myotonic dystrophy patients have been carried out. Decreased red blood cell and skeletal muscle membrane phosphorylation has been described as well as decreased calcium-stimulated potassium efflux from intact red blood cells (39,45). Although neither the abnormality of membrane phosphorylation nor that of potassium efflux has been shown to be of etiologic significance in myotonic dystrophy, these findings do support the hypothesis that an abnormal membrane is present in this disease. Other investigations offer further evidence for membrane abnormalities in this disease. These studies have demonstrated abnormalities in skeletal muscle electrophysiologic properties and muscle membrane composition (31,33).

In my other chapter in this volume, additional support is given to the membrane etiology of myotonic dystrophy. Evidence has been presented indicating decreased skeletal muscle membrane sensitivity to insulin in myotonic dystrophy patients. Insulin is a hormone known to produce its physiologic action by attaching to the cell surface, and it can be postulated that an abnormality in the cell membrane would hamper its effectiveness in regulating intracellular metabolic events. If subsequent research demonstrates the presence of skeletal muscle insulin insensitivity in most myotonic dystrophy patients, this would have important therapeutic implications. For example, myotonic dystrophy patients might be given a pharmacologic agent that would enhance their sensitivity to endogenous insulin; alternatively, administration of exogenous insulin might prove helpful.

VASCULAR SUPPLY TO NERVE AND MUSCLE

Lower Motor Neuron Disorders

The importance of nutrient supply by intraneural arterioles and capillaries within a peripheral nerve has been demonstrated recently by the investigations of Dyck (16) and his associates. Part of these data are presented in Dyck's chapter (*this volume*). Microinfarction in a peripheral nerve secondary to damage to the nutrient blood vessel has been a pathophysiologic mechanism long hypothesized to be operative in diabetes mellitus and many of the collagen vascular diseases (50). It may also be of importance in the etiology of certain types of infectious polyneuropathies (5). Some animal studies have revealed an increased permeability of intraneural capillaries in diphtheric and allergic neuritis (51). Such an abnormality in capillary membrane permeability may serve as an important initiating event in the poorly understood mechanism by which inflammatory cells attack peripheral neuron myelin sheaths.

Practical application of this type of research is not yet available, but with a greater understanding of intraneural circulation certain possibilities for the future can be suggested. If a greater clarification of microinfarction can be gained, then specific therapeutic agents to aid in increasing intraneural blood flow or in an enhancing the extent of the capillary network may be developed. With an increased understanding of the factors that regulate intraneural capillary permeability, more effective treatment for certain demyelinating peripheral neuropathies, such as Landry-Guillain-Barré syndrome, may be developed.

Duchenne Dystrophy

Over the past few years, investigations by Engel and co-workers (20,26) have suggested that the pathogenesis of certain muscular dystrophies or inflammatory myopathies may be related to inadequate blood supply to specific muscle groups. Histochemical changes resembling those seen in progressive muscular dystrophy and dermatomyositis have been produced by these investigators in rats by embolization and in other studies by combined aortic ligation and simultaneous administration of serotonin (20,26).

More recent studies by Engel and his co-workers (*this volume*) reflect a change in their thinking about the pathophysiology of Duchenne dystrophy.

Before the experiments of Engel noted above, Demos (10) had found slowed arm-to-tongue circulation times in patients with Duchenne dystrophy. This work and the investigation of Engel have prompted Bradley et al. to search for a vascular cause of muscular dystrophy in selected muscular dystrophy patients, as well as dystrophic mice (6). These investigators have found no abnormalities in intramuscular blood flow in patients with Duchenne dystrophy, in patients with other muscular dystrophies, or in mice with hereditary muscular dystrophy. Morphometric analysis by other investigators (28) of small blood vessels in patients with progressive muscular dystrophy has shown no quantitative abnormalities. These findings have cast considerable doubt on the vascular theory of muscular dystrophy, but continued investigation will be needed before final conclusions can be made.

AXONAL TRANSPORT

Lower Motor Neuron Disorders

In addition to the obvious importance of capillary blood supply in bringing nutrients to nerve and muscle cells, recent investigations (41) have revealed another important mechanism for nutrient supply within each individual nerve fiber. Evidence from animal studies now indicates that there is a flow of nutrients within an axon at both slow and fast rates going centrifugally from the nerve cell body to the periphery of the nerve fiber (41). This flow has been demonstrated to be important in carrying certain intracellular organelles as well as enzymes from the cell body to the periphery (41). More recent research has shown still another type of flow of materials within the nerve fiber. These data have suggested a flow from the periphery centripetally toward the cell body (21).

The physiologic significance of these different types of axonal flow patterns remains to be clarified. However, most researchers believe that these intracellular transport mechanisms are important in the supply of nutrients and in the intracellular regulation of the peripheral nerve cell metabolism. There is strong speculation that the axonal flow mechanisms may be of considerable importance in the trophic influence of motor nerve cells on the peripheral skeletal muscle that they supply. Further speculation has suggested that abnormalities in axonal flow may be responsible for many of the sensory as well as sensorimotor polyneuropathies that have their primary symptoms at the furthermost portion of the axon (5). The longer the axon and the larger the nerve fiber, the greater its metabolic demands. If the cell body has some compromise in its metabolic function, the flow of materials from the cell body to the periphery may be hampered only enough to show symptoms in the most vulnerable portions in the nerve fiber. Additional experimentation evaluating the various types of axonal transport noted above may prove to be of considerable interest in determining the etiology of many of the peripheral neuropathic or even myopathic disorders. Identification of an abnormality in axonal transport that correlates with a specific clinical disease state should encourage the development of new therapeutic approaches in managing peripheral neuropathy.

Myasthenia Gravis

Prior to the immunologic investigations suggesting a postjunctional etiology to myasthenia gravis (discussed in the section on myasthenia gravis under Nerve-Muscle Cell Interaction), most researchers (18,19) felt that the cause of this disorder resided in the prejunctional motor neuron. A decreased size of the miniature end-plate potential, characteristically seen in myasthenia gravis intercostal muscle, had been interpreted to be owing to decreased amounts of acetylcholine being packaged in the synaptic vesicles or incomplete release of acetylcholine after nerve stimulation (18,19). Presynaptic pathology is still a consideration and axonal transport is an issue. Intracellular organelles as well as various enzymes responsible for the synthesis and packaging of acetylcholine at the nerve terminals are carried from the cell body to the periphery by axonal transport (41). Although the most recent studies favor a postjunctional etiology for myasthenia gravis, investigations of axonal transport in this disease will be of considerable interest.

SUMMARY

Recent research investigations have provided important new insights into the management of several of the major neuromuscular disorders, but no major clarification of the exact cause for the muscular dystrophies or various neuropathic diseases has emerged. The discovery of circulating acetylcholine receptor antibodies in myasthenia gravis patients is an example of a potential breakthrough in the management of individuals with this disorder. Serial evaluations of such antibody titers may prove extremely helpful in predicting the clinical course of the disease as well as evaluating the effectiveness of any pattern of therapy. The red cell membrane abnormalities, in particular, the calcium-stimulated potassium efflux in patients with Duchenne and myotonic muscular dystrophy, may allow for the development of more sensitive methods for detecting the presence of either of these diseases. Such a greater sensitivity in disease detection should allow a more precise identification of disease carriers and thereby provide a more effective preventive medical approach to controlling both disorders. The *in vitro* immunologic techniques presently being used to evaluate lymphocyte toxicity or muscle cells offer still another type of potential assistance in the management of patients. In the future, patients with inflammatory muscle diseases, such as dermatomyositis and polymyositis, may be followed by serial evaluations of lymphocyte toxicity in blood samples from patients with these diseases. Lymphocyte-muscle tissue cultures may also be used to evaluate the effectiveness of various medications in decreasing lymphocyte toxicity and in this way guide the clinician to select the best possible therapeutic agent for a specific patient's disease. Less immediately applicable treatment advances may occur as greater clarification of the vascular etiology to nerve or muscle cell disorders evolves. If such primary vascular abnormalities can be demonstrated to be present in specific diseases, various vasoactive medications as well as other therapeutic measures designed to increase blood flow through intraneural and intramuscular blood vessels will be obvious therapeutic considerations.

REFERENCES

1. Almon, R. R., and Appel, S. H. (1976): Serum acetylcholine-receptor antibodies in myasthenia gravis. *Ann. N.Y. Acad. Sci.,* 274:235–243.
2. Appel, S. H. (1976): Membranes and muscular dystrophy. In: *Pathogenesis of the Human Muscular Dystrophies. Fifth International Congress,* edited by L. P. Rowland. Excerpta Medica, Amsterdam (*in press*).
3. Appel, S. H., Almon, R. R., and Levy, N. (1975): Acetylcholine receptor antibodies in myasthenia gravis. *N. Engl. J. Med.,* 293:760–761.
4. Axelsson, J., and Thesleff, S. (1959): A study of supersensitivity in denervated mammalian skeletal muscle. *J. Physiol.,* 149:178–193.
5. Bradley, W. G., and Thomas, P. K. (1974): The pathology of peripheral nerve disease. In: *Disorders of Voluntary Muscle,* edited by J. N. Walton, pp. 234–273. Churchill Livingstone, Edinburgh.
6. Bradley, W. G., O'Brien, M. D., and Walder, D. N. (1975): Failure to confirm a vascular cause of muscular dystrophy. *Arch. Neurol.,* 32:466–473.
7. Buchthal, F., and Engbaek, L. (1948): On the neuromuscular transmission in normal and myasthenic subjects. *Acta Psychiatr. Neurol.,* 23:3–11.
8. Buller, A., Eccles, J. C., and Eccles, R. M. (1960): Interactions between motor neurones and muscles in respect of the characteristic speeds of their responses. *J. Physiol.,* 150:417–439.
9. Dawkins, R. L., and Mastaglia, F. L. (1973): Cell-mediated cytotoxicity to muscle in polymyositis. *N. Engl. J. Med.,* 288:434–438.
10. Demos, J. (1961): Mesure des tempsde circulation chez 79 myopathies. *Rev. Fr. Etud. Clin. Biol.,* 6:876–887.
11. Desmedt, J. E., and Borenstein, S. (1976): Diagnosis of myasthenia gravis by repetitive stimulation. *Ann. N.Y. Acad. Sci.,* 274:174–188.
12. Douglas, W. B., and Cosmos, E. (1974): Histochemical responses of dystrophic murine muscles cross-innervated by sciatic nerves of normal mice. In: *Exploratory Concepts in Muscular Dystrophy, II,* edited by A. T. Milhorat, pp. 374–380. Excerpta Medica, Amsterdam.
13. Drachman, D. B. (1974): The role of acetylcholine as a neurotrophic transmitter. *Ann. N.Y. Acad. Sci.,* 228:160–176.
14. Drachman, D. B., and Fambrough, D. M. (1976): Are muscle fibers denervated in myotonic dystrophy? *Arch. Neurol.,* 33:485–488.
15. Drachman, D. B., and Witzke, F. (1972): Trophic regulation of acetylcholine sensitivity of muscle: Effect of electrical stimulation. *Science,* 176:514–516.
16. Dyck, P. J. (1975): Pathologic alterations of the peripheral nervous system of man. In: *Peripheral Neuropathy,* edited by P. J. Dyck, P. K. Thomas, and E. H. Lambert, pp. 296–336. W. B. Saunders Co., Philadelphia.

17. Elliott, H. C. (1945): Studies on the motor cells of the spinal cord. III. Position and extent of lesions in the nuclear pattern of convalescent and chronic poliomyelitis patients. *Am. J. Pathol.*, 21:87.
18. Elmqvist, D. (1965): Neuromuscular transmission with special reference to myasthenia gravis. *Acta Physiol. Scand. Suppl. 249*, 64:1–34.
19. Elmqvist, D., Hofmann, W. W., Kugelberg, J., and Quastel, D. M. J. (1964): An electrophysiological investigation of neuromuscular transmission in myasthenia gravis. *J. Physiol.*, 174:417–434.
20. Engel, W. K., and Derrer, E. C. (1975): Drugs blocking the muscle damaging effects of 5-HT and noradrenaline in aorta-ligatured rats. *Nature*, 254:151–152.
21. Griffin, J. W., Price, D. L., Drachman, D. B., and Engel, W. K. (1976): Axonal transport to and from the motor nerve ending. *Ann. N.Y. Acad. Sci.*, 274:31–45.
22. Grampp, W., Harris, J. B., and Thesleff, S. (1972): Inhibition of denervation changes in skeletal muscle by blockers of protein synthesis. *J. Physiol.*, 221:743–754.
23. Grob, D., and Namba, T. (1976): Characteristics and mechanism of neuromuscular block in myasthenia gravis. *Ann. N.Y. Acad. Sci.*, 288:143–173.
24. Guth, L. (1968): "Trophic" influences of nerve on muscle. *Physiol. Rev.*, 48:645.
25. Haas, D. C., and Arnason, B. G. W. (1974): Cell mediated immunity in polymyositis. *Arch. Neurol.*, 31:192–196.
26. Hathaway, P. W., Engel, W. K., and Zellweger H. (1970): Experimental myopathy after arterial embolization: Comparison with childhood X-linked pseudohypertrophic muscular dystrophy. *Arch. Neurol.*, 22:365–377.
27. Heilbronn, E., Mattsson, C., Thornell, L., Sjostrom, M., Stalberg, E., Hilton-Brown, P., and Elmqvist, D. (1976): Experiment myasthenia in rabbits: Biochemical, immunological, electrophysiological and morphological aspects. *Ann. N.Y. Acad. Sci.*, 274:337–353.
28. Jerusalem, F., Engel, A. G., and Gomez, M. R. (1974): Duchenne dystrophy: Morphometric study of the muscle microvasculature. *Brain*, 97:115–122.
29. Johns, T. R., and Thesleff, S. (1961): Effect of motor inactivation on the chemical sensitivity of skeletal muscle. *Acta Physiol. Scand.*, 51:136–141.
30. Johnson, R. L., Fink, C. W., and Ziff, M. (1972): Lymphotoxin formation by lymphocytes and muscle in polymyositis. *J. Clin. Invest.*, 51:2435–2449.
31. Kuhn, E. (1973): Myotonia. In: *New Developments in Electromyography and Clinical Neurophysiology, Vol. I*, edited by J. E. Desmedt, pp. 413–417. Kargel, Basel.
32. Lentz, T. L. (1974): Neurotrophic regulation at the neuromuscular junction. *Ann. N.Y. Acad. Sci.*, 228:323–337.
33. Lipicky, R. J., and Bryant, S. H. (1973): A biophysical study of the human myotonias. In: *New Developments in Electromyography and Clinical Neurophysiology, Vol. I*, edited by J. E. Desmedt, pp. 451–463. Karger, Basel.
34. Lomo, T., and Rosenthal, J. (1972): Control of Ach sensitivity by muscle activity in the rat. *J. Physiol.*, 221:493–513.
35. Mastaglia, F. L., Dawkins, R. L., and Papadimitriou, J. M. (1974): Lymphocyte muscle cell interactions *in vivo* and *in vitro*. *J. Neurol. Sci.*, 22:261–268.
36. McComas, A. J., Sica, R. E. P., and Campbell, M. J. (1971): "Sick" motor neurones: A unifying concept of muscle disease. *Lancet*, 1:321–325.
37. McComas, A. J., Sica, R. E. P., and Upton, A. R. M. (1974) Multiple muscle analysis of motor units in muscular dystrophy. *Arch. Neurol.*, 30:249–251.
38. McComas, A. J., Sica, R. E. P., Upton, A. R. M., and Petits, F. (1974): Sick motor neurons and muscle disease. *Ann. N.Y. Acad. Sci.*, 228:261–279.
39. Miller, S. E., Roses, A. D., and Appel, S. H. (1975): Erythrocytes in human muscular dystrophy. *Science*, 188:1131.
40. Neerunjun, J. S., and Dubowitz, V. (1974): Muscle transplantation and regeneration in the dystrophic hamster. Part 2. Histochemical studies. *J. Neurol. Sci.*, 23:521–536.
41. Ochs, S. (1974): Systems of material transport in nerve fibers (axoplasmic transport) related to nerve function and trophic control. *Ann. N.Y. Acad. Sci.*, 228:202–223.
42. Patrick, J., and Lindstrom, J. (1973): Autoimmune response to acetylcholine receptor. *Science*, 18:871–872.
43. Pennington, R. J. (1971): Biochemical aspects of muscle disease. In: *Advances in Clinical Chemistry*, edited by O. Bodansky and A. L. Latner, pp. 410–439. Academic Press, New York.

44. Romanul, F. C. A., and VanDer Meulen, J. P. (1967): Slow and fast muscles after cross innervation. Enzymatic and physiologic changes. *Arch. Neurol.,* 17:387–402.
45. Roses, A. D., Herbstreuth, M. H., and Appel, S. H. (1975): Membrane protein kinase alteration in Duchenne muscular dystrophy. *Nature,* 254:350–351.
46. Salafsky, B. (1971): Functional studies of regenerated muscles from normal and dystrophic mice. *Nature,* 229:270.
47. Stalberg, E., Trontelj, J. V., and Schwartz, M. S. (1976): Single-muscle fiber recording of the jitter phenomenon in patients with myasthenia gravis and in members of their families. *Ann. N.Y. Acad. Sci.,* 274:189–202.
48. Thesleff, S. (1974): Physiological effects of denervation of muscle. *Ann. N.Y. Acad. Sci.,* 228:89–104.
49. Thiele, B., and Stalberg, E. (1975): Single fibre EMG findings in polyneuropathies of different etiology. *J. Neurol. Neurosurg. Psychiatry,* 38:881–887.
50. Thomas, P. K., and Eliasson, S. G. (1975): Diabetic neuropathy. In: *Peripheral Neuropathy,* edited by P. J. Dyck, P. K. Thomas, and E. H. Lambert, pp. 956–981. W. B. Saunders Co., Philadelphia.
51. Waksman, B. H. (1961): Experimental study of diphtheric polyneuritis in the rabbit and guinea pig II. The blood-nerve barrier in the rabbit. *J. Neuropathol. Exp. Neurol.,* 20:35.
52. Walton, J. N., and Gardner-Medwin, D. (1974): Progressive muscular dystrophy and the myotonic disorders. In: *Disorders of Voluntary Muscle,* edited by J. N. Walton, pp. 561–613. Churchill Livingstone, Edinburgh.

Advances in Neurology, Vol. 17, edited by
R. C. Griggs and R. T. Moxley, III. Raven Press,
New York © 1977.

Clinical Examination of Patients with Neuromuscular Disease

Michael H. Brooke

*Department of Neurology and Jerry Lewis Neuromuscular Research Center,
Washington University School of Medicine, St. Louis, Missouri 63110*

INTRODUCTION

The physical examination in patients with neuromuscular disease often perplexes those who are unfamiliar with these illnesses. Such perplexity is unnecessary since the examination is basically very simple. There are four aspects to it. These are inspection, palpation, examination of reflexes, and evaluation of muscle strength. It is also convenient to take the various parts of the body in sequence. The head and neck, the shoulders, the arms, the torso, hips and the legs are all separately examined. If one conscientiously does this, it is difficult to miss significant findings.

INSPECTION

Inspection of the muscles reveals the presence or absence of wasting as well as the occurrence of any spontaneous movements such as fasciculations or myokymia. Weakness of muscles also alters a patient's resting posture in some quite characteristic fashions. These postural alterations are often far more helpful in determining the extent of weakness than is the more formal evaluation of a patient's strength. Due to space limitations, the abnormalities produced by weakness of the muscles of the head and neck will be ignored.

Wasting of the muscles around the shoulders is usually easily seen. The bony prominences become more noticeable. Posteriorly, the spine of the scapula juts out, no longer hidden by the supraspinatus above and the infraspinatus below. The deltoid may be wasted and a marked "step" is formed at the point of the shoulder. As the shoulders become weak, the scapulae tend to slide laterally and upwards on the thorax as the muscle tone is no longer sufficient to brace them backwards. When this happens, the points of the shoulders tend to fold anteriorly rather as if one were folding over the corner of a piece of paper in a dog-eared fashion. Since there is often associated pectoral muscle wasting, a crease is formed which runs diagonally from the axilla towards the neck. Winging of the scapula, in which the lower medial corner or sometimes the entire medial border of the scapula juts backwards, may also be noticed. In slender people it may be difficult to determine whether or not this winging is of pathological significance. Many physicians employ the technique of having the patient push against the wall in order to determine whether winging is real or not. I have found the following maneuver more reliable: the patient is asked to raise his arms outstretched in front of him until they are horizontal. He is then told to bring the arms slowly down again until the hands are at his side. In patients with winging of the scapula, this downward movement always exacerbates the winging and very often during the maneuver the medial inferior corner of the scapula pops backwards with a sudden rotary movement. Another sign of shoulder weakness which is extremely useful is the "trapezius hump." This is a prominence in the mid portion of the belly of the trapezius which is easily seen from in front. It is probably due to the activity of this muscle in trying to provide some support in fixation of the scapula. It is especially prominent during abduction of the arms but may also be noticeable at rest. In extreme weakness the upper border of the scapula itself may override the shoulder and be visible from in front. A secondary effect of shoulder weakness is on the position of the hands. In the normal standing posture the hands are held with the thumbs facing forward. Weakness of the shoulder, with the attendant displacement of the scapula, causes the arms to turn so that the back of the hand now faces forwards. This is an extremely sensitive sign of shoulder weakness.

Inspection of the arms and hands is relatively straight-forward. One looks for wasting in the biceps, triceps, and in the forearm muscles. As a practical tip, it is easy to look for wasting of the forearm muscles when the patient holds the arms forward with the elbows flexed, putting the forearms in a vertical position, a posture similar to that used in boxing at the turn of the century. The bellies of the muscles on the medial and lateral side of the forearms may then be compared easily and any wasting detected.

In examining the muscles of the hands the signs of flattening of the thenar and hypothenar eminence and of "guttering" of the interossei muscles are well known. One maneuver which is useful in patients who are suspected of having wasting of the first dorsal interosseous is to ask them to abduct the thumb to the first finger. Normally this results in a prominent belly of the first dorsal interosseous muscle. In patients with wasting, the belly does not develop and palpation of the muscle reveals it to be flabby. Weakness of the muscles of the hand cause characteristic changes in the posture of the hand. Ordinarily a hand's normal posture is with the fingers semiflexed at all joints and the thumb held in a plane at right angles to the fingers (so that the thumbnail faces forwards when the hands are held by the side). In weakness of muscles of the thenar eminence the thumb rotates so that it lies in the same plane as the fingers — the so-called simian or ape-like hand. An additional abnormality is associated with weakness of the other small muscles of the hand. The fingers are held loosely, neither adducted nor abducted, and the fingers, although remaining flexed at the interphalangeal joints, become extended at the metacarpophalangeal joints producing the "claw" hand.

The quadriceps femoris, above all other muscles in the body, are most susceptible to wasting, and it is the vastus lateralis and medialis that bear the brunt of this wasting. The diagnosis of disuse atrophy should always be made with some reluctance since focal atrophy of muscle groups is generally due to disease of the neuromuscular system rather than disuse, but it is remarkable how rapidly the quadriceps will waste following even a brief period of bedrest or as a result of pain occurring in the hip or knee. Quadriceps wasting can be noticed more easily if the patient is asked to tense the thigh by making the knee stiff or fixing the kneecap. When this is done, the bellies of the normal medial and lateral vasti are prominent just above the knee. A wasted thigh is not only slender but tapers perceptibly towards the knee.

When the muscles of the anterior tibial and peroneal groups are lost, the tibia assumes a "knife-edge" configuration due to the prominence of its anterior border. A groove is seen immediately lateral to this knife-edge border. Sometimes a similar groove is seen in normal people of slight build, but if the patient is asked to dorsiflex the foot a distinction between the normal and abnormal can be made. Normally during such dorsiflexion the bulge of the anterior tibial muscle obliterates this groove. In abnormal wasting the muscle belly is not prominent and the groove persists. Loss of the gastrocnmeii causes the medial and lateral bellies of this muscle to change from their normally rounded configuration to a tapering and rather flabby appearance. We have also found it useful to inspect the size of the extensor digitorum brevis. Both myopathies and neuropathies may cause a foot drop but if the cause be due to a disease of the peripheral nerve, the extensor digitorum brevis is usually reduced in size. In a foot drop caused by a myopathy, such as in the scapulo peroneal syndrome, the extensor digitorum brevis is often hypertrophied, perhaps because this small muscle is used in a futile attempt to dorsiflex the feet by pulling up on the toes.

Finally, all the muscle groups should be examined to look for the presence or absence of fasciculations or other involuntary movements. One of the many unanswered questions in neuromuscular disease is how to differentiate benign fasciculations from those of pathological significance. Some have maintained that the benign fasciculation is a brief repetitive twitch of the same group of muscle fibers occurring over a period of two to three minutes, whereas pathological fasciculations appear in many muscle groups in a random fashion. Watching a patient with diffuse fasciculations is reminiscent of watching the surface of a pond in summer when the fish are rising, the ripples arise here and there with no seeming pattern. Unfortunately, there is no hard and fast differentiation of benign from pathological fasciculations. It has been our experience that perfectly normal people without any neuromuscular disease have periods of time when fasciculations may be quite intense and diffuse. Isolated fasciculations may last for many days in a patient who fails to develop any sign of neuromuscular disease when followed over many years. Fasciculations are exacerbated by many factors, such as fatigue, both physical and mental, cigarette smoking, and the consumption of coffee or other caffeine containing drinks. There is perhaps one clue to the fact that a fasciculation is of pathological significance, and this is related to the size of the fasciculation. A fasciculation is an involuntary discharge of one motor unit generally arising close to the nerve cell body and resulting in the contraction of all the muscle fibers supplied by that nerve cell. When denervation occurs, the several hundred muscle fibers supplied by a particular nerve may become devoid of their nerve supply. Ordinarily they atrophy, but, reinnervation from a neighboring nerve cell may occur. This results in the accumulation of additional muscle fibers within the newly formed motor unit. By a constant process of denervation and reinnervation, motor units may come to contain several thousand muscle fibers rather than a few hundred. If such a large motor unit is the site of a fasciculation, a large part of the muscle may be involved in a single fasciculation so that the twitch extends across a good portion of the muscle belly. In my experience this has a clinical correlation with the large fasciculations seen in denervating disease. Thus, the presence of a sizable fasciculation may be some indication of organicity. Unfortunately, this is less useful in practice since by the time denervation and reinnervation is extensive and the fasciculations are large, the disease is clinically apparent by other criteria.

A fasciculation is a brief twitch of a small portion of the muscle and should be differentiated from the phenomenon of myokymia. Some confusion has arisen in the literature and, on occasions, the differentiation is obscured. As opposed to a fasciculation, myokymia is a repetitive train of action potentials causing a brief tetanic contraction of the muscle fibers of a motor unit. Because of the repetitive nature of the discharge, the visible contraction is much longer in its time course. The twitchlike characteristic of a fasciculation can be differentiated from the more sinuous movement of myokymia. Moreover, myokymia seldom involves one nerve fiber alone. The same abnormality affects many motor units and their contraction and relaxation gives an undulating character to the whole muscle which resembles the movement seen in a field of wheat as the wind blows across it. Myokymia is also more apt to move the joint across which the muscle acts than are fasciculations.

PALPATION

After the muscles have been examined, additional information may be obtained by palpating the muscle and by percussing it. There is really no way of describing the texture of normal muscle except to say that it has a certain resilience; it is equally difficult to describe the abnormal. However, the physician who learns to tell the difference between a rather flabby, atrophic, denervated muscle and the peculiar rubbery consistency of muscle in Duchenne's dystrophy will find that palpation is a useful means of examination. One of the most characteristic signs is the feeling of the gastrocnemius muscle of a patient with the pseudohypertrophic form of muscle dystrophy (Duchenne's). The children's stores often carry a type of toy fashioned after the nature of spiders, snakes, or monsters of various kinds. They are made of a plastic which has a jelly like consistency and shakes and trembles in an all too lifelike fashion. I bring this up only to point out that the muscle of a patient with Duchenne's dystrophy has almost exactly the same kind of feel as the substance out of which these toys are made.

The evaluation of a patient's tone is more important in children than it is in adults. Even the concept of tone is a difficult one to explain. It means different things to physiologists, pediatricians, and neurologists. The word is used here to indicate the degree of resistance to movement that a limb has when the patient is relaxed. When the arm is picked up and the elbow flexed or the forearm gently shaken, the movements which occur at the elbow and the wrist are damped slightly by the normal tone in the muscles. The joints move freely and readily enough but a minimum amount of resistance can be perceived, even though it does not hamper the movement. In a patient who is hypotonic, the limb has all the resilience of overcooked spaghetti. It is impossible to describe in words the feeling that such a limb has, and only the examiner's experience with patients with varying degrees of tone will allow him to make an accurate assessment. In children, the degree of head lag and the position of the body in ventral suspension are examined in addition to passive movement of the limbs. To evaluate head lag, the baby lies on his back and his shoulders are raised by pulling his arms. Even in the newborn, the child will make some attempt to flex his neck and bring the head up with the shoulders. Head lag is a phenomenon in which the head droops passively backwards and no attempt is made to raise it. The degree of tone may also be evaluated by holding the child under the trunk and lifting him clear of the surface in the supine position. In hypotonic conditions the body will assume the posture of an inverted U, whereas in a normal child, shortly after birth, the back will be relatively straight and the arms and legs flexed.

Very often in hypotonic children the joints are hyperextensible; for example, the fingers may be bent backwards to touch the forearms, or the feet dorsiflexed so that the toes can be made to touch the shins. Although the term hypotonic is sometimes used for such joints, it is better to name them hyperextensible or hypermobile.

Causes of increased tone in neuromuscular diseases are usually associated with contractures of the muscles. A contracture is a shortening which occurs in the muscle in the absence of any voluntary activity or any electrical signs of muscle activity. It is most often associated with a fibrotic shortened muscle. The muscles around any joint may be involved and usually shorten into the position which the patient adopts at rest. Thus, a patient confined to a wheelchair will have flexion contractures of the hips, knees, and elbows.

Percussion of the muscle should also be carried out and may reveal the presence of myotonia, of myoedema, or of other abnormal direct percussion responses. Percussion myotonia is the sustained and uncontrollable contraction, associated with a delay in relaxation, which is produced by a sharp blow. It is characteristically sought in the thenar eminence, percussion of which causes an abrupt abduction and flexion of the thumb. The patient then struggles to get his hand back into the normal relaxed position. However, myotonia should also be looked for in muscles other than those of the hand. Percussion of the extensor muscles of the fingers in the forearm may result in the abrupt extension of the fingers followed by a slow downward drift as the myotonia relaxes. Another way of detecting myotonia is to slant a light obliquely across the belly of a muscle such as the deltoid. Percussion will then cause the contraction of a strip of the muscle producing a depression which will be shadowed by the oblique light. This method is useful in eliciting myotonia of the tongue and muscles acting across large joints.

Myoedema is a phenomenon seen in hypothyroidism and in other metabolic abnormalities. Percussion of the muscle produces an initial depression which spreads outwards across the muscle rather like the ripples on a pond when a stone is thrown into the water. The initial depression then mounds upwards giving the appearance of a small hillock where the muscle was percussed. The hillock may last for many seconds to minutes. Some have used the term myoedema for actual swelling of the muscle, as in a patient with a tender, painful muscle during an acute attack of polymyositis or of rhabdomyolysis. I think these two usages should be carefully differentiated.

Normal muscle will also contract upon percussion, particularly over the thenar eminence and the muscles of the forearm. However, the normal response is a brief contraction which immediately relaxes. It is usually not very marked and the joint moves little if at all. Occasionally this percussion response may become quite brisk without having the characteristic delayed relaxation phase of myotonia. It is particularly seen in denervating illnesses and also in electrolyte imbalance in which the direct response to muscle percussion is augmented.

REFLEXES

Examination of the deep tendon reflexes is an important part of the muscle examination. The reflexes which are evaluated are those of any standard neurological examination and include the biceps, triceps, supinator, knee, and ankle jerks together with the superficial reflexes of the abdomen and the plantar responses. With regard to the deep tendon reflexes, I have never really understood the system of grading which is used by many. I refer to the +, ++, +++, etc. system. I would like to assume that there are others equally baffled by this system, and I would, therefore, make a plea that reflexes be described as either absent, diminished, normal, or hyperactive. If it is necessary to add the comment that there is associated clonus, then so be it. At least this has the advantage of clarity when others subsequently read the patient's notes. In judging whether a reflex is hyperactive, attention is paid to the spread of the reflex to neighboring muscle groups and most importantly to the degree of "snap" in the muscle contraction. Ordinarily when a tendon is tapped, the initial contraction of the muscle has a rather smooth quality before relaxing. If a tension recording were taken from the muscle, the familiar curve would be seen. In a hyperactive reflex, the initial upsweep of such a curve is very steep. This gives the appearance of a distinct snap to the muscle contraction. The tendon jerk becomes more jerky than usual, so to speak.

MUSCLE STRENGTH

The evaluation of muscle strength is at the heart of the examination of the neuromuscular system. For the detailed evaluation of individual muscles, the classical monograph "Aids to the Investigation of Peripheral Nerve Injuries" by the Medical Research Council is enthusiastically recommended. The grading system which is used therein is most useful. Strength is evaluated in the following categories: 0 — no movement of the muscle, 1 — flicker or trace of contraction, 2 — active movement when gravity is eliminated, 3 — active movement against gravity, 4 — active movement against gravity and resistance, and 5 — normal power. This elegant system of grading has been corrupted by at least a generation of neurologists. All of us insist on grading muscle as 4+, 3±, and so on. The disadvantage inherent in the system is that once a muscle becomes weak (i.e. grade 4) there is a wide variation in the degree of strength until a muscle loses the ability to move the joint against any resistance and becomes grade 3. This dilemma is a difficult one to solve and attempts to quantitate muscle strength exactly by the use of dynamometers and so forth has not yet led to a more reliable method. This led us to adopt a system of functional muscle testing, a heresy which will be explained later. It is time consuming to examine every muscle in the body and most of us develop a shortened method. I think that an acceptable compromise is to examine the strength at each joint with all the movements possible at that joint. Thus, neck flexion, extension, and rotation is examined. Abduction, adduction, extension, and flexion of the shoulder, extension and flexion of the elbow is tested, and so on with all the joints of the body. This may not be pleasing to the purists, but it does have the advantage of allowing the examiner to see more than two patients in an afternoon.

It is important here to discuss another aspect of the evaluation of strength. It has been a frequent experience to see a patient whose weakness has been described as severe only to find that their trouble is more psychological than it is muscular. Organic weakness gives very characteristic signs. The examiner can overcome the patient's best efforts to resist him and the resistance which the muscle displays is uniform throughout the range of movement. Thus, if one is testing the abductors of the shoulders in a patient who is slightly weak, the patient is instructed to "make wings," the arms are held up horizontally and pressure on the elbow allows the examiner to push the patient's arms downwards towards his side. The resistance that the examiner feels is the same at the beginning of this movement as it is when the patient's elbows have been forced down to 45 degrees. This is quite different from the hysterical weakness in which there is a sudden "giving way" phenomenon. In the same situation of testing shoulder abduction, it may initially be quite difficult to depress the patient's elbow but then the muscle suddenly collapses and the arm falls down to the side. In fact a repetitive "catch and give" phenomenon may occur resulting in a feeling rather like cog wheel rigidity in which small contractions are succeeded by periods of relaxation. This is never due to muscle weakness. If the patient has pain in the joint being tested, however, this may give the same result. Thus, when the phenomenon of "sudden give" is detected in examining a muscle, the patient should be asked if the joint or the muscle hurts. If such pain is present, it is impossible to get an accurate assessment of muscular strength. This last point cannot be stressed too strongly.

If a patient is suspected of having hysterical weakness, he should be observed closely to see whether he makes movements with the limb when he is unaware of scrutiny which he denies being able to perform upon command; a patient who is totally unable to step onto a small stool may do so readily when he uses the stool to climb on to the examining couch. Another sign of value in the testing of a patient with suspected hysteria is to palpate the antagonist muscles while testing muscle strength. Thus, if one feels contraction of the triceps while the biceps is being examined, one may surmise that all is not well. Since this paragraph is degenerating into the nature of random thoughts, I will add one further which is of value. The presence of biceps weakness carries with it a useful clinical sign. The biceps strength is obviously tested with the wrists supinated. Patients with biceps weakness invariably use one of two tricks to try and overcome the examiner. The first is to rotate the forearm midway between pronation and supination in which position the added help of the brachioradialis comes into play. The other maneuver is to pull the elbow backwards. This is so like the movement used by a bartender in pulling up a pint of beer that we have used the term "the bartender's sign" for it.

If heresy is to be preached it might as well be florid heresy. That which follows will, I am sure, provoke disagreement. I have found that the formal examination of muscle strength in the fashion mentioned above has not been as useful as the functional evaluation of a patient's abilities. The whole concept of functional muscle testing is to determine in what way the patient's functional abilities such as stepping onto a stool, climbing, getting up from a chair, and so on are disturbed. It is remarkable how the way in which a patient walks and does certain tasks will allow a quite accurate deduction of the muscle groups that are weak. An evaluation of the functional disability of the patient also provides more accurate testing of the progression or improvement of an illness. A patient may be able to arise from the floor only with difficulty and with the support of both hands when first seen, but some months later may get up with transient hand support on one knee. The formal muscle strength testing in both these situations may reveal only grade 4 muscles. Thus the improvement cannot really be gauged from formal strength testing. I think we all find it difficult to put down in words how strong a muscle is and functional testing is an attempt to make the evaluation more accurate.

Functional evaluation begins with an examination of the gait. Consider what happens to the gait if the patient has progressive weakness of the hip muscles. In normal walking, as the heel hits the ground, and the weight of the body is transferred to that leg, the strain is taken up by those muscles which abduct the leg on the hip. Obviously, this does not cause an abduction of the leg while walking but, rather, prevents the pelvis from tilting sharply so that the opposite hip is dropped. This function of the hip abductors is best thought of as a shock absorbing mechanism which smooths out the shock transmitted from the leg to the pelvis. In minimal hip weakness, this action is lost. The patient's heel frequently hits the ground with a quite audible thud and the pelvis tilts slightly to the opposite side. When this trouble is bilateral, as it usually is, this produces a heavy footed gait and a mild waddle. As the hip weakness becomes worse, other muscle groups are involved, particularly those of the hip and back extensors. This spreading weakness adds another characteristic to the walk. One normally stands with the back straight and the body's weight acts through the center of gravity in a line which lies anterior to the hip joints. Thus without the help of any muscle tone, the body would jack-knife forward at the hips. The hip and back extensors prevent such a collapse. When these muscles become weak, the patient develops a compensatory posture. The shoulders are thrown backwards and a lumbar lordosis becomes apparent. This enables the body's weight to be thrown on a line behind the hip joints, further accentuating the backward lean. The body cannot collapse from this position since it is supported as much by bony and ligamentous structures as it is by muscle. The walk in such circumstances has the previous waddling characteristic, superimposed on which is a lumbar lordosis and an associated protrusion of the abdomen. This walk in which the patient waddles gently down the street, arms thrown back and belly thrust forward, has been termed the aldermanic posture, a term which will become obsolete as the literature of Dicken's gives way to video tapes of Westerns.

Weakness of the quadriceps muscles gives rise to a phenomenon called "backkneeing." During normal walking, the quadriceps act to stabilize the knee joint. There used to be an old schoolboy trick, and I doubt that the practice has disappeared, in which one approached the victim from behind and tapped sharply on the backs of the knees. In the unwary, this resulted in a sudden collapse of the knees causing the victim some momentary panic before the quadriceps took up the strain. It is exactly this collapse of the knee joint that the patient with quadriceps weakness fears most. To protect himself against this, he will lock the knee backwards in a position of hyperextension. He does this while standing and also with each step that he takes. At the same time that his heel hits the ground the knee is thrust backwards and the joint is stabilized mechanically by this thrust.

At first one might think that shoulder weakness would give little abnormality in the way a patient walks. However, we have already alluded to the abnormal posture of the shoulder during shoulder weakness and this is easily noticed during walking. The scapulae are allowed to slide forward and laterally when the muscle tone is no longer sufficient to keep them braced backwards. This causes the shoulders to hunch and allows the arms to rotate so that the backs of the hands are facing forward. As the patient walks, an odd floppiness of the arms is added to his hunched appearance. The floppiness is due to the lack of stabilization of the upper arm by normal muscle tone. With each step the arm swings passively to and fro, a pendulum suspended from the shoulder.

Distal weakness of the legs causes another characteristic abnormality of gait. Weakness of the peroneal and anterior tibial groups hinders dorsiflexion of the foot. Walking is not easy for a patient with this problem; as the heel is lifted off the ground, the foot hangs limply from the ankle. The patient is in danger of tripping over any object which catches his toes, a danger which can be avoided only by lifting the knee high in the air. The patient is now faced with another problem. If he brings his foot downwards in a normal fashion, the toe will hit first and, because of weakness of eversion, he may well sprain his ankle as the foot collapses under him. Somehow or other he has to dorsiflex the foot and since he cannot do this under muscular control he uses a short flinging movement of the lower leg in order to throw the toes upwards. He must get the foot quickly down on the ground following this, lest it passively falls back into plantar flexion. This quick throw and rapid descent produces the foot slapping gait. The sight of the high stepping walk with the foot being slapped onto the ground producing a noise like a clapperboard is almost unmistakable. Perhaps the word "almost" should be emphasized because there is another gait that is superficially similar. Patients with loss of position sense in the feet also raise the legs high and stamp the feet on the ground, since they are not quite sure where the feet are nor yet where the ground is. They like to make firm contact with the foot not only so that the forcible shock of the foot hitting the ground will force proprioceptive impulses through a somewhat jaded nervous system, but also so that they may hear the comforting sound of foot upon path. This results in a stamping gait as the patient goes on his uncertain way. The essential difference between these two kinds of walk is that in the stamping gait of a patient with position sense loss, the foot is dorsiflexed when the knee is high, whereas in the steppage gait of a patient with anterior tibial or peroneal weakness the foot dangles limply from the leg. In weakness of the muscles of the posterior aspect of the calf the spring to the step is lost and the patient may walk with a shuffle. It should be stressed that a significant amount of gastrocnemius weakness may be present without any detectable abnormality of gait. In patients with weakness of the muscles of both anterior and posterior compartments of the leg the ankle joint is unstable in quiet standing and the patient may shift his weight uneasily from foot to foot.

There are, of course, other abnormalities which may be seen when a patient walks. It is beyond the scope of this paper to describe the walk in upper motor neuron illnesses, the gait of a patient with Parkinsonism, or of those with cerebellar disorders. Each have their own characteristics and these are well described in the standard neurological texts. Perhaps brief mention should be made of the hysterical abnormalities of gait. These are always difficult to evaluate and the patient's disturbance is usually a bizarre one. All varieties are seen from the patient whose every step is a slow and cautious exploration into unknown territory to those whose wild and acrobatic movements seem to bring them to the brink of disaster. It is interesting that if the physician can forebear to hold out the helping hand when the patient seems imminently on the point of collapsing to the floor, the hysteric will miraculously regain his balance and proceed unsteadily to some new predicament.

Observation of a patient while he is carrying out some simple tasks is an important part of the examination. The activities which are most useful to watch are arising from a sitting position on the floor, arising from a chair, stepping onto a chair, stepping onto a foot stool, walking on the heels, hopping on the toes, and raising the arms above the head. Weakness of muscles produces definite alterations in the way in which these are carried out. The fact that it is easier to get the cooperation of young patients with this series of tests than in attempting a more formal evaluation of strength is an added advantage.

ARISING FROM THE FLOOR

Ordinarily, a patient can arise from a sitting position on the floor swiftly and easily. He flexes his legs, drawing the feet under him, one hand may be transiently placed on the floor to provide an added push, and he then adopts a squatting position. From this position he stands, keeping the trunk erect, simply by straightening the legs. Children usually dispense with any hand support and bounce to their feet before one really has time to analyze the movement. With the development of hip weakness, there is a rather systematic deterioration in this performance. Starting from the same position, sitting on the floor with legs outstretched, the patient with proximal hip weakness will start by making a quarter turn of the trunk, usually to the weaker side. The hand towards which he is turning is then placed on the floor and simultaneously the knees are drawn up under the body. The whole weight is then shifted so that the patient is either resting on hands and knees or on one hand and one knee. In the next movement the patient straightens his knees raising his hips in the air. Colloquially, I know this as the "butt first" maneuver and the patient forms an arch with the buttocks at the apex. It is much easier for a patient to stand upright by straightening at the hips from this position than it is for him to arise from a squatting position. When the weakness is mild, a patient may arise readily from the floor when asked to do so, only the fact that he hoists his hips in the air before the rest of his body gives the clue to his loss of strength. When the weakness of the hips is severe, the patient adopts the butt first posture more laboriously and, indeed, the arch that the body forms is rather precariously balanced. The feet are wide spread and the hands firmly planted on the ground. One hand is then placed upon the thigh, leaving the body supported on both feet and one hand. This is the "tripod sign" so called because of the three point base upon which the patient rests. A firm thrust of the hand which is resting on the knee is sufficient to brace the trunk upwards and to allow some patients to stand. In others, both hands must be placed on the thighs to support the weight of the trunk. When viewed from the side, the body forms the shape of a capital A on its side with the apex being the hips and the cross bar the arms. The trunk is then inched laboriously upwards by the hands walking up the thighs. This entire maneuver is often known as the Gower's sign. Because the hand support on the thighs is crucial to the performance of this movement it should be noted that variations exists.

Some patients, particularly children with mild weakness, bend the arm and rest the elbow on the thigh when assuming the upright position. In others with very mild weakness the hand may touch the thigh only transiently in a rather fluid movement as the patient stands. Some patients adopt a maneuver which is slightly different from the Gower's maneuver. They find it easier to arise from a sitting position by first placing both hands slightly behind them flat upon the floor. The knees are then drawn up and the initial few inches of movement are obtained by a push from both arms. The patient then arises from a squatting position in the usual fashion. This initial bilateral arm push is another indication of mild hip weakness.

In analyzing the various ways in which patients arise from the floor, each component movement should be noted. These are as follows: hand support on the floor, either unilateral or bilateral; the quarter turn movement of the trunk; the butt first maneuver; and hand support on the thighs, either unilateral or bilateral, transient or laboured. If all these aspects are noted during a course of an illness, there will be a change in the performance which will be noted easily. This change may well occur at a time when formal testing of muscle strength does not show any difference.

ARISING FROM A CHAIR

The patient is asked to stand up from a chair, most standard kitchen chairs are about 18 inches high. This is ordinarily done without any assistance from the hands. Various changes are produced by different degrees of hip weakness. In early hip weakness the patient may need to put one hand on his knee or on the side of the chair and push briefly with this hand while standing. As the weakness becomes more severe, it may be necessary to use both hands for support. Finally, not only must both hands be used for support on the chair, but the patient climbs up his thighs with his hands in the typical fashion described under the Gower's maneuver. The patient may also begin the task by rocking the trunk. The trunk is rocked backwards and forwards in order to gain the momentum to enable the patient to stand.

STEPPING ONTO A CHAIR

Stepping up onto a chair between 18 and 20 inches high is a difficult task and unless the patient feels secure in doing it, the examiner should not insist. Anyone who can do this movement quickly without hand support and without pulling himself up on neighboring objects, has fairly good muscle strength. Early weakness of the hips results in a slight "pause" during the step. The patient places one foot on the chair and seems to gather himself for the effort. This hesitation is one of the earliest signs of hip weakness. The patient bends the knee of the leg which is still standing on the ground and then thrusts himself upwards. He now has to transfer his weight to the foot which is on the chair and in patients with some hip weakness, this is very often a moment of difficulty. Patients who are unable to do the task will fall back to stand on the other leg. Other patients may start to fall backwards momentarily but then catch themselves and are able to pull themselves up onto the chair. This results in a sag of the hip in mid movement, known as the "hip dip." Both the hesitation and the hip dip are indications of proximal weakness.

STEPPING ONTO A STOOL

We use a stool about 8 inches high for evaluating the stepping power of patients who are unable to step up onto a chair. This movement is usually an easy one and should be within the capabilities of even the elderly or the debilitated patient. Abnormalities in this movement associated with mild hip weakness are very similar to those described when the patient steps onto a chair. There may be a slight hesitation at the beginning of the movement. The hip dip presents often as a wobble in mid movement, almost as if the leg is about to give way. In addition, patients who have hip weakness may attempt to "throw" themselves up onto the foot stool. It is as if the whole body takes part in the movement upwards in a "throwing" motion, in which the shoulders seem to take as great a part as the hips. When the weakness becomes more severe, the patient may place one hand upon his knee in order to straighten the knee out and brace the trunk upwards, rather in the fashion that he does when arising from the floor. As the loss of strength progresses, the patient may have to use both hands, one on the knee and one on a nearby support to pull himself up onto the stool. The movement is evaluated for both legs individually and is graded as to whether there is hesitation, a hip dip, an upward throw, and unilateral or bilateral hand support.

WALKING ON THE HEELS

Normally one can walk on the heels of either foot with the feet dorsiflexed. This is done with no alteration in the posture of the trunk. Weakness of the anterior tibial muscles impedes this movement. It may be severe enough that the toes cannot be lifted from the ground at all. But in mild weakness the patient uses an alteration in his posture to enable him to do this. The knees are held stiffly and the hips are thrust backwards while the trunk is slightly flexed, so that the trunk counterbalances the change in the weight distribution. This new posture results in the legs slanting backwards when viewed from the side and gives the weakened anterior tibial muscles additional help in pulling the toes off the ground. Persons with normal strength never need to use this additional backward thrust of the hips to dorsiflex the feet.

HOPPING ON THE TOES

The patient is asked to hop on the toes of one foot and then the other. Some patients whose walk is almost normal are not able to do this at all. This is one of the few sensitive tests to bring out weakness of the plantar flexors of the feet. The test should be interpreted with caution in those with severe thigh and hip weakness since the performance may be hampered by the patient's real fear of the leg collapsing at the knee. In such cases the patient can be asked simply to walk on his toes.

RAISING THE ARMS ABOVE THE HEAD

Ordinarily there is no difficulty in holding the arms straight and abducting them from the sides to bring them up above the head until the hands touch. When viewed from in front, the hands follow the circumference of a semi-circle from the sides of the body to the mid line above the head. Patients with shoulder weakness adopt several tricks to try and overcome their difficulty. One of the earliest is a tendency to flex the elbows during the maneuver. A moment's reflection on the nature of levers and fulcrums will reveal that if the elbow is flexed the shoulder muscles have less work to do in supporting an arm abducted to 90 degrees. The second abnormality that may occur in the movement is the use of the trapezius and other accessory muscles during the movement. This results in a shoulder shrug as the movement is attempted. The last abnormality which is seen in severe weakness, is found when a patient is unable to get the arms above the head unless he clasps his hands in front of him and pulls. I am not sure what the mechanism is, but this makes it easier for the patient to get his hands above his head.

The preceding series of tests can be done quite quickly and will give much useful information with regard to proximal weakness of the hips and shoulders and distal weakness of the legs. It is also obvious that these maneuvers will not give information with regard to the strength in the hands, forearms, and upper arms. This means that formal examination of the biceps and triceps, of the forearm extensors and flexors, and of the small muscles of the hands must be carried out.

ACKNOWLEDGMENT

This work was supported in part by a grant from the Muscular Dystrophy Association.

The preceding is excerpted with permission from a forthcoming book *A Clinicians View of Neuromuscular Disease* to be published by The Williams & Wilkins Co.

Advances in Neurology, Vol. 17, edited by
R. C. Griggs and R. T. Moxley, III. Raven Press,
New York © 1977.

Myasthenia Gravis, Dermatomyositis, and Polymyositis: Immunopathological Diseases

Audrey S. Penn

H. Houston Merritt Clinical Research Center for Muscular Dystrophy and Related Diseases, Department of Neurology, College of Physicians and Surgeons, Columbia University and the Neurological Institute of the Presbyterian Hospital, New York, New York 10032

Accumulating evidence continues to suggest that myasthenia gravis, dermatomyositis, and polymyositis are immunopathological diseases. Yet the initiating events and the sequence in the production of disease are still far from being completely understood. In order to assess properly the methodology and the significance of the evidence used, it is important to review pertinent aspects of the immune response and current investigative methods before reviewing studies of the diseases.

The normal immune system functions primarily as our major line of defense against invading microorganisms (1). It requires the cooperative interaction of cells (lymphocyte, macrophages, leukocytes), products of these cells, and the complement system.

Both normal immune defenses and reactions against "self"-components (autoimmunity) are mediated by a dual system of immunocompetent lymphocytes: B cells and T cells (2). B cells are derived from the bone marrow stem cells, which are processed, in the chicken, by a separate central lymphoid organ, the bursa of Fabricius, and by an equivalent area not yet anatomically defined in man. They then migrate to the spleen and the lymph nodes, where they constitute the germinal centers and differentiate further into plasma cells, which synthesize and secrete immunoglobulins of all classes and antibody of defined specificity for antigen. The size of the germinal center is proportional to the intensity of antigenic stimulation (3).

T cells (thymic-dependent lymphocytes) are also derived from bone marrow stem cells but differentiate through several steps within the thymus gland. Mature T cells migrate to the spleen and lymph nodes where they occupy the so-called thymic-dependent areas or circulate as "memory" cells to participate, after antigenic stimulation, in cell-mediated reactions. Only peripheral circulating lymphocytes are immunocompetent; the central organs do *not* contain such cells.

Humoral immunity, which acts primarily against bacterial pathogens, depends on the production and action of antibodies with or without the contribution of complement. Antibodies coat the surface of bacteria or other toxic elements and immobilize motile forms allowing for agglutination, adherence to macrophages and polymorphonuclear leukocytes, phagocytosis, or lysis. Lysis is mediated by complement, a system of non-antibody serum β-globulins that is sequentially activated by reaction of antigen with antibody (4). Activated complement factors bind, also in sequence, to membrane-bound antigen, ultimately causing membrane lysis. Individual complement factors function in phagocytosis, immune adherence, and chemotaxis for leukocytes, much as do T-cell products, described below.

T cells are responsible for cellular immunity: delayed hypersensitivity, graft-versus-host reactions, rejection of allografts, and defense against viral and fungal pathogens. By an unknown mechanism, T cells recognize and process antigens so that sensitized T cells proliferate into lymphoblastic forms when they encounter that specific antigen. These lymphoblasts may cause direct lysis of tissue cells bearing the offending antigen, or they may be cytotoxic by producing a series of factors known as lymphokines. Lymphokines attract and immobilize macrophages, are chemotactic for eosinophils and neutrophils, attract and induce proliferation of other lymphocytes, and may be directly toxic. One lymphokine, transfer factor, has been demonstrated to transfer delayed hypersensitivity to purified protein derivative (tuberculin) (PPD) in humans (2).

Another extremely important T-cell function is cooperation with B cells for maximal antibody production. Antibody synthesis by B cells against most antigens is severely curtailed if T cells are absent (3). Indeed B cells recognize determinants on complex antigens which by size and location are essentially equivalent to haptenes, whereas T cells recognize the major carrier protion of the molecule (3). The exact mechanism for this type of cooperation, particularly the nature of the T-cell surface receptor and the contribution of macrophages, is still unknown. Equally important may be a class of T cells capable of suppression of antibody synthesis by B cells. Both thymectomy and antithymocyte serum, which eliminate T cells, paradoxically increase antibody production against some antigens (5).

T cells and B cells cannot be distinguished from each other by the light microscope or by ultrastructure. Accordingly, identification relies on functional characteristics. Until recently, assessment of functional status of the humoral immune system relied on measurements of immunoglobulin levels and response to immunization (vaccines, toxoids). Skin tests (delayed hypersensitivity), survival of isogeneic and allogeneic skin grafts (graft-versus-host), tested cellular mechanisms, and levels of total hemolytic complement and C-1 esterase (C-1s) could be measured (1). At present, B cells are identified and can be enumerated by detection of surface immunoglobulin (IgM and IgD), surface receptors for F_c immunoglobulin fragments and complement, as well as by their capacity to form complement-dependent sheep red cell rosettes. T cells are identified by surface alloantigens (such as the θ antigen on mouse cells), by capacity to bind spontaneously to sheep RBC (E rosettes), and through their ability to undergo blastic transformation and proliferation after incubation with plant lectins or mitogens [phytohemagglutinin, pokeweed (PWM), concanavalin A], ubiquitous antigens such as PPD, Candida or streptococcal derivatives or with allogeneic lymphocytes in the mixed-lymphocyte culture (MLC). Other lymphokines produced by sensitized T cells include the migration inhibition factor (MIF) (6) and lymphotoxin, which is assayed by quantitative cytotoxic effects on cultured cell lines of fibroblasts, L cells, or fetal muscle cells that bear the offending initiating antigen (7). The components of complement may also be measured individually (4).

The immune system may fail to function normally (7) because of deficiencies of one or more of the major components (8), but misdirected (autoimmunity) or excessive (hypersensitivity) activity of the system can also be destructive. Hypersensitivity is an amplification of normal defense mechanisms that causes tissue destruction as well as obliteration of the offending antigen. In autoimmunity, the same destructive phenomena are directed against self-antigens. Hypersensitivity reactions may also be mediated by antibody or by sensitized T lymphocytes. Four basic types were classified by Coombs and Gell (9). Reactions that depend on antibody overactivity include anaphylactic reactions (type 1) and immune-complex diseases (type 3), in which circulating antigen-antibody complexes block filters such as kidney glomeruli or lung, or bind complement and result in lytic lesions. The antigen may be virus, malarial parasite, Australia antigen, or foreign serum (serum sickness). Hemolytic anemia or tissue cytotoxicity may occur because the antigen binds to surface tissue antigens and coats the surface of cells, rendering them targets for complement-dependent or direct killer cell lysis (type 2). Similarly, cell-mediated hypersensitivity (type 4) may result in tissue damage by direct cytotoxic action of killer T cells or participation of mediators such as lymphotoxin. Special immunocytochemical detection (fluorescein or peroxidase) of bound antibody or complement demonstrates the underlying pathogenesis in types 2 and 3 in which the pathologist is likely to see a typical "inflammatory infiltrate."

In autoimmune diseases, the mechanisms that are responsible for self-tolerance and normally prevent recognition of self-components as antigens are disrupted and produce harmful antibodies or cells sensitized against self-components (red cells, nuclei, DNA, thyroid cells, or muscle elements) (10). The self-component may be altered by binding of a drug [demonstrated for alpha-methyldopa in hemolytic anemia or for apronalide (Sedormid ®) in thrombocytopenic purpura] or a virus (3). In normal individuals, there may be nanogram amounts of circulating thyroglobulin to which autologous B cells react without production of large amounts of antibody or thyroid disease (11). Tolerance here has been postulated to be mediated by the absence of reactive "helper" T cells, normally required to recognize specific antigen and cooperate with B cells in production of antibody.

In experimental thyroiditis, these T cells can be nonspecifically activated by the use of adjuvants (12). Alternatively, specific suppressor T cells may hold to a minimum the production of antibody by B cells against a particular antigen or completely suppress immunoglobulin production, as in common variable hypogammaglobulinemia (13). Inadequate or absent suppressor T-cell activity may be responsible for allowing B cells to produce antibody to self-antigens. Suppressor cells are deficient in the New Zealand black or black/white hybrid mice, which display a variety of autoantibodies (14).

Immune response (IR) is under genetic control. An immune response gene, linked on the chromosome to the major histocompatibility locus, determines a genetic predisposition to certain diseases (15). Well-studied murine examples include viral-induced lukemias and experimental auto-immune murine thyroiditis, readily acquired by certain inbred strains bearing specific H2 types whereas other strains respond poorly to thyroglobulin immunization (16). The cells that mediate the genetic control in this model are T cells (17).

MYASTHENIA GRAVIS

Myasthenia gravis must now be regarded as one of the major autoimmune diseases because of the recent demonstrations (18–20) that the characteristic defect in neuromuscular transmission results from partial blockade of acetyl-choline receptors by a circulating autoantibody.

Since the original suggestions by Nastuk and co-workers (21) and Simpson (22), it has been appreciated increasingly that many features of myasthenia suggest an immunopathological pathogenesis. The thymus gland is abnormal in 70 to 90% of patients. Lymphoid follicles in the form of germinal centers occur in the medulla of the gland in approximately 70%, a lesion known as hyperplasia; thymoma is found in 10% (23). Muscle may show lymphorrhages, foci of lymphocytes in muscle, or, less commonly, overt necrosis and inflammation (24). Myasthenia is also associated with auto-allergic disorders such as systemic lupus erythematosus, rheumatoid arthritis, and thyroid disorders (hypo- and hyperthyroidism, thyroiditis). Circulating autoantibodies are also found. Approximately 20 to 40% of the patients have antinuclear antibodies; 30% thyroglobulin; and 5 to 6% rheumatoid factor (25). Antimuscle antibodies, which can be detected by immunohistochemical techniques, occur in 30% of myasthenics, 20% of those with thymoma alone, and 95% of patients with myasthenia and thymoma. The presence of these antibodies is absolutely concordant with the immunofluorescence staining of thymic "myoid" cells, epithelioid species that represent remnants of striated fetal myoid elements (25,26).

Muscle antigens, implicated by careful comparison of phase and fluorescence photographs or ultrastructural analysis, include myosin, the major A-band protein; tropomyosin, troponin, or other I-band species; and membrane proteins of the sarcoplasmic reticulum (25,27). Direct immunochemical analyses (immunodiffusion, complement fixation, tanned red cell hemagglutination) employing crude muscle fractions as antigen confirmed the presence of antigen-antibody reactions but did not identify the specific antigen in mixtures. Immunodiffusion and complement fixation techniques demonstrated reactions with purified human skeletal muscle myosin in a few patients, especially those with myasthenia, thymoma (28), and a high titer of immunofluorescence staining of the A band. Yet muscle antibodies, present in only 30% of patients, have no obvious direct role in inhibiting neuromuscular transmission. Indeed, no staining of end plates could be detected by careful immunofluorescence examination of cholinesterase-localized end plates (29).

Transient neonatal myasthenia (6 to 8 weeks duration) of infants born to myasthenic mothers is another well-known and immunologically intriguing facet of myasthenia. Placentally transferred maternal IgG is one of the infant's major lines of defense until age 3 to 4 months, when the infant's own immunoglobulin G titer reaches adequate levels. This phenomenon strongly supports the hypothesis that a circulating factor, possibly IgG antibody, is involved in production of disease.

Humoral and Cellular Immunity

In spite of the multiplicity of autoantibodies and their suspected causal role, there has been little evidence of major derangements of the two arms of the immune system in patients. In one report (30) complement levels of myasthenics were found frequently with low levels, implying complement consumption by an antigen-antibody reaction, during exacerbation and high levels during remission. However, low complement levels may be the exception so that measurements of total hemolytic complement may not have much predictive value (31). Levels of the major classes of immunoglobulin, except for those reported in one study indicating depressed IgA content (31), are normal or slightly above normal (32). Investigations searching for depressed cellular immunity by testing the ability of myasthenics to be sensitized to dinitrochlorobenzene (DNCB), a universal antigen, were contradictory (33,34). In recent studies, overt skin test anergy did not occur to the routine battery (mumps, Candida, PPD, streptokinase/streptodornase [SK/SD]) or to DNCB (31).

In vitro studies of cellular immunity used the blastogenic response of isolated peripheral blood lymphocytes to mitogens and antigens, variations of the macrophage migration inhibition assay, assays of circulating B and T cells, and assays of cytoxic effects of isolated lymphocytes on fetal muscle or thymic cells in culture. Most workers have not demonstrated any accelerated or suppressed response of myasthenic lymphocytes to mitogens (PHA, PWM, concanavalin A, antithymocyte globulin); to streptococcal, tuberculin, or staphylococcal antigens; or to crude muscle or thymic antigens (35–38). The migration inhibition assay, which employs leukocytes (macrophages, polymorphonuclear leukocytes, and lymphocytes), demonstrated as much inhibition to central nervous system antigens as to muscle homogenate and muscle proteins, and results were inconclusive (39). Macrophage migration inhibition by autologous muscle and thymus did not differ from that of controls (31). The B-cell/T-cell composition of peripheral myasthenic lymphocytes was normal in one study of active myasthenics performed at thymectomy (37). In three studies (40–42), there was a modest depression of circulating T cells, especially in those post-thymectomy (from 4 months on), whereas a fourth study found normal E rosettes 8 years after thymectomy (31).

Hyperplastic thymus glands contain excessive numbers of B lymphocytes, as detected by surface immunoglobulin staining and sheep red cell antibody-complement (EAC) rosettes (37,30). Indeed, cytochemical assay of EAC binding to frozen thymic sections indicated that the reactive cells were located in the germinal centers in the medulla of the glands, the phenomenon regarded as "hyperplasia" (43). In addition, thymocytes from hyperplastic glands stimulated autologous peripheral blood lymphocytes (PBL) to transform in a one-way mixed-lymphocyte reaction system, implying an antigenic difference between the two cell populations. This was not a reflection of differences in surface HL-A antigenic species (40), and the basis for the antigenic disparity remains unclear.

In contrast, lymphoepithelial thymomas associated with myasthenia did not include excessive numbers of B cells and did not stimulate in the mixed-leukocyte reactions. After PHA stimulation, both thymoma cells and cells from hyperplastic glands produced a cytotoxic effect on cultured human fetal muscle cells (44). However, in a study designed to detect cytotoxic effects of isolated mononuclear cells in polymyositis by release of creatine phosphokinase into the culture media, four myasthenics were studied as controls (45). Their cells had no effect on the fetal rat cultures.

Histocompatibility

The unexpected frequency of certain HL-A types in certain groups of myasthenics strongly suggests a genetic predisposition even though familial incidence is uncommon (46). Data from six studies indicate that young female myasthenics, with hyperplastic thymus glands, carry the HL-A8 antigen in disproportionate numbers (46–51). Older males with myasthenia or with a thymoma and myasthenia and a high incidence of antimuscle antibodies appear to show an excessive frequency of HL-A3 (48) or HL-A2

(49) antigens and less frequent HL-A8. In addition, further MLC studies, using cells of patients homozygous for both HL-A and lymphocyte-defined (LD) antigens, indicate an unusual frequency of an LD antigen, similar to LD-8a in myasthenics (46,52). However, HL-A8 was more frequent than LD-8a in females with myasthenia. This suggests that the putative IR gene may be closer to the SD-2 locus of the chromosome (which bears HL-A8 and other HL-4 alleles) than it is to the LD-1 locus, which includes the LD-8a allele. HL-A and LD determinants are presumed to be markers for the IR gene itself. Indeed, the LD-MLC gene may itself be an IR gene. Clustering of HL-A or LD determinants in a disease may, therefore, be an indicator of a genetically instructed mechanism for antigen recognition mediated via the protein product of the IR gene. That protein is presumed to be on T cells but does not appear to be responsible for the autologous MLC reaction between thymic lymphocytes and peripheral blood lymphocytes in patients with thymic hyperplasia since HLA types on the two populations of cells were identical. Rather, the IR gene product might serve as an attachment site for virus or allow reaction to an altered self-antigen.

Reactions to self-antigens might also develop if the suppressor T-cell population were lost or functioned inadequately. Adequacy of the function of such cells in myasthenics has not yet been tested. Instead, thymectomy of some patients either reduces or reduces further the function of such a T-cell population since these myasthenics demonstrated an increased reaction to alloantigens, post-thymectomy, as tested by the MLC technique (42).

The Experimental Model

A major breakthrough occurred when the venom of certain elapid snakes, including cobras and the multibanded krait, *Bungarus multicinctus,* proved to contain α-neurotoxins, which bound specifically and with high affinity to the nicotinic acetylcholine receptor (53,54). The radiolabeled toxin provided a specific marker to follow during isolation and purification of receptor from the rich sources provided by the electric fish and electric eel, long employed for isolation and investigation of acetylcholinesterase. The other major technical advances were the use of nonionic detergents for solubilization of membrane proteins without denaturation and the development of affinity chromatography, a technique in which specific ligands, covalently attached to an inert solid carrier, are used to capture compounds to which they have high affinity from a crude mixture. The desired protein can then be desorbed by a second ligand of higher affinity. Purified cobra toxins and synthetic quaternary ammonium ligands have been employed for the affinity chromatography of acetylcholine receptor, which may then be eluted with Bis-Q (55), gallamine (56), carbamylcholine (57), or similar compounds.

RABBITS

The first attempts to produce an antibody to isolated electric eel receptor, by Patrick and Lindstrom (58) and Changeux et al. (59), yielded precipitating antibody; moreover, as soon as the titer rose significantly, the immunized rabbits became severely ill with flaccid paralysis. Detailed studies of the clinical, electrical, and immunochemical characteristics of the rabbit model indicated that the severity of the limb, respiratory, and ear muscle weakness and the degree of reversibility of weakness with anticholinesterases were directly related to the antibody titer (60). The antibody titer usually rises within 2 to 6 days of a boosting injection that has been administered from 7 to 28 days after the immunizing injection (61,62). The antibody is an IgG (61).

Electrophysiological studies on the rabbits and *in vitro* studies on isolated intercostal muscle demonstrated all of the parameters of myasthenia, including decremental responses to low rates of stimulation, postactivation exhaustion, post-tetanic potentiation, and a 50% reduction in the amplitude of the miniature end-plate potentials (MEPPs) (61). Rabbits, boosted 28 days after immunization, developed decremental responses of up to 90% and a reduction in MEPP amplitudes to approximately 50%. In many rabbit intercostal muscle fibers, no MEPPs could be detected (60–62). The degree of decrement, the MEPP amplitude, and the *in vitro* binding of α-bungarotoxin to intercostal fibers correlated well with the antibody titer (60). Importantly, careful administration of α-cobratoxin to rats with reduction of available end plates to 70% (63) demonstrated the same electrophysiological features, indicating that the antibody interferes with the same receptor determinants that contribute to electrogenesis and to which α-toxins bind. Current evidence indicates that the effect of antibody is indirect, probably via steric hindrance of the access of small molecules such as acetylcholine since the α-toxin and the antibody do not bind to the same determinants (19,60).

Histochemical (61,62) and ultrastructural examination of muscle and end-plate regions of immunized rabbits did not demonstrate any degree of inflammation or foci of lymphocytes suggesting lymphorrhages. End plates of immunized animals demonstrated an accumulation of dense material in the synaptic clefts not found in controls. There were a few foci of muscle fiber necrosis.

RATS

Both the clinical and morphological features of the model in rats differed from those in rabbits. When conventionally immunized with complete Freund's adjuvant and electric fish receptor, rats did not become paralyzed (60–64). Only a few became detectably weak, although antibody titers were often as high as in rabbits, and there were typical decremental responses and reduced MEPP amplitudes, repaired by anticholinesterases. Rats also showed these electrophysiological abnormalities approximately 10–14 days after receiving only one injection of receptor-plus-adjuvant (64) when they were not obviously weak.

Another version of the rat model was studied by Lennon et al. (65). The animals received eel receptor plus complete Freund's adjuvant supplemented with extra *Mycobacterium butyricum* and *M. tuberculosis* plus 10^{10} *Bordetella pertussis* organisms. A single injection produced two phases of weakness, an acute phase at 7 to 12 days and a chronic phase at 26 to 35 days. In the early phase, most rats receiving higher doses of receptor were obviously weak, but not paralyzed, with modest antibody titers. Electrical features were characteristic.

Morphological studies (66) indicated degeneration of tips of the synaptic fold with disruption and splitting off of the postsynaptic areas and invasion and removal of the split-off areas by macrophages. In the chronic phase the rats were progressively weak but there were no decremental responses unless challenged with curare. However, MEPP amplitudes were typically reduced and the titer of antibodies was higher than in acute-phase rats. At this stage, ultrastructural changes were similar to those found in myasthenia, with simplified postsynaptic folds.

The model has also been successfully produced in guinea pigs, goats, sheep, and monkeys (65,67). Guinea pigs develop a mild form, whereas monkeys develop a severe form of the experimental disease. Antigenic determinants, among those shared by Torpedo and eel receptor (only approximately 50% of determinants are identical) (61), seem also to be phylogenetically conserved in receptors from rabbits, monkeys, and rats. In spite of producing a very high titer of antibody against Torpedo receptor in rats, detectable titers of reaction against isolated rat receptor are 1,000 times less (20). Disease is produced at this low level of reaction of anti-Torpedo antibodies with common determinants of the rat receptor. Mice receptors share so few determinants with Torpedo and eel that immunization with fish receptors produces a high titer of antibody but no clinical effect, and production of the model disease requires the use of rat receptor (68).

IMMUNOLOGY

Results from rabbit studies strongly suggest a causative role for circulating antireceptor antibodies induced by immunization. Direct application of antibody to the electroplax preparation and to rat diaphragm (61) and frog muscles (60) resulted in reduced MEPPs and reduced carbamylcholine depolarization (61) to approximately 40% of normal. Cytotoxic T cells may also contribute to the pathogenesis or even initiate the process. The inflammatory reaction found in the acute phase of the rat model of Lennon and colleagues suggests that T cells play a major role. However, the extra adjuvants they used are known to potentiate the effects of muscle membrane antigens in the production of experimental myositis (69), and may have modified this rat model by invoking cytotoxic T cells. Cellular immunity to receptor has been demonstrated through delayed hypersensitivity in rats and guinea pigs (65) and transformation of lymphocytes from immunized rabbits when incubated with receptor *in vitro*. Also, the model disease produced in inbred histocompatible rats and guinea pigs has been passively transferred with lymph node cells. Recipient rats demonstrated mild weakness, electrophysiological signs, and delayed hypersensitivity but no detectable antibody (70,71).

It would appear that both cellular and humoral mechanisms are involved in the model disease. At the least, T cells are involved in instructing B cells to recognize the antigen to allow production of antibodies of the IgG class. Alternatively, antibody-dependent cytotoxicity or opsonization of end plates, with contributions from complement fixed by tissue-bound receptor-antibody reactions, may be an important mechanism.

TREATMENT OF THE MODEL

The model disease in rats has been successfully prevented by thymectomy before immunization but not by thymectomy 35 days after immunization (64,70). In rabbits, however, preimmunization thymectomy had no obvious clinical or electrophysiological effects, nor did the antibody titer change significantly (G. Toufexis, K. Brockbank, R. E. L. Lovelace, H. W. Chang, and A. S. Penn, *unpublished results*). Administration of azathioprine to rabbits prevented the appearance of the disease and suppressed cellular immunity for at least 4 months. Hydrocortisone administered in gradually increasing doses from the day of immunization also suppressed the development of disease after the booster injection (72).

Reaction with Acetylcholine Receptor in Myasthenia

The first demonstrations of an effect of factors in myasthenic sera on receptors were indirect. Autoradiography of radioiodinated α-bungarotoxin binding sites was used to assess the numbers of receptors at myasthenic neuromuscular junctions in deltoid biopsies (73). These biopsies proved to contain only 11 to 30% of binding sites found in control muscles, and myasthenic junctions were elongated and less folded. An increased extrajunctional binding was also demonstrated. Globulin fractions of 5 of 15 myasthenics inhibited α-bungarotoxin binding to a crude receptor preparation isolated from denervated rat muscle (74). However, neither the serum, the globulin fraction, nor the active IgG isolated from one serum similarly blocked binding to crude receptor from normal human muscle. However, serum IgG inhibition of α-bungarotoxin binding to normal human muscle end plates was demonstrated using an antibody to toxin and immunoperoxidase detection of antitoxin antibody (75).

These experiments are predicated on the specificity of α-bungarotoxin binding and on the demonstration that toxin does not occupy sites bound by antibody. The specificity of binding to normal and denervated rat muscle has been examined in detail by Brockes and Hall (76) and shown to be equivalent, although receptors from the two muscles differ slightly on isoelectric focusing and in curare binding. If a saturating amount of toxin is allowed to bind to electric fish receptors before application of antibody, then specific anti-eel or anti-torpedo receptor antibodies precipitate receptors as well as toxin. If antibody, in excess, is allowed to bind completely before addition of toxin, toxin will be completely excluded (61). This has also been shown using denervated rat muscle receptor and myasthenic globulin (60).

Recently, the sensitive double-antibody radioimmunoassay has been used to demonstrate reactions directly between myasthenic serum globulin fraction, or IgG, and crude acetylcholine receptor preparations from denervated rat and human muscle, solubilized with detergent and labeled with radioiodinated α-bungarotoxin. Serum antibody activity was demonstrated in approximately 70% of patients using rat receptor (19) and 95% with human receptor (20). Also, 80% of patients have serum antibody activity to purified and well-characterized electric fish receptors as assessed by microcomplement fixation (18) and by double-antibody radioimmunoassay (A. S. Penn, H. W. Chang, D. L. Schotland, and S. Lammé, *unpublished results*). All of these assays indicated some degree of correlation of antibody titer with severity of the disease in the total of approximately 175 patients studied so far. A few patients with ocular myasthenia do have antibody, but those who do exhibit a lower titer than patients with generalized myasthenia. Nine of the eleven patients with myasthenia and a thymoma had antibody (20). Presence of antibody did not correlate with the presence or absence of any HL-A phenotype (19). Steroid therapy was demonstrated to reduce antibody titers in two or three patients (20). The role of circulating antibodies in myasthenia was also evaluated by passive transfer of myasthenic IgG to cyclophosphamide-treated mice by 9 to 14 daily injections (77). These mice demonstrated reduced MEPP amplitudes, reduced radioiodinated α-bungarotoxin–detectable sites, and, in some cases, decremental responses.

Cellular immunity to acetylcholine receptor in myasthenic patients has also been demonstrated using isolated peripheral blood lymphocytes. In one study, a crude water-soluble receptor-enriched fraction of electric eel organ membranes was employed. Lymphocyte transformation after 5 days of incubation with antigen was assessed by ^{14}C-thymidine incorporation.

Ratios of uptake with or without added antigen indicated a modest uptake by myasthenic lymphocytes in a range that was barely significant (78). Patients who improved after at least 10 days of prednisone therapy demonstrated reduced lymphocyte responses (79). A careful investigation using purified eel receptor, in a detergent that did not damage lymphocytes, indicated impressive responses in older males and patients with thymomas, with a positive correlation between the degree of lymphocyte stimulation and severity of symptoms (80). Thymocytes from two young female myasthenics out of seven studied responded to receptor but failed to stimulate autologous lymphocytes; one other stimulated autologous lymphocytes but did not react to receptor.

Possible Mechanisms and Relation to Therapy

The finding of humoral and cellular reactions to receptor indicates that antibody is not produced simply because of lack of thymic control. There is little evidence of defective cellular mechanisms even though humoral systems are quite active, with excessive B cells in the thymus and production of a multiplicity of autoantibodies. Indeed, sensitized T cells may initiate the lesion or contribute to it. There seems to be a loss of tolerance in myasthenia that originates in the thymic control stage. A population of suppressor T cells may be lacking or there may be excessive helper cell activity, but the well-known beneficial response to thymectomy (25,81) would then be paradoxical since by removing suppressor T cells thymectomy tends to increase the production of autoantibodies (5,82). Other evidence indicates that the myasthenic thymus contains the offending receptor and muscle antigens within its myoid cell population (26,83, and A. S. Penn, H. W. Chang, D. L. Schotland, and S. Lammé, *unpublished results*) and, at some stages, may also contain the antibody (83,84). Consequently, tolerance to self-antigens has clearly been breached. This suggests that there may have been an alteration in the normal thymic myoid components prominent in fetal life, so that they become antigenic. The acquisition of a viral antigen is one possibility or another alteration in some way related to possession of certain HL-A types.

Except for anticholinesterases, the other current modes of therapy are immunosuppressive. Thoracic duct drainage (85,86) and antithymocyte globulin (ATG) directly deplete T cells. Both have been effective in myasthenia if therapy is prolonged to the point of skin test anergy, but side effects of ATG may be intolerable (87). Prednisone inhibits the model disease, especially when given with the immunizing dose of antigen (72), and appears to suppress both humoral and cell-mediated immunity to receptor in myasthenics (79,80). The sites of steroid action on the immune system are still largely unknown and there are species variations, so that no conclusions can be drawn as to the primary site of steroid action. Thymectomy, which is beneficial in approximately 75% of patients (81), may simultaneously remove antigen, B-cell precursors involved in antibody formation, and regulating immune cell populations. It has not been effective in the model disease unless timed correctly, but the response in myasthenia is often delayed and its role in the treatment of myasthenia appears secure. The unimpressive and uncertain effects of immunosuppressive agents (azathioprine, cyclophosphamide, methotrexate) (88) most probably reflect the inability to time therapy appropriately with initiating events in the disease and its exacerbations as well as the dread of serious side effects.

DERMATOMYOSITIS AND POLYMYOSITIS

Although dermatomyositis (DM) and polymyositis (PM) probably do not represent the same disease, recent work strongly suggests that they are immunopathological entities with a similar, if not identical, final common injury to muscle.

Viral Etiology

A direct viral etiology is unlikely although myxovirus-like filamentous-tubular structures were demonstrated in five patients by Chou (88) and Sato and colleagues (89). In other patients with PM and fatal DM, intra-cytoplasmic particles were present, with a triangular lattice crystalline array felt to be consistent with one of the picornavirus group (polio, echo, coxsackie, or encephalomyocarditis virus) (90–92). Other investigators doubt that this material is virus since immunofluorescence demonstration and viral isolation have been unsuccessful. A recent case where coxsackie A9 was isolated did not have classic PM but had slowly progressive weakness and wasting, present from infancy, with a sudden fatal acute febrile illness at age 11 (93).

Antibody Etiology

Another possible pathogenic mechanism considered for these diseases is participation of antigen-antibody immune complexes with or without fixation of complement (type III hypersensitivity). This pathogenesis would be similar to that of systemic lupus erythematosus (SLE) where circulating DNA–anti-DNA complexes are responsible for the glomerular disease. Antibodies to breast tumor homogenates were demonstrated in a few patients with associated dermatomyositis (94,95), but they appear to be tumor specific and unrelated to the development of DM since eight other patients without any evidence of DM had similar immediate type skin sensitivity and complement-fixing antibody (96). Appropriate autoantibodies reflecting the primary disease may also be seen when polymyositis complicates SLE or rheumatoid arthritis. Antibodies to muscle antigens have not been convincingly demonstrated, although a series of evaluations has employed most classic methods (25). Titers were similar in patients and controls or equal in dystrophic and neurogenic diseases. Careful immunofluorescence analysis employing human myofibrils, which readily detect antimuscle antibodies in myasthenia, have consistently failed to detect antibodies in serum from DM or PM patients (25,97).

The major recent study that suggested a role for immune-complex deposition or complement-dependent cytophilic antibodies, which might cause antibody-dependent cytotoxicity to muscle membrane targets, is the investigation by Whitaker and Engel (98). This study demonstrated bound IgM in the wall of a muscle vessel from a child with DM, using fluorescein-tagged IgM. Deposits of IgG, IgM, and C-3 complement component were detected especially in children with DM, but also in 33 to 50% of patients with PM and an associated collagen-vascular disease. The independent study by Fessel and Raas (99) did not confirm this, but details of the type of disease and age of their eight patients are not available. Recently, Dawkins and Mastaglia (100) reported their failure to demonstrate IgG and C-3 deposits in one adult PM patient with clear-cut lymphocyte-mediated cytotoxicity, whereas Griggs et al. (101) found such deposits in several children with DM. The positive results in children with DM tend to emphasize that the juvenile form of this disease may be a consequence of widespread vasculitis, as strongly suggested by the studies of Banker (102,103). The offending antigen remains unknown—although the contribution of a virus such as coxsackie or herpes zoster (104) must be considered and pursued. Similarly, the contribution of Australia antigen to the immune complex deposition in vessel walls in periarteritis nodosa (105) suggests that detection of bound immunoglobulin in PM associated with collagen-vascular disease may represent a clue to the pathogenesis of both processes. Since DM may occur in patients who lack complement factors (102) or who are agammaglobulinemic (106) and since total serum complement is usually normal, more questions than answers remain.

Experimental Myositis

Attempts to produce an experimental model of myositis have still not successfully reproduced a progressive clinical myopathy but have contributed evidence of abnormal cell-mediated immunity to muscle. Several original studies simply produced adjuvant arthritis (25,107) with a few inflammatory lesions remote from joints or injection sites. Injection of heterologous muscle plus complete Freund's adjuvant into rats produced foci of inflammation, and isolated lymphocytes from immunized animals were cytotoxic against fetal muscle cultures and caused similar lesions in isogeneic recipient animals after passive transfer (108–110). Recipient animals also developed antibodies that bound to alternate striations of isogeneic muscle (111).

However, application of these sera to monolayer cultures of chick embryo skeletal muscle did not produce cytotoxicity as assessed by release of ^{51}-Cr and CPK (112). More widespread and intense myositis was produced in certain rat strains by using a mitochondrial-sarcotubular fraction of homologous muscle, reducing the tubercle bacilli in the adjuvant and increasing the amount of protein injected (69,113). Affected recipients had elevated serum enzymes (CPK, aldolase, GOT), and the disease could be passively transferred with lymphocytes. In another recent investigation, the myofibrillar fraction of heterologous muscle consistently produced a more severe myositis, with more impressive CPK elevations in recipients than mitochondrial or microsomal fractions. Sera from immunized animals stained A-bands and Z-line regions of stretched myofibrils (114). Thus more convincing experimental models of myositis are under investigation and the results so far suggest a primary role for sensitized cytotoxic T lymphocytes, although antibodies to skeletal muscle components are also produced.

Cellular Immunity in Patients

Lymphocytes isolated from patients with PM and DM have been examined for cytotoxic effects. Johnson and colleagues (115) demonstrated production of the T-cell lymphokine, lymphotoxin, when patient lymphocytes were cultured with their own (autochthonous) muscle in medium free of immunoglobulin (fetal calf serum). The supernatants of these cultures were cytotoxic to human fetal muscle culture monolayers by both histological criteria and inhibition of incorporation of ^{14}C-labeled amino acids. The supernatants contained lymphotoxin with the chromatographic characteristics of a standard lymphotoxin preparation. This study also demonstrated clearly that methylprednisolone, at a concentration nearly that of normal plasma cortisol, markedly suppressed the cytotoxic effects when added to a supernatant sample before application to the cultures.

Similarly, lymphocytes from patients with polymyositis proved cytotoxic to chick embryo muscle cultures as assessed by release of ^{51}-Cr (100). Serum or serum plus complement had no effect, indicating the absence of circulating complement-dependent antibody. Immunosuppression, with prednisone or azathioprine, to the point of skin test anergy to ubiquitous antigens (PPD, mumps, SK/SD) depressed this cell-mediated cytotoxicity. Importantly, alternate-day prednisone, even at 100-mg levels (or daily <10 mg), did not. In another study by Haas and Arnason (45), using a similar design, lymphocytes from patients produced muscle fiber destruction of rat fetal cultures as well as CPK release into the culture medium. Serum caused no detectable change. The ultrastructure of such muscle cultures and of muscle from patients with DM may demonstrate close apposition of lymphocytes and muscle membranes plus evidence of emperipolesis (the ability of lymphocytes to enter and move around in other cells without disrupting the cell membrane) (116).

Other attempts to demonstrate cell-mediated hypersensitivity of lymphocytes from patients with myositis to mitogens and muscle homogenate antigens have not been entirely convincing. Lymphocyte transformation assays, assessing incorporation of tritiated thymidine, were very modestly different from results using control lymphocytes in two studies (117,118), and normal in a third recently published (119). It therefore appears that cytotoxic T cells and their products may be responsible for induction of the inflammatory infiltrate and necrosis of muscle in many cases of adult DM and PM. The initiating event that results in sensitization of T cells remains obscure. Possibilities include an exogenous viral infection (88–92, 104) with secondary alteration of muscle proteins so that they become antigenic. Another pathogen that may be involved is *Toxoplasma gondii*. Kagen and colleagues (120) found a striking incidence of positive Sabin-Feldman dye tests and complement-fixation tests in PM and DM of recent onset, but no organism could be isolated from muscle.

Investigations in patients suggest that immunosuppressive therapy, including that with corticosteroids and antimetabolites, should be used in doses adequate to suppress cellular immunity and at appropriate times in the course of the disease. Therapy for these diseases is discussed further by Rowland et al. (*this volume*).

CONCLUSIONS

Current evidence supports an immunopathological pathogenesis for myasthenia gravis, polymyositis, and dermatomyositis. The humoral arm of immune defense appears to be directly responsible for the lesion in myasthenia gravis, but cellular mechanisms, at the thymic regulatory level, are also involved. Cytotoxic T cells seem to produce the lesions of experimental myositis, in which antimuscle antibodies can be detected, and those of polymyositis and dermatomyositis, in which antibodies have not been convincingly shown. Childhood dermatomyositis is probably an exception in which antibodies and complement contribute to an underlying vasculitis. Immunosuppressive measures can modify or prevent the disease in experimental models, and the evidence indicates a solid rationale for their use in human diseases, although much more information is required as to the site of action and appropriate therapeutic timing.

ACKNOWLEDGMENT

Supported by center grants from the Muscular Dystrophy Association and the National Institute of Neurological and Communicative Diseases and Stroke (NS 11766).

REFERENCES

1. Roitt, I. (1974): *Essential Immunology*. Blackwell Scientific Publications, London.
2. Craddock, C. G., Longmire, R., and McMillan, R. (1971): Lymphocytes and the immune response. *N. Engl. J. Med.*, 285:324–331, 378–384.
3. Eisen, H. (1974): *Immunology*. Harper & Row, Hagerstown, Maryland.
4. Müller-Eberhard, H. J. (1971): The molecular basis of the biological activities of complement. *Harvey Lect.*, 66:75–104.
5. Gershon, R. K. (1974): T-cell control of antibody production. *Contemp. Top. Immunobiol.*, 3:1–40.
6. David, J. R. (1973): Lymphocyte mediators and cellular hypersensitivity. *N. Engl. J. Med.*, 288:143–149.
7. Granger, G. A., Daynes, R. A., Runge, P. E., Prieur, A. M., and Jeffes, E. W. B., III (1975): Lymphocyte effector molecules and cell-mediated immune reactions. *Contemp. Top. Mol. Immunol.*, 4:205–241.
8. Good, R. (1971): Disorders of the immune system. In: *Immunobiology*, edited by R. A. Good and D. W. Fisher, Sinauer Associates, Stamford, Conn.
9. Coombs, R. R. A., and Gell, P. G. H. (1968): Classification of allergic reactions responsible for clinical hypersensitivity and disease. In: *Clinical Aspects of Immunology*, edited by P. G. H. Gell and R. R. A. Coombs. Blackwell Scientific Publications, Oxford.
10. Stiller, C. R. (1975): Autoimmunity: Present concepts. *Ann. Intern. Med.*, 82:405–410.
11. Bankhurst, A. D., Torrigiani, G., and Allison, A. C. (1973): Lymphocytes binding human thyroglobulin in healthy people and its relevance to tolerance for auto antigens. *Lancet*, 1:226–230.
12. Allison, A. C., Denman, A. M., and Barnes, R. D. (1971): Cooperating and controlling functions of thymus-derived lymphocytes in relation to autoimmunity. *Lancet* 2:135–140.
13. Waldman, T. A., Broder, S., Blaese, R. M., Durm, M., Blackman, M., and Strober, W. A. (1974): Role of suppressor T-cells in pathogenesis of common variable hypogammaglobulinemia. *Lancet*, 2:609–613.
14. Steinberg, A. B. (1974): Pathogenesis of autoimmunity in New Zealand mice. V. Loss of thymic suppressor function. *Arthritis Rheum.*, 17:11–14.
15. Benacerraf, B., and McDevitt, H. O. (1972): Histocompatibility-linked immune response genes. *Science*, 175:273–279.
16. Vladutiu, A. O., and Rose, N. R. (1974): Autoimmune murine thyroiditis. Relation to histocompatibility (H-2) type. *Science*, 174:1137–1139.
17. Vladuti, A. O., and Rose, N. R. (1975): Cellular basis of the genetic control of immune responsiveness to murine thyroglobulin in mice. *Cell. Immunol.*, 17:106–113.
18. Aharanov, A., Abramsky, O., Tarrab-Hazdai, R., and Fuchs, S. (1975): Humoral antibodies to acetylcholine receptor in patients with myasthenia gravis. *Lancet*, 2:340–342.
19. Appel, S. H., Almon, R. R., and Levy, N. (1975): Acetylcholine receptor antibodies in myasthenia gravis. *N. Engl. J. Med.*, 293:760–761.
20. Lindstrom, J. M., Lennon, V. A., Seybold, M. E., and Whittingham, S. (1976): Experimental autoimmune myasthenia gravis and myasthenia gravis. *Ann. N.Y. Acad. Sci.*, 274:254–274.
21. Nastuk, W. L., Strauss, A. J. L., and Osserman, K. E. (1959): Search for a neuromuscular blocking agent in the blood of patients with myasthenia gravis. *Am. J. Med.*, 26:394–409.
22. Simpson, J. A. (1960): Myasthenia gravis. A new hypothesis. *Scot. Med. J.*, 5:419–436.
23. Castleman, B. (1966): The pathology of the thymus gland in myasthenia gravis. *Ann. N.Y. Acad. Sci.*, 135:496–505.
24. Russell, D. S. (1953): Histological changes in striped muscles in myasthenia gravis. *J. Pathol. Bacteriol.*, 65:279–289.
25. Penn, A. S., Schotland, D. L., and Rowland, L. P. (1971): Immunology of muscle disease. *Res. Publ. Assoc. Res. Nerv. Ment. Dis.*, 49:215–240.
26. Töro, I., Gazsó, L., Török, R. O., and Oláh, I. (1968): Myogenese in gewebekülturen des thymus electronen mikroskopische untersuchung. *Z. Zellforsch*, 89:241–249.
27. Mendell, J. R., Whitaker, J. N., and Engel, W. K. (1973): The skeletal muscle binding site of antistriated muscle antibody in myasthenia gravis: An electron microscopic immunohistochemical study using peroxidase conjugated antibody fragments. *J. Immunol.*, 111:847–856.

28. Penn, A. S., Schotland, D. L., and Rowland, L. P. (1969): Antibody to human myosin in man. *Trans. Am. Neurol. Assoc.,* 94:48–53.
29. Engel, W. K., and McFarlin, D. E. (1966): Muscle lesions in myasthenia gravis. Discussion. *Ann. N.Y. Acad. Sci.,* 135:68–78.
30. Nastuk, W. L., Plescia, O. J., and Osserman, K. E. (1960): Changes in serum complement activity in patients with myasthenia gravis. *Proc. Soc. Exp. Biol. Med.,* 105:177–184.
31. Simpson, J. A., Behan, P. O., and Dick, H. M. (1976): Studies on the nature of autoimmunity in myasthenia gravis. Evidence for an immunodeficiency type. *Ann. N.Y. Acad. Sci.,* 274:382–389.
32. Lisak, R. P., and Zweiman, B. (1976): Serum immunoglobulin levels in myasthenia gravis, polymyositis and dermatomyositis. *J. Neurol. Neurosurg. Psychiatry,* 39:34–37.
33. Adner, M. M., Sherman, J. D., Ise, C., Schwab, R. S., and Damashek, W. (1964): An immunologic survey of forty-eight patients with myasthenia gravis. *N. Engl. J. Med.,* 271:1327–1333.
34. Kornfeld, P., Siegal, S., Weiner, L. B., and Osserman, K. E. (1965): Immunologic response in the thymectomized and non-thymectomized patients. *Ann. Intern. Med.,* 63:416–428.
35. Houseley, T., and Oppenheim, J. J. (1967): Lymphocyte transformation in thymectomized and nonthymectomized patients with myasthenia gravis. *Br. Med. J.,* 2:679–681.
36. Lisak, R. P., and Zweiman, B. (1975): Mitogen and muscle extract induced *in vitro* proliferative responses in myasthenia gravis, dermatomyositis and polymysitis. *J. Neurol. Neurosurg. Psychiatry,* 38:521–524.
37. Adou, N. I., Lisak, R. P., Zweiman, B., Abrahamsohn, I., and Penn, A. S. (1974): The thymus in myasthenia gravis. Evidence for altered cell populations. *N. Engl. J. Med.,* 291:1271–1275.
38. Kalden, J. R., Lohmann, E., Peter, H. H., and Hilger, C. (1976): Antibody-dependent cellular cytotoxicity and B- and T-cell activity in the peripheral blood of myasthenia gravis patients. *Ann. N.Y. Acad. Sci.,* 274:421–433.
39. Albert, L. I., Rule, A., Norio, M., Kott, E., Kornfeld, P., and Osserman, K. E. (1972): Studies in myasthenia gravis: Cellular hypersensitivity to skeletal muscle. *Am. J. Clin. Pathol.,* 58:647–653.
40. Lisak, R. P., Abdou, N. I., Zweiman, B., Zmijewski, C., and Penn, A. S. (1967): Aspects of lymphocyte function in myasthenia gravis. *Ann. N.Y. Acad. Sci.,* 274:402–410.
41. Koziner, B., Bloch, K. T., and Perlo, V. P. (1976): Distribution of peripheral blood latex-ingesting cells, T-cells, and B-cells in patients with myasthenia gravis. *Ann. N.Y. Acad. Sci.,* 274:411–420.
42. Brinbaum, G., and Tsairis, P. (1976): Suppressor lymphocytes in myasthenia gravis and effect of adult thymectomy. *Ann. N.Y. Acad. Sci.,* 274:527–535.
43. Staber, F. G., Fink, U., and Sack, W. (1975): B lymphocytes in the thymus of patients with myasthenia gravis. Letter. *N. Engl. J. Med.,* 292:1032–1033.
44. Armstrong, R. M., Nowak, R. R., and Falk, R. E. (1973): Thymic lymphocyte function in myasthenia gravis. *Neurology (Minneap.),* 23:1078–1083.
45. Haas, D. C., and Arnason, B. G. W. (1974): Cell-mediated immunity in polymyositis. Creatine phosphokinase release from muscle cultures. *Arch. Neurol.,* 31:192–196.
46. Pirskanen, R. (1976): Genetic associations between myasthenia gravis and the HL-A system. *J. Neurol. Neurosurg. Psychiatry,* 39:23–33.
47. Dick, H. M., Behan, P. O., Simpson, J. A., and Durward, W. F. (1974): The inheritance of HL-A antigens in myasthenia gravis. *J. Immunogenet.,* 1:401–412.
48. Fritze, D., Herrmann, C., Jr., Naeim, F., Smith, G. S., and Walford, R. L. (1974): HL-A antigens in myasthenia gravis. *Lancet,* 1:240–242.
49. Feltkamp, T. E. W., Van den Berg-Loonen, P. M., Nijenhuis, L. E., Engelfreit, C. P., Van Rossum, A. L., Van Loghem, J. J., and Oosterhuis, H. J. G. H. (1974): Myasthenia gravis, autoantibodies and HL-A antigens. *Br. Med. J.,* 1:131–133.
50. Säfwenberg, T., Lindblom, J. B., and Osterman, P.-O. (1973): HL-A frequencies in patients with myasthenia gravis. *Tissue Antigens,* 3:465–469.
51. Müller-Eckhardt, C., Gross, W., Friedrich, F., Krüger, J., and Kunze, K. (1974): HL-A antigen-frequenzen und zellvermittelte immunreaktionen bei myasthenia gravis. *Z. Immunitaetsforsch,* 147:331 (abstract).

52. Möller, E., Hammarström, L., Smith, E., and Matell, G. (1976): HL-A8 and LD-8a in patients with myasthenia gravis. *Tissue Antigens*, 7:39–44.
53. Chang, C. C., and Lee, C. Y. (1963): Isolation of neurotoxins from the venom of Bungarus multicinctus and their modes of neuromuscular blocking action. *Arch. Int. Pharmacodyn. Ther.*, 144:241–257.
54. Changeux, J.-P., Kasai, M., and Lee, C. Y. (1970): Use of snake venom toxin to characterize the cholinergic receptor protein. *Proc. Natl. Acad. Sci. U.S.A.*, 67:1241–1247.
55. Chang, H. W. (1974): Purification and characterization of acetylcholine receptor-I from Electrophorus electricus. *Proc. Natl. Acad. Sci. U.S.A.*, 71:2113–2117.
56. Meunier, J.-C., Sealock, R., Olsen, R., and Changeux, J.-P. (1974): Purification and properties of the cholinergic receptor protein from Electrophorus electricus electric tissue. *Eur. J. Biochem.*, 45:371–394.
57. Karlsson, E., Heilbrun, F., and Widlund, L. (1972): Isolation of the nicotinic acetylcholine receptor by biospecific chromatography on insolubilized Naja naja neurotoxin. *FEBS Lett.*, 28:107–111.
58. Patrick, J., and Lindstrom, J. (1973): Autoimmune response to acetylcholine receptor. *Science*, 180:871–872.
59. Sugiyama, H., Benda, P., Meunier, J.-C., and Changeux, J.-P. (1973): Immunological characterization of the cholinergic receptor from Electrophorus electricus. *FEBS Lett.*, 35:124–128.
60. Green, D. P. L., Miledi, R., and Vincent, A. (1975): Neuromuscular transmission after immunization against acetylcholine receptors. *Proc. R. Soc. Lond. (Biol.)*, 189:57–68.
61. Penn, A. S., Chang, H. W., Lovelace, R. E., Niemi, W., and Miranda, A. (1976): Antibodies to acetylcholine receptors in rabbits: Immunochemical and electrophysiological studies. *Ann. N.Y. Acad. Sci.*, 274:354–376.
62. Heilbronn, E., Mattsson, C., Thornell, L.-E., Sjöström, M., Stalberg, E., Hilton-Brown, P., and Elmquist, D. (1976): Experimental myasthenia in rabbits. Biochemical, immunological, electrophysiological, and morphological aspects. *Ann. N.Y. Acad. Sci.*, 274:337–353.
63. Satyamurti, S., Drachman, D. B., and Slone, F. (1975): Blockade of acetylcholine receptors: A model of myasthenia gravis. *Science*, 187:955–957.
64. Sanders, D. B., Schleifer, L. S., Eldefrawi, M. E., Norcross, N. L., and Cobb, E. E. (1976): An immunologically induced defect of neuromuscular transmission in rats and rabbits. *Ann. N.Y. Acad. Sci.*, 274:319–336.
65. Lennon, V. A., Lindstrom, J., and Seybold, M. E. (1975): Experimental autoimmune myasthenia: A model of myasthenia gravis in rats and guinea pigs. *J. Exp. Med.*, 141:1365–1375.
66. Engel, A. G., Tsujihata, M., Lindstrom, J. M., and Lennon, V. A. (1976): The motor end-plate in myasthenia gravis and in experimental autoimmune myasthenia gravis. *Ann. N.Y. Acad. Sci.*, 274:60–79.
67. Tarrab-Hazdai, R., Aharonov, A., Silman, I., Fuchs, S., and Abramsky, O. (1975): Experimental autoimmune myasthenia induced in monkeys by purified acetylcholine receptor. *Nature*, 256:128–130.
68. Fulpius, B. W., Zurn, A. D., Granato, D. A., and Leder, R. M. (1976): Acetylcholine receptor and myasthenia gravis. *Ann. N.Y. Acad. Sci.*, 274:116–129.
69. Morgan, G., Peter J. B., and Newbould, B. B. (1971): Experimental allergic myositis in rats. *Arthritis Rheum.*, 15:599–609.
70. Lennon, V. A., Lindstrom, J., and Seybold, M. E. (1976): Experimental autoimmune myasthenia gravis: Cellular and humoral immune responses. *Ann. N.Y. Acad. Sci.*, 274:283–299.
71. Tarrab-Hazdai, R., Aharonov, A., Abramsky, O., Yaar, I., and Fuchs, S. (1976): Passive transfer of experimental autoimmune myasthenia by lymph node cells in inbred guinea pigs. *J. Exp. Med. (in press)*.
72. Abramsky, O., Tarrab-Hazdai, R., Aharonov, A., and Fuchs, S. (1976): Immunosuppression of experimental myasthenia gravis. *J. Immunol.*, 117:225–228.
73. Fambrough, D. M., Drachman, D. B., and Satyamurti, S. (1973): Neuromuscular junction in myasthenia gravis: Decreased acetylcholine receptors. *Science*, 182:293–295.
74. Almon, R. R., Andrew, C. G., and Appel, S. H. (1974): Serum globulin in myasthenia gravis: Inhibition of α-bungarotoxin binding to acetylcholine receptors. *Science*, 186:55–57.

75. Bender, A. N., Ringel, S. P., Engel, W. K., Daniels, M., and Vogel, Z. (1975): Myasthenia gravis: a serum factor blocking acetylcholine receptors of the human neuromuscular junction. *Lancet,* 1:607–609.

76. Brockes, J. P., and Hall, Z. W. (1975): Acetylcholine receptors in normal and denervated rat muscle. I. Purification and interaction with ^{125}I-α-bungarotoxin. II. Comparison of junctional and extrajunctional receptors. *Biochemistry,* 14:2092–2106.

77. Toyka, K. V., Drachman, D. B., Pestronk, A., and Kao, I. (1975): Myasthenia gravis: Passive transfer from man to mouse. *Science,* 190:397–399.

78. Abramsky, O., Aharanov, A., Teitelbaum, D., and Fuchs, S. (1975): Cellular immune response to acetylcholine receptor-rich fraction in patients with myasthenia gravis. *Clin. Exp. Immunol.,* 19:11–16.

79. Abramsky, O., Aharanov, A., Teitelbaum, D., and Fuchs, S. (1975): Myasthenia gravis and acetylcholine receptor. *Arch. Neurol.,* 32:684–687.

80. Richman, D., Patrick, J., and Arnason, B. G. W. (1976): Cellular immunity in myasthenia gravis. *N. Engl. J. Med.,* 294:694–698.

81. Perlo, V. P., Arnason, B. G. W., Poskanzer, O., Castleman, B., Schwab, R. S., Osserman, K. I., Papatestis, A., Alpert, L., and Kark, A. (1971): The role of thymectomy in the treatment of myasthenia gravis. *Ann. N.Y. Acad. Sci.,* 183:308–315.

82. Okumura, K., and Tada, T. (1971): Regulation of homocytotropic antibody formation in the rat. III: Effect of thymectomy and splenectomy. *J. Immunol.,* 106:1019–1025.

83. Mittag, T., Tormay, A., Woo, C., and Kornfeld, P. (1976): Acetylcholine receptors and anti-receptor globulins in myasthenic thymus. *Fed. Proc.,* 35:292.

84. Mittag, T., Kornfeld, P., Tormay, A., and Woo, C. (1976): Detection of anti-acetylcholine receptor factors in serum and thymus from patients with myasthenia gravis. *N. Engl. J. Med.,* 294:691–694.

85. Bergström, K., Franksson, C., Matell, G., and von Reis, G. (1963): The effect of thoracic duct drainage in myasthenia gravis. *Eur. Neurol.,* 9:157–167.

86. Tindall, S. C., Peters, B. H., Caverley, J. R., Sarles, H. E., and Fish, J. C. (1973): Thoracic duct lymphocyte depletion in myasthenia gravis. *Arch. Neurol.,* 29:202–203.

87. Pirofsky, B., Beaulieu, R., Bardana, E. J., and August, A. (1974): Antithymocyte antiserum effects in man. *Am. J. Med.,* 56:290–296.

88. Chou, S. M. (1968): Myxovirus-like structures and accompanying nuclear changes in chronic polymyositis. *Arch. Pathol.,* 86:649–658.

89. Sato, T., Walker, D. L., Peters, H. A., Reese, H. H., and Chou, S. M. (1971): Chronic polymyositis and myxovirus-like inclusions: electron microscopic and viral studies. *Arch. Neurol.,* 24:409–418.

90. Chou, S. M., and Gutmann, L. (1970): Picornavirus-like crystals in subacute polymyositis. *Neurology (Minneap.),* 20:205–213.

91. Mastaglia, F. L., and Walton, J. N. (1970): Coxsackie-like particles in skeletal muscle from a case of polymyositis. *J. Neurol. Sci.,* 11:593–599.

92. Ben-Bassat, M., and Machtey, I. (1972): Picornavirus-like structures in acute dermatomyositis. *Am. J. Clin. Pathol.,* 58:245–249.

93. Tang, T. T., Sedmak, G. V., Siegesmund, K. A., and McCreadie, S. R. (1975): Chronic myopathy associated with Coxsackie virus type A9. *N. Engl. J. Med.,* 292:608–611.

94. Curtis, A. C., Heckaman, J. H., and Wheeler, S. H. (1961): Study of the autoimmune reaction in dermatomyositis. *J.A.M.A.,* 178:571–573.

95. Alexander, S., and Forman, L. (1968): Dermatomyositis and carcinoma. *Br. J. Dermatol.,* 80:86–89.

96. Grace, J. R., Jr., and Kondo, R. (1958): Investigations of host resistance in cancer patients. *Ann. Surg.,* 148:633–641.

97. Strauss, A. J. L., Van der Geld, H. W. R., Kemp, P. G., Jr., Exum, E. D., and Goodman, H. O. (1965): Immunological concomitants of myasthenia gravis. *Ann. N.Y. Acad. Sci.,* 124:744–766.

98. Whitaker, J. N., and Engel, W. K. (1972): Vascular deposits of immunoglobulin and complement in idiopathic inflammatory myopathy. *N. Engl. J. Med.,* 286:333–338.

99. Fessel, W. J., and Raas, M. C. (1968): Autoimmunity in the pathogenesis of muscle disease. *Neurology (Minneap.),* 18:1137–1139.

100. Dawkins, R. L., and Mastaglia, F. L. (1973): Cell-mediated cytotoxicity to muscle in polymyositis. *N. Engl. J. Med.,* 288:434–438.

101. Leddy, J. P., Griggs, R. C., Klemperer, M. R., and Frank, M. M. (1975): Hereditary complement (C2) deficiency with dermatomyositis. *Am. J. Med.*, 58:83–91, 1975.
102. Banker, B. Q., and Victor, M. (1966): Dermatomyositis(systemic angiopathy) of childhood. *Medicine*, 45:261–289.
103. Banker, B. Q. (1975): Dermatomyositis of childhood. Ultrastructural alterations of muscle and intramuscular blood vessels. *J. Neuropathol. Exp. Neurol.*, 34:46–75.
104. Norris, F. H., Jr., Dramov, B., Calder, C. D., and Johnson, S. G. (1969): Virus-like particles in myositis accompanying herpes zoster. *Arch. Neurol.*, 21:25–31.
105. Decker, J. L., Steinberg, A. D., Gershwin, M. E., Seaman, W. E., Klippel, J. H., Plotz, P. H., and Paget, S. A. (1975): Systemic lupus erythematosus. Contrasts and comparisons. *Ann. Intern. Med.*, 82:391–404.
106. Gotoff, S. P., Smith, R. D., and Sugar, O. (1972): Dermatomyositis with cerebral vasculitis in a patient with agammaglobulinemia. *Am. J. Dis. Child.*, 123:53–56.
107. Pearson, C. M. (1956): Development of arthritis, periarthritis and periostitis in rats given adjuvants. *Proc. Soc. Exp. Biol. Med.*, 91:95–100.
108. Kakulas, B. A. (1966): Destruction of differentiated muscle cultures by sensitized lymphoid cells. *J. Pathol. Bacteriol.*, 91:495–503.
109. Takayanagi, T. (1967): Immunohistological studies of experimental myositis in relation to human polymyositis. *Folia Psychiatr. Neurol. Jpn.*, 21:117–127.
110. Esiri, M. M., and MacLennon, I. C. M. (1974): Experimental myositis in rats. I. Histological and creatine phosphokinase changes, and passive transfer to normal syngeneic rats. *Clin. Exp. Immunol.*, 17:139–140.
111. Dawkins, R. L., Eghtedari, A., and Holborow, E. J. (1971): Antibodies to skeletal muscle demonstrated by immunofluorescence in experimental autoallergic myositis. *Clin. Exp. Immunol.*, 9:329–337.
112. Dawkins, R. L., and Loewi, G. (1973): Cytotoxic effect of antisera on ^{51}Cr-labelled monolayers of skeletal muscle. *J. Pathol.*, 110:67–74.
113. Kalden, J. R., Williamson, W. G., and Irvine, W. J. (1973): Experimental myasthenia gravis, myositis and myocarditis in guinea pigs immunized with subcellular fractions of calf thymus or calf skeletal muscle in Freund's complete adjuvant. *Clin. Exp. Immunol.*, 5:319–340.
114. Manghani, D., Partridge, T. A., and Sloper, J. C. (1974): The role of the myofibrillar fraction of skeletal muscle in the production of experimental polymyositis. *J. Neurol. Sci.*, 23:489–503.
115. Johnson, R. L., Fink, C. W., and Ziff, M. (1972): Lymphotoxin formation by lymphocytes and muscle in polymyositis. *J. Clin. Invest.*, 51:2435–2449.
116. Mastaglia, F. L., Dawkins, R. L., and Papadimitriou, J. M. (1974): Lymphocyte muscle cell interactions *in vivo* and *in vitro*. *J. Neurol. Sci.*, 22:261–268.
117. Saunders, M., Knowles, M., and Currie, S. (1969): Lymphocyte stimulation with muscle homogenate and other muscle-wasting disorders. *J. Neurol. Neurosurg. Psychiatry*, 32:569–571.
118. Esiri, M. M., MacLennan, I. C. M., and Hazelman, B. L. (1973): Lymphocyte sensitivity to skeletal muscle in patients with polymyositis and other disorders. *Clin. Exp. Immunol.*, 14:25–35.
119. Lisak, R. P., and Zweiman, B. (1975): Mitogen and muscle extract induced in vitro proliferative responses in myasthenia gravis, dermatomyositis and polymyositis. *J. Neurol. Neurosurg. Psychiatry*, 38:521–524.
120. Kagen, L. J., Kimball, A. C., and Christian, C. L. (1974): Serologic evidence of toxoplasmosis among patients with polymyositis. *Am. J. Med.*, 56:186–191.

Advances in Neurology, Vol. 17, edited by
R. C. Griggs and R. T. Moxley, III. Raven Press,
New York © 1977.

Therapy for Dermatomyositis and Polymyositis

Lewis P. Rowland, Christopher Clark, and Marcelo Olarte

H. Houston Merritt Clinical Research Center for Muscular Dystrophy and Related Diseases, Department of Neurology, College of Physicians and Surgeons, Columbia University and the Neurological Institute of the Presbyterian Hospital, New York, New York 10032

CONCEPTS OF DERMATOMYOSITIS AND POLYMYOSITIS

Our assignment in this volume is to discuss the treatment of polymyositis. There are problems, however, in evaluating both "treatment" and "polymyositis." It therefore seems appropriate to begin by consideration of this group of disorders, because this influences evaluation of therapy.

Polymyositis is a conceptual problem, and the modern version of the problem may be said to have started in 1954 with the seminal paper of Lee M. Eaton (46). He indicated that the word "dermatomyositis" is inappropriate to describe a condition if the rash is lacking, and since similar myopathy might occur without rash, the proper term would be "polymyositis." Subsequently, leading investigators of muscle disease wrote about dermatomyositis and polymyositis as though the terms were interchangeable (8,83,117,165). Their papers, however, included personal classifications of the several related syndromes, each classification implying a multiplicity of disorders that were lumped together. In the classification of Walton, Bradley, and their colleagues (42,124), the myopathy is placed in a central position, and cases of dermatomyositis are included under three separate categories: (a) myopathy with "minor skin changes" or "minor collagen-vascular disease"; (b) myopathy with florid skin changes and severe collagen-vascular disease; and (c) myopathy with malignancy. In evaluating their cases, it is therefore not possible to separate, for example, cases of dermatomyositis from those of rheumatoid arthritis with myopathy or of systemic lupus erythematosus with myopathy. In contrast, some authors explicitly exclude patients with a myopathy associated with any collagen-vascular disease other than dermatomyositis (95,96,123). Pearson (116,117) and Bohan and Peter (15) separated typical polymyositis and dermatomyositis for general analysis but joined the two titles for cases associated with malignancy. This tendency to amalgamate dermatomyositis and polymyositis permeates the literature. In the analysis of some series of cases, no distinction is made between patients with and without rash in regard to prognosis, response to treatment of various kinds, or malignancy.

It is our view (128) that this confuses both clinical analysis and evaluation of therapy.

For instance, Medsger et al. (95,96) wrote about the epidemiology of polymyositis. They were careful to define terms and to establish criteria for diagnosis in making a regional survey by analysis of hospital records. It might be expected that in such a rigorous attempt it would be possible for the reader to determine how many patients had rash and how many did not, especially since the summary of one paper (95) stated that there was no difference in prognosis between polymyositis and dermatomyositis. However, it is not possible to discern how many patients were in each category. Nor is it possible to make this distinction in papers by other students (145). We believe it is important to make this distinction for several reasons (128). First, dermatomyositis is a recognizable syndrome, blurred only because it merges into scleroderma in approximately 10% of cases. Polymyositis, on the other hand, is impossible to define (if a definition includes characteristics that apply to every case) and is certainly a heterogenous group of conditions. Polymyositis is not a "disease" but a syndrome owing to diverse causes. Moreover, in some cases it is impossible to distinguish between polymyositis and sporadic cases of muscular dystrophy (72). Second, it is important to distinguish between polymyositis and dermatomyositis because myopathy in the latter tends to be more severe; more patients are unable to walk and the mortality rate is higher than in cases without rash (128). Third, cases with rash are much more likely to be associated with malignancy than cases with myopathy without rash (128). Each of these distinctions bears on evaluation of therapy, and it is therefore appropriate to state the basis for these assertions.

Dermatomyositis

The diagnosis of dermatomyositis is based on clinical criteria. There is no pathognomonic laboratory test; there is no critical need for muscle biopsy, electromyogram, or determination of serum enzymes—tests that merely establish the myopathic nature of the disease. What is required is weakness and a rash, an erythematous and edematous rash with predilection for certain anatomical areas: eyelids, malar region, anterior and upper chest, extensor surfaces of fingers, elbows and knees, and periungual areas. All or only some of these parts may be affected. The disease is almost always sporadic; familial cases are exceptional (82).

As for the myopathy, there are few distinguishing characteristics. The evolution of weakness is relatively rapid, measured in weeks or months as opposed to the years of muscular dystrophy. Weakness affects proximal limb muscles primarily, especially the legs, sometimes the neck, and often the muscles of deglutition, but eye movements are spared. [One case reported (152) to document ophthalmoplegia in dermatomyositis could have been myasthenia gravis.] Myalgia is present in fewer than half the cases. Reflexes may or may not be attentuated. In our first Columbia series, covering 15 years and ending in 1966, mortality was considerable, approaching 30% (128). Whether there has been improvement in recent years, with improved methods of respiratory support, remains to be seen. The disease occurs in all decades of life, and in our series most of the complete remissions occurred in children, who were also more susceptible to calcinosis. The incidence of associated malignant neoplasm varies from series to series but is approximately 10% of patients older than 40 (7,129), and the frequency of the site of primary tumors in these cases corresponds roughly to the frequency of malignancies in general, although tumors of the ovary may be overrepresented and colorectal malignancies disproportionately few (7).

It is noteworthy that in our series inflammatory cells were present in the muscle biopsy in only 75% of the cases. Rose and Walton (124) noted that inflammatory cells may be lacking in similar number. Munsat and Cancilla (106) also discussed this problem. It may be argued that the biopsy represents only a minuscule portion of the entire muscle mass and that inflammatory cells would be found if more muscles could be sampled. Nevertheless, it is difficult for those who insist on appropriate histological changes to define polymyositis in these terms (123) if the criteria are not always met in otherwise typical cases of dermatomyositis. Moreover, inflammatory cells may be seen in heritable muscular dystrophies, as in almost 50% of the cases of Dubowitz and Brooke (45) or 36% of the cases of Jerusalem (72). Inflammatory cells in a muscle biopsy do not necessarily differentiate polymyositis from dystrophy, and lack of inflammatory cells cannot, *per se,* exclude polymyositis. This creates problems in diagnosis and definition in cases without rash and does little to warrant use of "inflammatory myopathies" as a more precise term.

Whether dermatomyositis is one or several conditions cannot be resolved without knowing the pathogenesis. There is a growing tendency to regard the disease in children as distinct from the adult disease, based primarily upon the observation in childhood cases of zonal necrosis of muscle in the light microscope and in the electron microscope, endothelial lesions with tubular aggregates, and microinfarcts (5,6). Banker (5) stated that the vascular lesions are not observed in adult cases and establish the childhood form as a unique disorder. In a personal communication, she stressed the importance of analyzing childhood and adult cases separately, but such a comparison has yet to be done. Whether there are identifiable clinical differences remains to be established, and ultimate identification of two or more forms of dermatomyositis must await recognition of etiology and pathogenesis.

Polymyositis

Eaton was an astute observer and he was undoubtedly correct when he indicated that there must be cases of the same disease as dermatomyositis, but in which the rash is lacking. That is perhaps an incongruous statement, but we have seen several patients who illustrate the fact.

For instance, a 10-year-old girl with proximal limb weakness of relatively recent onset always looked as though she had been crying (Fig. 1). Her lids were always edematous and erythematous. We attempted to photograph this appearance and the print is not very convincing. If it is difficult to photo-

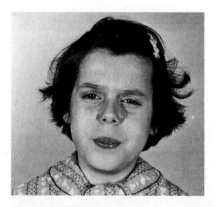

FIG. 1. A 10-year-old girl with proximal limb weakness. No rash. Eyelids slightly puffy and erythematous. The minimal cutaneous sign of dermatomyositis?

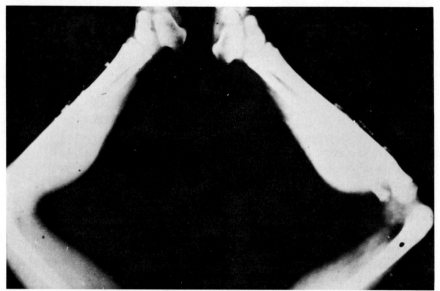

FIG. 2. Limb weakness without rash at age 5 led to diagnosis of Duchenne dystrophy, but strength improved and was followed by pretibial calcinosis at age 8.

graph this appearance, relatives and physicians might miss the sign. If lid edema is the minimal cutaneous expression of dermatomyositis, it will be difficult to distinguish between dermatomyositis and polymyositis.

In another case there probably was a rash that was never observed. This boy began to have limb weakness at age 5. An experienced neurologist made the diagnosis of Duchenne dystrophy, but instead of weakening as the years went by the boy regained strength completely. At age 9 there was no weakness whatsoever, but chalky material began to exude from his shins. Roentgenograms indicated that this was because of pretibial calcinosis (Fig. 2), which must mean that the skin and subcutaneous tissues had been involved at some time, presumably when he was weak, although the parents had never observed a rash.

In a more dramatic example, a preadolescent girl was ultimately encased

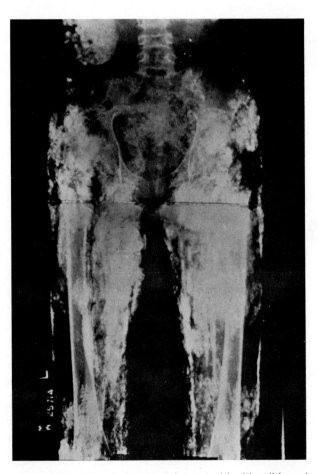

FIG. 3. Severe calcinosis universalis in preadolescent girl with mild weakness and no history of rash.

in calcinosis several years after a syndrome of relatively mild limb weakness with no discernible rash (Fig. 3). These examples happen to have been children, but presumably the same kind of mild and inconspicuous rash could occur in adults.

These three cases were probably cases of dermatomyositis, but cases in which the rash was inconspicuous. Cases of this kind suggest that the same disease, with the same etiology and pathogenesis, could occur without rash (polymyositis).

But if dermatomyositis is indeed a clinical diagnosis and if we then take away the rash, how are we to recognize polymyositis? Excluding the rash of dermatomyositis, Bohan and Peter (15) set four criteria: weakness, degeneration and regeneration of muscle fibers with inflammatory exudate, high serum enzymes, and myopathic EMG, with signs of irritability. Most of these criteria, however, establish merely myopathy, rather than a neurogenic disorder, as the cause of weakness. Devere and Bradley (42) used similar criteria and also emphasized myalgia, but analysis of their cases indicates the limitations of their suggestions: myalgia was lacking in 27%. The muscle biopsy was completely normal in 17% and lacked inflammatory cells in 35%. The EMG was normal in 11%, showed only myopathic abnormalities in 44%, and lacked evidence of abnormal irritability in 55%. Creatine phosphokinase (CPK) activity was normal in 35%. It is clear that there is no pathognomonic single test or sign, and that it is difficult to assign combinations of laboratory or clinical abnormalities that assure the diagnosis of polymyositis (157).

We have tried to establish criteria that would permit the identification of polymyositis (128), but some of these would not meet universal acceptance (Table 1):

TABLE 1. *Criteria for diagnosis of polymyositis*

---

1. Myopathy similar to myopathy of dermatomyositis
   a. Course: rapid progression (weeks or months); reversibility
   b. Distribution: dysphagia as well as proximal limb weakness
   c. Muscular pain and tenderness
   d. Laboratory: myopathic EMG; myopathic biopsy, inflammatory cells; serum enzymes; esophageal motility

2. Evidence of systemic disease
   a. Clinical: arthralgia, Raynaud's, fever
   b. Laboratory: ESR, γ-globulin, rheumatoid factor

3. No other diseases evident
   a. No family history (dystrophies)
   b. No rash, calcinosis, or palpebral edema (dermatomyositis)
   c. No other cranial muscles or cholinergic response (myasthenia gravis)
   d. No overt endocrine disorder
   e. No specific biochemical disorder in muscle biopsy (carnitine deficiency, acid maltase deficiency, phosphorylase deficiency)

Not *all* of these characteristics are present in every case. The essential elements are the major categories: myopathy similar to that of dermatomyositis and no clinical evidence of other disease.

First, the myopathy must resemble the myopathy of dermatomyositis. That is, it must evolve more rapidly than any kind of muscular dystrophy (from which it must be distinguished) and it may be reversible, either spontaneously or in apparent response to treatment. Reversibility, however, cannot be a criterion in the early stages, before a remission is observed, and not all cases of polymyositis improve.

Second, dysphagia is not a common symptom in limb-girdle dystrophy and is common in dermatomyositis, so that this symptom is helpful but not crucial. Myalgia and muscle tenderness are similarly helpful when present, but these criteria are not required because they are lacking so often in dermatomyositis.

Third, electrodiagnostic, clinical, and histological criteria should at least exclude neurogenic disease, and some abnormality of serum enzymes is to be expected, especially in the acute stages. That is, neurogenic disease should be excluded. (Polyneuropathy occurs in other collagen-vascular diseases, but not in dermatomyositis.)

Fourth, if there is widespread evidence of degeneration and regeneration of muscle, with prominent interstitial inflammatory response or other prominent abnormalities such as vacuolar change or cytoplasmic bodies, the diagnosis is easier. However, milder or minimal changes are not inconsistent with the diagnosis.

Fifth, the distribution of weakness is almost always most pronounced in proximal limb muscles, and the legs may be affected alone or with shoulder girdles; two cases of distal polymyositis have been recorded (9,68) and we have seen one. The face may be weak (125) and dysphagia is common, but other cranial muscles are only rarely affected. Weakness of neck flexor muscles is emphasized by some (15).

Sixth, clinical evidence of systemic disease helps: for instance, fever, arthralgia, Raynaud symptoms, or abnormally increased serum γ-globulin.

Seventh, some negative criteria are also necessary: no family history of similar disease to exclude muscular dystrophy; nothing to suggest a cutaneous disorder if the syndrome is to be separated from dermatomyositis; no cranial muscle symptoms other than dysphagia or facial weakness (especially no ophthalmoplegia), and no cholinergic drug response, because these manifestations would create a syndrome virtually impossible to differentiate from myasthenia gravis; and, finally, no overt evidence of thyroid or adrenal disease or other metabolic disorder.

What this means, in practice, is that if there are no signs of systemic illness, any patient over age 30 with a syndrome of myopathic weakness is deemed to have "polymyositis" until and unless some other diagnosis becomes evident. The age is important because the only muscular dystrophies that begin after age 30 are facioscapulohumeral and myotonic dystrophies, which are evident by virtue of the distribution of weakness and familial incidence. Although polymyositis of "facioscapulohumeral" distribution has been reported, some of these were familial and therefore impossible to distinguish from dystrophy (107). We have been able to find no reports of families with limb-girdle muscular dystrophy beginning after age 30, and this is the form of dystrophy that would be most confused with polymyositis. If the myopathy is accompanied by evidence of systemic lupus, rheumatoid arthritis, or some other collagen-vascular disease, the myopathy may be regarded as "polymyositis" but it is then one of several manifestations of the underlying disease. Unless there are signs of some identifiable collagen-vascular disease, it is very difficult to identify polymyositis (not dermato-myositis) in patients younger than age 30.

LIMITATIONS OF THE CRITERIA

These criteria serve to help identify "polymyositis," but aside from the acute or subacute characteristics of the myopathy and the negative considerations that exclude other diseases, none of the "criteria" is essential to the diagnosis. Even the acute or subacute nature of the myopathy may lead to confusion, for cases of chronic polymyositis have been reported. Also, it has not been our practice to include cases of acute myoglobinuria in the differential diagnosis, because so many of the acute cases are related to exertion or genetic disorder and because few progressive muscle diseases have been associated with myoglobinuria (127a). Walton and Adams (159) did include myoglobinuria as a form of polymyositis, however, and why not include them if the brief, acute myopathies associated with viral infection qualify?

The heterogeneity of polymyositis as defined by these criteria will be discussed in more detail later. Here, however, that heterogeneity must be considered in evaluating the criteria. When we applied these criteria in 1966 (28), "polymyositis" proved to include some disorders that were ultimately revealed by appropriate laboratory study. The reader may wonder why thyroid disorders and myositis ossificans were included (Table 2); identification of these cases was not immediate but required appropriate laboratory tests, and in the case of myositis ossificans, the characteristic radiographic abnormalities were lacking for several months while a 10-year-old girl was followed for stiff back and mild proximal limb weakness, with diffuse myopathic changes in muscle biopsy. We have described one of the cases of hyperthyroid myopathy, which was associated with prominent arthralgia and carcinoma of the lung (129). Muscle biopsy in thyrotoxic myopathy ordinarily shows little change, but extensive degeneration and inflammatory response have been described (154a). Is this an unusual manifestation of thyrotoxic myopathy? Or can polymyositis sometimes be a complication of thyrotoxicosis? Or can both polymyositis and thyrotoxicosis be manifestations of a common autoimmune disorder, with or without malignant disease?

It would be logical to exclude cases of "polymyositis" that ultimately prove to have some identifiable "cause." Then, however, decisions would have to be made about other "causes." According to conventional practices, "polymyositis" is a suitable designation for the myopathic syndromes that attend all collagen-vascular diseases. But what about sarcoid? This is identified by characteristic granulomas, but lesions in other organs may be lacking and other changes in muscle may be identical to those of derma-

TABLE 2. *Diseases associated with "polymyositis syndrome"*

	Number of patients	
	CPMC[a] (1958–1965)	HUP[a] (1967–1971)
Total patients	83	47
Idiopathic	46	25
Systemic lupus erythematosus	7	2
Sarcoidosis	4	2
Rheumatoid arthritis	3	4
Systemic sclerosis	3	5
Bone disease	2[b]	0
Macroglobulinemia	2	0
Alcoholism	2	2
Hyperthyroidism[c]	2[c]	0
Carcinoma	1[d]	2
Thymoma	1	1
Thyroiditis	0	1
Psoriasis	1	2
Possible drug reaction	0	1
Hypothyroidism,[c] periarteritis, Sjögren, temporal arteritis, toxoplasmosis, trichinosis, myositis ossificans,[e] malabsorption, myoglobinuria[f]	1 each	0

[a] CPMC, Columbia-Presbyterian Medical Center; HUP, Hospital of the University of Pennsylvania.
[b] Hypophosphatemia (1); bone infarcts (1).
[c] Endocrinopathies not clinically evident.
[d] Malignant carcinoid.
[e] Ossification not evident for 6 months.
[f] Pigmenturia associated with progressive myopathy.

tomyositis (65a). Myopathies associated with malignant neoplasms are permitted in most series; if so, why not the pharmacologically unresponsive syndrome associated with thymoma (127)? It is not clear which diseases should be included under the designation of polymyositis and which should not.

The problem has been further complicated by the recent interest in lipid storage myopathies, which are identified by a vacuolar myopathy that may be attended by perivascular inflammation (73a) and, clinically, may resemble polymyositis. Some but not all of these lipid storage myopathies are associated with abnormally low muscle content of carnitine (47a,b). For that reason, and because phosphorylase deficiency has also been mistaken for polymyositis (91a), we have added the final negative criterion in Table 2, excluding specific metabolic disease.

The lipid storage myopathies raise still another question about the criteria listed. In formulating these criteria in 1966, we were impressed that muscular dystrophies are presently irreversible and that when a myopathy improves spontaneously, or in apparent response to prednisone therapy, it would probably prove to be polymyositis. Although this is a retrospective criterion that is not applicable to cases of recent onset, the importance of reversibility was the central message of Nattrass (109a) in one of the earliest and most influential papers of the 1950s, when the modern concept of polymyositis was being formulated. However, cases of lipid storage myopathy may improve with prednisone therapy (47a,b,73a,120a). This may be still another reason to exclude all metabolic myopathies from considerations of polymyositis, but carnitine deficiency and lipid storage could be the result of an acquired rather than a genetic disorder, and therefore a form of polymyositis. Moreover, there are likely to be problems deciding how much lipid storage qualifies for this separate diagnosis. And if these cases are excluded, should any of the other causes be allowed to stand? Would that mean that polymyositis becomes a diagnosis of exclusion, comprising only cases in which no other cause is evident? Is there any reason to believe that the remaining cases are not also heterogeneous in cause? The only solution to this dilemma is to identify specific causes of these diseases and then to deal with each category separately. In the meantime, we proceed with imprecise criteria for diagnosis, and this must certainly affect evaluation of therapy.

DIFFICULTY DIFFERENTIATING POLYMYOSITIS FROM MUSCULAR DYSTROPHY

Even using these criteria, in some cases no distinction can be made between a presumably acquired disease, polymyositis, and an inherited disease, muscular dystrophy. A single example suffices: A boy began to have symptoms of pelvic girdle weakness at age 12. We first saw him at age 15 and there was pronounced proximal limb weakness. In the electromyogram there were myopathic signs, with evidence of hyperexcitability as in polymyositis, and in the muscle biopsy there was evidence of degeneration and regeneration with a mild inflammatory cellular response. He was treated with prednisone in the hope that this was a chronic form of polymyositis, but he did not respond. During the next few years he continued to become slowly weaker. There is no way to determine whether this was a sporadic case of limb-girdle dystrophy or polymyositis unresponsive to steroid therapy.

In another case three diagnoses were possible. Limb weakness became symptomatic for this woman at age 32, with no family history of similar disease. Aside from limb weakness, the only other abnormality on examination was a goiter, and biopsy revealed histological evidence of thyroiditis. The serum CPK was moderately increased (75 units, normal less than 45), the EMG myopathic, and there was no inflammation in the muscle biopsy. Serum T4 content was low normal. She was treated with thyroid extract for 6 months and was then clearly euthyroid, but the weakness did not change. Was this limb-girdle dystrophy, hypothyroid myopathy, or polymyositis? [Although hyperthyroid myopathy invariably improves when patients are rendered euthyroid, there have been reports of persistent weakness after hypothyroidism was cured (3).] Therefore, it is not possible to distinguish some cases of muscular dystrophy, genetic diseases not presently amenable to therapy, from cases of polymyositis, acquired conditions that are presumed to be reversible. If a series of cases labeled "polymyositis" includes some patients with "dystrophy," evaluation of therapy will be affected.

HETEROGENEITY OF "POLYMYOSITIS"

Next is the problem of heterogeneity among patients with the syndrome of polymyositis. In acute cases, polymyositis may be due to toxoplasmosis (27,76,126,130) or trichinosis (38,93), and there is increasing suspicion that viral agents may be responsible for some cases (10,16,20,22,26,28–30, 43,62,64,78,79,90–92,99,101,108,110,112,113,131,134,135,138,154–156, 166,169). In tropical countries, schistosomiasis (88) or cysticerosis (2,132) may be found. In one of our patients, a 50-year-old woman with weakness for 6 months, the muscle biopsy contained trichina. We discounted trichinosis as the cause of polymyositis because the symptoms are ordinarily acute and because asymptomatic infestation still occurs, but one woman (32) died of intestinal obstruction due to trichinosis, and encysted worms in muscle may have accounted for weakness during the preceding year.

As indicated by the analysis of our first Columbia series by Drs. David Sagman and Donald Schotland, many patients with syndromes of polymyositis have well-recognized collagen-vascular diseases (153,158), including rheumatoid arthritis, systemic lupus, Sjögren syndrome, progressive systemic sclerosis, and giant cell arteritis (Table 2). "Mixed connective tissue disease" (144), identified by the presence of antibodies to extractable DNA, was not recognized. One of our patients suffered severe weakness and wasting of limb muscles, Raynaud symptoms, and constipation but never had frank scleroderma. A dilated, aperistaltic esophagus, calcinosis circumscripta, and dilated colon (Fig. 4) indicated that this was progressive systemic sclerosis.

Some patients prove to have sarcoid (52,146). One man had severe proximal limb weakness associated with a malabsorption syndrome and calcific pancreatitis; at the time of our original report, we merely listed this

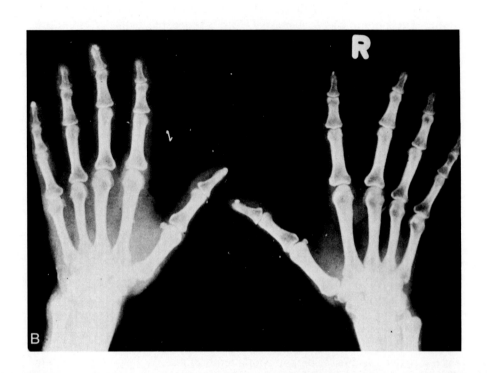

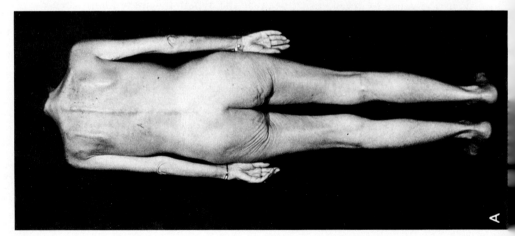

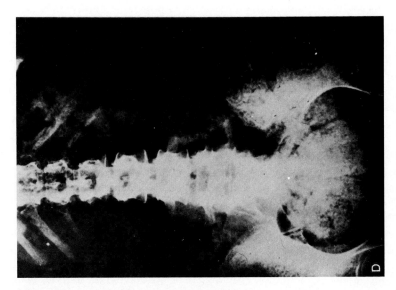

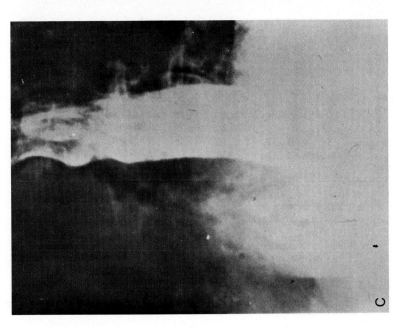

FIG. 4. A. Marked wasting and limb weakness in woman with Raynaud's syndrome and constipation but no frank scleroderma. Progressive systemic sclerosis. **B.** Calcinosis circumscripta evident in tips of left third and fifth fingers and right thumb and index finger. **C.** Aperistaltic dilated esophagus. **D.** Plain film of abdomen; colon distended by feces.

as one of the possible causes of "polymyositis," but it was probably related to the hypocalcemia-hypophosphatemia-osteomalacia-weakness syndrome recently emphasized (121,139,148,149). Steatorrhea may also lead to the vacuolar myopathy of hypokalemia (33). Alcoholism accounts for a significant number of cases of myopathy in any series (47,120); it sometimes causes an acute syndrome with or without myoglobinuria, and sometimes merely one of progressive chronic weakness. Some cases are associated with malignant tumors (129,147) or thymoma (127). Unrecognized endocrine disease can cause subacute weakness, including hyperthyroidism, hypothyroidism, hyperadrenalism, and hypercalcemia, so that these must be considered in any laboratory evaluation of weakness in adults. Similarly, sporadic cases of phosphorylase deficiency (15) and carnitine deficiency may simulate polymyositis. Increasingly, abuse of therapeutic drugs (especially steroids and kaluretic agents) causes weakness and sometimes the drug ingestion is surreptitious. A recent addition to the list of myotoxic drugs is penicillamine (12,111,140). We have had no patients with the myopathy of chronic renal disease (50b) or amyloidosis (23,53,80,89,168), but these myopathies could also present as "polymyositis." Sometimes the nature of the associated disease is not evident.

That the Columbia series is not totally unrepresentative is evident from cases seen in 4 years at the University of Pennsylvania (Table 2) and analyzed by Dr. G. Bhatt. One new diagnosis was "psoriatic myopathy" (70,103), called to our attention by Dr. Walter Shelley, Professor of Dermatology. Whether this is a casual relationship is an epidemiological question, but we have seen two cases.

These two series of cases attest to the heterogeneity of polymyositis.

TABLE 3. *Differential diagnosis of polymyositis*

Etiology unknown
Collagen-vascular diseases
   Systemic lupus, rheumatoid arthritis, periarteritis nodosa, systemic sclerosis, giant cell
   arteritis, Sjögren syndrome
Infections
   Toxoplasmosis, trichinosis, schistosomiasis, cysticercosis
   Virus: Clinical or serological (influenza, rubella); ultrastructure
Drug-induced disorders
   Systemic: alcohol, penicillamine, clofibrate, steroids, emetine, chloroquin
   Intramuscular injections: meperidine, pentazocine
Other systemic diseases
   Carcinoma, thymoma, sarcoid, amyloid, psoriasis
Endocrine diseases
   Hyperthyroidism, hypothyroidism, hyperadrenocorticism, hyperparathyroidism,
     hypoparathyroidism
Metabolic diseases
   Hypocalcemia, osteomalacia, chronic renal disease
   Chronic K^+ depletion
   Carnitine deficiency in muscle
   Lack of acid maltase, phosphorylase

The name of some recognized syndrome can be attached to approximately half the cases if appropriate studies are performed (Table 2). The remainder are "idiopathic" and they, too, are probably heterogeneous in origin, which must affect evaluation of therapy. It may be more appropriate to discuss the differential diagnosis of polymyositis (Table 3) than the "classification."

PROBLEM OF NOMENCLATURE

If "polymyositis" encompasses so many diverse conditions, and if it is so difficult or impossible to define, it would be more appropriate to use some less precise term. "Myopathy" is often substituted. Some prefer the term "inflammatory myopathy," but that is merely a translation and, since it sounds even more specific, it depends on the demonstration of inflammatory cells in muscle. "Polymyositis" seems so entrenched at the moment that lexicographers are not apt to change it by fiat. It is probably acceptable so long as it is recognized that this is no more a diagnosis than "polyneuritis," "headache," or "epilepsy," each of which permits diverse etiology. Whatever term is used, it seems important to recognize that the myopathy is due to one of numerous known causes and that the idiopathic cases are probably also due to more than one cause. "Polymyositis" cannot be regarded as a unique disease. In the collagen-vascular diseases individual cases may be difficult to categorize, but that does not obliterate the unique features of the major categories: rheumatoid arthritis, systemic lupus erythematosus, and the several forms of arteritis (153). Myopathy is occasionally a manifestation of all of these. So, also, are rashes, fever, and increased erythrocyte sedimentation rate. It does not seem logical to equate these conditions just because myopathy is an inconstant manifestation of all. Whether dermatomyositis is really a "collagen-vascular" disease remains to be demonstrated. There is no evidence that collagen is affected, and the case for angiitis is just beginning to be documented (5,6,73).

Differences Between "Polymyositis" and Dermatomyositis

Is there any sense in trying to differentiate between polymyositis and dermatomyositis? Is this merely nit-picking, an exercise in futility and of no consequence? From the first Columbia series, we analyzed three groups of patients, 48 with unequivocal dermatomyositis and approximately equal numbers of patients with polymyositis associated with named syndromes or with idiopathic polymyositis (Table 4). There were no differences in clinical or laboratory data between the two groups of patients with polymyositis, and they were therefore considered as one, to contrast with dermatomyositis. Then there were significant differences.

First, there were cases of dermatomyositis in the first decade, the well-known syndrome of childhood dermatomyositis (5,13,21,50,67,100,151, 161). But there were very few cases of polymyositis without rash in children. This may be, in part, an artifact. An adult, especially after age 30, with

TABLE 4. *Dermatomyositis and polymositis: comparison of some clinical features*

	Dermatomyositis (no. of patients)	Polymyositis (no. of patients)		
		"Named"	"Idiopathic"	Total
Total	58	37	46	83
Onset first decade	16(28%)	2	0	2 (2%)
Onset after 40	28 (40%)	23	31	54 (65%)
Fatal	18 (31%)	4	1	5 (4%)
Contemporary malignancy	4 (14%)	2	0	2 (2.4%)
Unable to walk	15 (26%)	2	2	4 (5%)
Muscle tenderness	23	12	6	18
Dysphagia	31	9	17	26
Dysarthria	13	2	4	6
Arthralgia	13	15	10	25
Raynaud's	6	5	5	10
ESR increased	33/47	24/36	28/44	52/80
γ-globulin > 1.5 g/dl	12/34	12/32	15/38	27/70
LE cells	0/39	3/27	0/35	3/62
Esophagus (X-ray)	9/36	4/16	6/25	10/41

proximal myopathic weakness of recent onset is assumed to have polymyositis or a related syndrome. A child with similar weakness that is not congenital is assumed to have either Duchenne or limb-girdle dystrophy, depending on gender, even if there is no family history of similar disease. Onset after age 40, in our series and perhaps for similar reasons, was more common in polymyositis than in dermatomyositis.

A more significant difference was related to the severity of the myopathy. More patients were unable to walk when the syndrome was dermatomyositis; the fatality rate was 31% for dermatomyositis, and only 4% when the rash was lacking (128). Similarly, the association with contemporary malignancy was 14% among adults with dermatomyositis but only 4% when there was no rash. This kind of analysis has not been undertaken in other series, and it is not possible to know if these differences are peculiar to our series. None of the other characteristics of the syndromes was significantly different in the two groups.

Finally, the heterogeneity of polymyositis is itself evidence of difference from dermatomyositis. Although "polymyositis" is associated with all forms of collagen disease, dermatomyositis is linked only to scleroderma and to none of the others. For instance, arthralgia is common in dermatomyositis, but rheumatoid arthritis has not been reported and the visceral lesions of systemic lupus erythematosus are lacking in dermatomyositis.

If these differences are real, and if dermatomyositis is homogeneous and polymyositis heterogeneous, it does not make much sense to evaluate the results of therapy in groups of patients that include both dermatomyositis and polymyositis. Yet that is exactly what has been done in many published series.

Pathogenesis

As discussed elsewhere in this volume by Dr. Penn, dermatomyositis has been regarded as an autoimmune disease, but there is virtually no evidence of abnormal humoral antibodies (119). The disease has been recorded in patients genetically lacking components of complement (81) or with hypogammaglobulinemia (54,58,168), but this question is still being raised (162). Even the statistical relationship to malignant disease has not been explained (4,129,163). Attention is therefore directed to the lymphocytes, and there have been reports of abnormal transformation of lymphocytes exposed to muscle antigens, or to destruction of muscle cultures by lymphocytes from affected patients (24,25,36,39,40,49,50,61,74), but the results are not entirely consistent (24,25,84).

During the past few years there have been several reports of structures resembling virions in muscle from patients with dermatomyositis (10,78,79, 110,113,122) and polymyositis (22,28–30,50a,92,101,131,138), but no virus has been isolated, and similar particles have been seen in muscle from patients with other disorders (2a,20,26,108,112,134,135,166). Coxsackievirus (154) was isolated from muscles of a girl who died at age 11 and who seemed to have had a congenital myopathy, with an apparent acceleration at age 10 and fatal pneumonia. Whether the virus in muscle was part of a terminal infection or was associated with the myopathy was not clear. Even so, persistent viral infection is suspected in many diseases of uncertain etiology, including the collagen-vascular disorders, and it could be the agent that alters cell surfaces to trigger destructive autoimmune processes in subacute or chronic polymyositis or dermatomyositis. In acute cases, a more direct effect of virus is suspected in cases of polymyositis-associated infection with influenza virus (42,91,94a,99) or rubella (79), or after rubella vaccination (62). That this is possible is suggested by cases of acute polymyositis owing to toxoplasmosis or trichinosis.

A diffuse angiopathy has been incriminated, especially in childhood dermatomyositis (5,6,17). Although the light microscopic lesions present in postmortem examination (6) are less commonly seen in biopsies (5,13), Banker (5) believes that the endothelial lesions are characteristic of childhood cases. Less consistently, endothelial lesions of capillaries have also been reported in adults, with or without rash (57,73). Unlike the collagen-vascular diseases with which it is usually grouped, dermatomyositis is rarely associated with visceral disease. Overt joint changes of rheumatoid arthritis or renal failure have not been reported in dermatomyositis. Gastrointestinal bleeding may occur in children (6). Pulmonary fibrosis may occur in dermatomyositis (19,115,141a) but is seen more often in cases lacking rash (17,44,141a,160), suggesting a relationship to systemic sclerosis. The heart is almost never symptomatically involved in dermatomyositis, and in cases of cardiac disorder with limb weakness (66,85,133,146a,167) it has usually not been possible to exclude muscular dystrophy because the patients have been young, the disease has been measured in years rather than months, and inflammatory cells have been scanty, as in the following case.

W. R. (CPMC 158–00–43) began to have difficulty climbing stairs and rising from chairs at age 34. Two years later he was treated with prednisone, 10 mg daily, for several months, with no effect. At age 39 he became dyspneic. The gait was waddling. There was weakness against gravity of proximal leg muscles, less weakness of shoulder muscles, and normal strength distally. Knee jerks were not elicited; other myotatic reflexes were normal. There was no fever but the pulse was 120 and the respiratory rate 22. There was a gallop rhythm but no murmurs. The EKG showed left axis deviation, conduction defect, and premature ventricular contractions. SGOT was 70 units; SGPT, 60 units. Biopsy showed myopathic changes. Urinary creatine excretion was 431 mg/day. The following were normal: erthyrocyte sedimentation rate, lupus erythematosus (LE) cell preparations, latex fixation, protein bound iodine, calcium, phosphate, γ-globulin. After 1 month in the hospital, he died of intractable congestive heart failure. At autopsy, there was widespread degeneration of skeletal and cardiac muscle with no inflammatory response.

TREATMENT

Steroids

The view that corticosteroid therapy is virtually specific and effective for all forms of polymyositis and dermatomyositis stems in part, from the immunosuppressive actions of these hormones (4,31) but primarily, from the authoritative reports of Pearson (116), Walton and coworkers (8,124, 159), and Mulder and associates (105,165) between 1963 and 1968, a view buttressed by a later report from Newcastle (42). Yet these reports are intrinsically limited, and there are discrepancies among them and with some other reports.

The most important limitation is the total lack of any prospectively controlled evaluation of therapy. Everywhere it has become routine practice to treat patients with dermatomyositis or polymyositis with corticosteroids. Therefore, the natural history of the untreated conditions in contemporary times is not known. Before the introduction of steroids, the mortality rate from dermatomyositis was 50% among 38 patients seen at the Mayo Clinic prior to 1940 (114), and the mortality rate of 291 patients collected from the literature was 60% (142). However, antibiotics, respirators, and other general medical advances would also affect mortality rates, so it is not appropriate to compare modern series with the earlier ones. Even so, in some centers the mortality rates of patients with untreated dermatomyositis were significantly less than 50% in some reports. Rose and Walton (124) compared their results in 1963 to those of O'Leary and Waisman in 1940

(114), although many innovations—including antibiotics and respirators—had been introduced in the interim. Mulder, Winkelmann, et al. (105,165) compared treated and untreated patients at the Mayo Clinic, but the groups were not matched in relation to age, sex, complicating disease, or year of observation; their untreated patients presumably also included the early patients reported by Waisman and O'Leary. There has been no adequately controlled evaluation of therapy.

The need for controls can be illustrated. In one collection of cases of dermatomyositis before the introduction of steroids, 33% of patients enjoyed spontaneous remission, 33% were left with some disability (but may have improved), and 33% died (13). It is now difficult to encounter untreated patients, but the following episode indicates the need for controlled observations: In mid-December 1975, during an influenza epidemic, an 18-year-old college student had symptoms of respiratory infection for 2 weeks. At Christmas she began to have leg weakness, and by January 14 she was having much difficulty walking. The SGOT was 88 units, and CPK 679 units (normal less than 125). On February 21 she could walk only with great difficulty and could not rise from a chair without assistance. In the supine position she could not lift her feet from the bed. SGOT was 90, lactic acid dehydrogenase 209, and CPK 388 (normal less than 50 units). The EMG pattern was myopathic. In the muscle biopsy there were cytoplasmic inclusions (18,22) in virtually all muscle fibers; there was evidence of degeneration and regeneration, but no inflammatory cellular response. No virus-like particles were seen in the electron microscope. The electrocardiogram was compatible with myocarditis. Without specific therapy she rapidly began to improve. Serum enzymes were normal by March 1 and the EKG was almost normal. By mid-April she had resumed almost all normal activities, although she still had difficulty climbing stairs and there was slight weakness against resistance of the deltoids and psoas muscles against firm resistance. The EKG was entirely normal. In June, there was no weakness at all. Had she been treated with prednisone, she would have been a therapeutic triumph.

Even without appropriate controls, the results of the original reports vary. Pearson (116) reported "fair to excellent" improvement in all but 1 of 21 cases of polymyositis and all of 10 patients with dermatomyositis and no tumor. The only treatment failures were those cases associated with malignancy (9 cases) or Sjögren syndrome (2 cases). Later, however, there were reports of immunosuppressive therapy from the same center, describing "steroid-resistant" cases (97,150). Wedgewood et al. (161) also reported uniform improvement in 10 cases of childhood dermatomyositis, although 2 of them subsequently died. Rose and Walton (124) reported benefit in significantly fewer patients, but still in enough for a strong endorsement of steroids; improvement was seen in 58% of 51 patients with polymyositis alone or "polymyositis with minor evidence of dermatomyositis or other collagen disease." In the later paper from Newcastle (42), the results were similar in a larger number of patients. Of 105 adequately treated patients, 29 died and 14 were disabled, accounting for 41%, and improvement of the other 59% was attributed to steroid therapy. Vignos et al. (156) reported improvement in approximately half of 30 cases.

Reports from the Mayo Clinic were couched in different terms. In two reports (105,165) investigators found essentially no difference in the numbers of remissions or deaths in 119 patients treated with high-dose steroids and in 122 patients not treated, including patients with or without rash. Improvement or remission occurred in 69% of treated patients and in 64% of those not treated in the earlier series (105), but the corresponding numbers changed to 64% and 50% in the later report (165). They stated that there was no difference between cases of dermatomyositis and polymyositis, although the data were not given. They favored steroid treatment because calcinosis and contractures occurred in only 1 of 19 treated patients in contrast to 9 of 20 untreated. Hill (67) also found less calcinosis in treated patients. In the later Mayo series, improvement short of remission occurred in more treated patients, and worsening short of death occurred more often in the untreated group. The same authors described "cyclic myositis" (164), a syndrome relapsing when the dosage of steroids was reduced.

In contrast, some less favorable reports have had much less impact. Everett and Curtis (50) stated that steroids might reduce fever and erythema but did not affect the myopathy in five children with dermatomyositis. Ziegler and Hamilton (167) found improvement in only 4 of 13 treated cases. Riddoch and Morgan-Hughes (123) restricted analysis to cases with inflammatory cells in muscle and found sustained improvement in only 3 of 18 cases. In 1 case (55), there was no response to prednisone although triamcinolone was beneficial, yet Mollaret et al. (102) described a patient who was already being treated with triamcinolone for psoriatic rheumatoid arthritis when polymyositis supervened; the muscle lesions differed from those of steroid myopathy because there was a prolific inflammatory cellular response. In children with dermatomyositis, Bitnum et al. (13) found a mortality rate of 37.5% in 35 treated children and 39% in 65 cases without treatment. Medsger et al. (95,96) stated that corticosteroids did not affect outcome in cases collected from several hospitals. Favorable results have also been reported with drugs that are no longer used, including para-aminobenzoic acid (59) and salicylates (104) without corticosteroids.

These negative reports, including our own data, are liable to the same fundamental criticism as the favorable reports: not one was a prospective, randomized, controlled study. For that reason, we have not previously reported our own experience. In our first Columbia series (128), improvement was observed in 33% of 58 cases of dermatomyositis. And our more recent experience did not differ much. In a review of records, not a formal follow-up examination of patients, Dr. Christopher Clark found that 7 of 23 patients with dermatomyositis improved with cortocosteroid therapy

TABLE 5. *Outcome of (uncontrolled) steroid therapy of dermatomyositis and polymyositis neurological institute 1967–1975*

	Dermatomyositis (23)		Polymositis[a] (24)	
	(7) Improved	(16)[b] Unimproved	(8) Improved	(16)[b] Unimproved
Age < 40 yr	4	3	1	8
> 40 yr	3	13	7	8
Malignancy	0	2	0	0
Duration before therapy:				
< 6 mo	5	13	4	5
6–12 mo	1	1	1	3
> 1 year	1	2	3	8
Able to walk	5	14	6	16
Not	2	2	2	0
CPK > 500 units	5	11	3	8
< 500 units	2	5	5	7
Not done	0	0	0	1
Fall in enzymes:				
> 50%	5	8	6	9
No fall	0	3	0	3
No data	0	4	0	2
Normal at onset	2	1	2	2
Interval to improvement:				
< 1 mo	6		4	
1–3 mo	1		1	
> 3 mo	0		3	
Complications of steroids				
Gastrointestinal hemorrhage:				
Not fatal	2	0	0	0
Fatal	0	2	0	1
Psychosis	2	0	0	0
Delayed wound healing	0	0	1	0
Treatment[c]				
Corticosteroids	7	16	8	16
Methotrexate	1	1	1	4
Azathioprine	1	1	1	4
Cyclophosphamide	0	0	0	1
Nitrogen mustard	0	1	0	0

[a] All cases were "idiopathic," without evidence of collagen-vascular or other diseases.
[b] Some patients improved transiently.
[c] Some patients received more than one drug.

during the years 1967–1975, and 8 of 24 patients with polymyositis syndromes improved in the years 1967–1975 (Table 5). Most of the patients who improved had been treated within 6 months after onset, but some improved even if therapy had been delayed for more than a year. Patients in either category improved whether they were able to walk or not, and whether the serum CPK was initially more or less than 500 units. Serum enzymes fell by more than 50% whether there was clinical improvement or not. In both dermatomyositis and polymyositis, improvement was likely to occur within 1 month after treatment was begun, but for some patients improvement was delayed for 3 months of treatment. The data do not indicate how long apparently ineffective treatment should be continued in the hope that prolonged therapy will ultimately be beneficial. The incidence of serious complications was 8% for patients with polymyositis and 26% for those with dermatomyositis.

The mortality rates in different series of steroid-treated patients also vary dramatically (Table 6). Divergencies of this magnitude suggest that the comparisons are not based on the same criteria. For instance, dermatomyositis and polymyositis were separated in some series but not in others; collagen diseases were included in some but not others; children and adults were included in some, only children in others; criteria for the diagnosis of "polymyositis" varied and so did the years of study or the duration of observation. One major difference might be the frequency of malignancy, 14% in cases of dermatomyositis after age 40 in the first Columbia series (128) and only 2.4% in cases without rash. In no other series was this comparison made, although it would clearly affect mortality rates and effects of treatment.

If not all patients improve with steroid therapy, it would be important to identify favorable prognostic features. In several reports (42,116,117, 118,124), more favorable outcome seemed related to treatment within 2 months of onset and children fared better than adults. Some authors believe

TABLE 6. *Mortality rates in steroid-treated dermatomyositis and polymyositis*

Author (ref.)	Years of study	No. of patients	Diagnostic categories	% Dead
Pearson (116)	1957–1963	21	PM[a]	0
Pearson (116)	1957–1963	10	DM[a]	0
Logan et al. (83)	1950–1963	49	DM	35
Winkelmann et al. (164)	Onset before	119	Both PM and DM	24
	1959, follow to 1967	9	DM and malignancy	66
Rowland et al. (128)	1951–1965	53	DM	25
	1957–1965	83	PM	5
Degos et al. (41)	1952–1970	31	Adult DM	48
Riddoch and Morgan-Hughes (123)		22	"Inflammatory" only; no collagen diseases	40
Devere and Bradley (42)	1954–1974	42	PM	17
		67	DM-collagen diseases	31
		9	DM or PM and malignancy	66
Bitnum et al. (13)	1947–1962	7	Childhood DM only	30
Sullivan et al. (151)	1960–1969	18	Childhood DM only	0
Miller (100)	1958–1972	23	Childhood DM only	26

[a] PM, polymyositis; DM, dermatomyositis.

that prognosis is better in acute cases rather than subacute or chronic syndromes. Myopathies with rheumatoid arthritis, systemic sclerosis, and Sjögren syndrome are said to respond poorly, but dermatomyositis and polymyositis are said not to differ. Although the mortality rate of patients with dermatomyositis with malignancy is high in all series, it is the tumor that is likely to cause death, and the dermatomyositis may respond to therapy. Muscle biopsy abnormalities, magnitude of serum enzyme abnormality, and EMG pattern seem to bear no relation to outcome.

If not all patients improve, it is important to know how long to treat with large amounts of prednisone (at least 50 mg daily according to consensus). We have arbitrarily set 1 to 2 months as this time, but there is no evidence in the literature to accept this or any other period of treatment. If the patient improves, when should the dose be reduced? Pearson has advocated use of serum enzyme activity as a guide (117), but we and others (41,156) find that enzyme activity may fall without clinical improvement. Devere and Bradley (42) related most relapses to decreasing dosage. It seems reasonable, however, to decrease the dosage as promptly as the patient's clinical state warrants.

In surviving patients, it is difficult to determine whether the disease is still "active." Everett and Curtis (50) stated that there was rarely clinical evidence of progressive disease after 2 years, and most observers would accept progressive weakness as the most reliable sign. Devere and Bradley (42) took increased serum enzyme activity or erythrocyte sedimentation rate as a sign of "activity," but enzymes may be normal or only slightly increased before therapy, may not increase with clinical relapse, and may remain high even though there is no progression of weakness. Lymphocyte stimulation may prove to be a guide; in one series (40) abnormal responses were more common in untreated patients, but this was not true in another series (61). However difficult it is to ascertain "activity" of the disease, there seems to be growing recognition that dermatomyositis and most polymyositis syndromes have a finite duration. Although Devere and Bradley's use of serum enzymes as a measure may be debated, half of their surviving cases were "inactive" within 2 years of treatment, and only one-third were "active" 5 years after treatment was started.

The complications of steroid therapy also have to be considered (4). In the combined series from UCLA (116), Newcastle (42), and Mayo (105, 165), the incidence of serious complications was only 5%. In the first Columbia series, however, 18% experienced serious complications. Among 10 patients, equal numbers with systemic lupus erythematosus and polymyositis, Fries et al. (51) reported two psychoses and two serious infections, and Hill and Wood (67) also reported fatal infections. Gardner-Thorpe (52) reported serious side effects in all of 5 patients with sarcoid myopathy. Riddoch and Morgan-Hughes (123) encountered complications in 7 of 18 treated patients.

One possible complication warrants special attention. On the basis of an analysis of a large number of prospectively controlled evaluations of steroid therapy in different conditions, investigators have declared the risk of peptic ulcer a "myth" (34). Nevertheless, gastrointestinal hemorrhage occurred in 4 of our 23 patients with dermatomyositis treated in the past decade, and in 1 of 24 patients with polymyositis. Gastrointestinal hemorrhage occurred in 7 of 49 treated patients in the series of Logan et al. (83). This complication is doubly important, not only because of practical considerations, but also because pathological examination of the gastrointestinal tract has provided the main evidence that there are systemic vascular lesions in dermatomyositis. However, in the two postmortem cases reported by Boylan and Sokoloff (17), in two by Malkinson and Rothman (87), and in seven of the eight cases described by Banker and Victor (6), the patients had been treated intensively with steroids before the fatal gastrointestinal hemorrhage or perforation. Banker and Victor (6) and Boylan and Sokoloff (17) attributed these disasters to the endarteritis they consider fundamental in the disease. Although other authors have rarely found similar vascular lesions (151), gastrointestinal lesions were occasionally reported before the use of steroids (13,142), and Banker (5) also found endothelial lesions in muscle of patients who had not received steroids or other treatment. However, arteritic lesions in rheumatoid arthritis have been linked to corticosteroid therapy (14,48,63, 65,71,75,77,137). It is possible that the risk of steroid-induced gastrointestinal ulceration and perforation is greater in some diseases than in others, and that among the former are dermatomyositis or other collagen-vascular diseases associated with polymyositis.

Immunosuppressive Therapy

De facto testimony to the frequently unsatisfactory outcome of steroid therapy in these diseases is provided by the recent proliferation of papers describing immunosuppressive drug therapy (1,11,37,50,86,94,136,141, 150). As with corticosteroid therapy, the initial reports are all very favorable

TABLE 7. *Immunosuppressive drug treatment of polymyositis and dermatomyositis*

Author (ref.)	No. patients better/ treated
Schirren (136)	$4/5$
McFarlin and Griggs (94)	$3/3$
Malaviya et al. (86)	$4/4$
Sokoloff et al. (150)	$5/7$
Currie and Walton (37)	$3/7$
Haas (60)	$3/8$
Benson and Aldo (11)	$4/4$
Metzger et al. (97)	$17/22$
Schrago and Miescher (141)	$5/6$
Total	$48/66$

(Table 7) but there has been no controlled trial. And, also as without cortico-steroids, results in our patients have been disappointing in comparison to those in published reports. Two patients with polymyositis improved on immunosuppressive therapy (although still disabled) after steroid therapy had failed, and two patients with dermatomyositis also improved, but no benefit at all was encountered in 3 other patients with dermatomyositis or in 9 with polymyositis. We have not encountered serious side effects with methotrexate or azathioprine (56), although treatment had to be discontinued because of abnormal liver function tests in one patient when she was given methotrexate and then again when she received azathioprine. No serious side effects were documented in reports of these drugs in poly-myositis alone, but Fries et al. (51) mentioned aphthous ulcers, hemorrhagic cystitis, and Aspergillus infection in patients receiving cyclophosphamide. Whether immunosuppressive drugs are safer or more dangerous than corti-costeroids in these patients has not been established.

Dermatomyositis and Malignancy

The inordinately frequent association of dermatomyositis with ma-lignancy, especially after age 40, seems to be well established (7). Because the tumors may not be discovered until an autopsy examination is per-formed, and because it is widely believed that removal of the tumor will ameliorate the myopathy, the diagnosis of dermatomyositis regularly sets off a "search for occult malignancy." However, if the patient has been properly examined (including pelvis and rectum), and if chest film and routine blood studies have been performed, the "search" boils down to upper and lower gastrointestinal roentgenograms and urogram. These studies are almost never fruitful in the absence of appropriate symptoms or other laboratory abnormalities, and we have encountered one patient who was subjected to exploratory laparotomy in such a search, which seems to be carrying the notion too far. If a tumor is discovered, it should be man-aged according to oncologic principles. We have previously (129) docu-mented the numerous variations in the relation between dermatomyositis and malignancy (Table 8).

TABLE 8. *Dermatomyositis and maligancy: course of myopathy*

1. DM usually precedes symptoms of tumor.
2. DM may improve after tumor treated.
3. DM, after improvement, may not relapse when tumor reappears.
4. DM may follow treatment of tumor.
5. DM may improve spontaneously.
6. DM may improve with steroid therapy.
7. DM may improve after adrenalectomy or hypophysectomy.
8. DM may be fatal itself, or death may result from tumor.

These statements are based on cases cited in several reports (7,67,69,83,116,129,143).

Recommendations for Therapy

Given the present state of uncertainty about drug therapy for these diseases, it is difficult to be forthright in recommending therapy. We try to balance the severity of disability against the risks of therapy. Unless disability is severe, we have found it difficult to describe the risks of therapy to patients in a way that would allow truly informed consent and make the risks acceptable. If the patient's incapacity is severe enough and if the risks are understood, 60 to 100 mg prednisone daily is given for the most severe cases and 100 mg on alternate days is used for less-severe cases. Patients with slight disability may elect to defer treatment. If there is no response in a period of 1 to 2 months, the dosage is gradually reduced over the next few months. If serious disability persists, treatment with oral azathioprine is then instituted, with an arbitrary dose of 150 mg daily for adults. Oral azathioprine therapy seems more convenient than intravenous methotrexate, and there is no evidence that any one of the several immunosuppressive drugs is better than the others. When immunosuppressive drugs are used, it is uncertain whether steroid therapy should also be continued or in what dosage.

This is not a satisfactory state of affairs for a group of diseases that cause serious disability and may be fatal. A measure of the uncertainty is provided by contradictory views of experienced and thoughtful investigators on the need for a controlled trial. Bohan and Peter (15) expressed the need for such and we concur. Yet it has not been done for a variety of reasons; perhaps most important is the widespread belief that steroids provide effective treatment. For this reason, Devere and Bradley (42) believe there would be no moral basis for a controlled trial.

Calcinosis

Among survivors of dermatomyositis, especially children, calcinosis is a frequent problem. This may be mild and only a radiographic observation of little consequence to the patient. Often enough, however, it is cosmetically disfiguring or causes pain, ulceration, or infection. It was therefore welcome news when diphosphonates were reported to decrease these deposits (35), but later experience cast doubt on the value of this approach (98). Aluminum hydroxide was also reported to be beneficial in one case (109). Occasionally, surgical excision of calcium deposits is necessary because of pain or infection. Surgery should not be approached casually, however, since the trauma may induce deposits of calcium.

SUMMARY

Beneficial effects of corticosteroid therapy in dermatomyositis and polymyositis vary in different published reports from 25% to virtually all patients treated, with approximately 60% improving in the largest series. Mortality rates vary from 0 to 41% among treated patients. The incidence of serious complications of steroid therapy varies from 5 to 50% of patients treated. *De facto* evidence of the limitations of steroid therapy is provided by recent reports of benefit achieved by use of several different immunosuppressive drugs in "steroid-resistant" patients. As with the initial reports of steroid therapy, the first reports of immunosuppressive drug therapy are all favorable.

Numerous factors seem to account for these discrepancies. Foremost is the total lack of any prospectively controlled evaluation of drug therapy. Our experience provides evidence for several other causes of inconsistent experiences in different reports. Dermatomyositis is a reasonably homogeneous syndrome, but polymyositis is not. It is not possible to define "polymyositis" without the rash. What is called "polymyositis" is a heterogeneous group of disorders that range from acute infections by viruses, toxoplasmosis, or trichinosis to chronic disorders associated with numerous other diseases. It seems erroneous to consider polymyositis a "disease" when it is so often a symptom of a specific disorder, such as rheumatoid arthritis, systemic lupus erythematosus, other collagen-vascular disorders, or sarcoidosis. Even when no specific disorder can be identified, the varied clinical course of "polymyositis" suggests heterogeneous etiology. Some cases cannot be distinguished from sporadic instances of heritable disease, the muscular dystrophies. In our series, there were significant differences between polymyositis and dermatomyositis in course, outcome, age distribution, and association with malignancy. In other published reports, however, dermatomyositis and polymyositis are sometimes linked together in evaluation of outcome. In some series collagen-vascular diseases are included, whereas other investigators exclude them. In some series dermatomyositis is equated with polymyositis associated with systemic lupus erythematosus or another collagen-vascular disease. Because of these inconsistencies, it is difficult to compare results from different centers.

Some investigators believe that a controlled evaluation is necessary; others believe that the efficacy of steroid therapy is demonstrated and that there is no moral basis for controlled trial. The diffusion of medical excellence has led to treatment of many patients by their personal physicians, who are not likely to encounter sufficient numbers of patients to generate series that can be evaluated. It would be reasonable to advocate referral of these patients to regional academic centers for evaluation if the academic centers had shown some evidence that they could resolve the issues. Under these circumstances, it is difficult to provide specific recommendations for therapy. The practitioner is confronted by several choices. Many patients, even if not all, benefit when prednisone therapy is given in a dose of at least 50 mg daily (or 100 mg on alternate days). It is not known how long this dose should be continued before considering the disorder "steroid resistant."

In cases that do not respond to steroid therapy, immunosuppressive therapy is justified when the disease is incapacitating or life-threatening. Methotrexate, azathioprine, cyclophosphamide, and nitrogen mustards have all been used, but it is not known which drug is most effective, if arbitrary doses can be used, if peripheral leukopenia is a desired end point, or if steroids should be continued when immunosuppressive drugs are used.

ACKNOWLEDGMENT

The authors are indebted to Drs. A. S. Penn, D. Sagman, and other clinicians for access to cases. Dr. G. Bhatt analyzed the cases at the University of Pennsylvania. Electrodiagnostic studies were performed by Drs. R. E. Lovelace, P. V. DeJesus, and their associates. Histological studies were performed by Drs. D. L. Schotland, A. R. Hays, A. Eastwood, and their associates.

Supported by center grants from the Muscular Dystrophy Association and the National Institute of Neurological and Communicative Diseases and Stroke (NS 11766).

REFERENCES

1. Arnett, F. C., Whelton, J. C., and Zlizic, T. M. (1973): Methotrexate therapy in polymyositis. *Ann. Rheum. Dis.*, 32:536–546.
2. Armbrust-Figueriredo, J., Speciali, J. G., and Lison, M. P. (1970): Forma miopatica da cisticercose. *Arq. Neuropsiquiatr.*, 28:385–390.
2a. Astrom, E., Friman, G., and Pilstrom, L. (1975): Effects of viral and mycoplasma infection on the ultrastructure of human skeletal muscle. *Scand. J. Infect. Dis.*, 1:273–276.
3. Astrom, K. E., Kugelberg, E., and Muller, R. (1961): Hypothyroid myopathy. *Arch. Neurol.*, 5:474–482.
4. Azarnoff, D. L. (Ed.) (1975): *Steroid Therapy*. W. B. Saunders, Philadelphia.
5. Banker, B. Q. (1975): Dermatomyositis of childhood. Ultrastructural alterations of muscle and intramuscular blood vessels. *J. Neuropathol. Exp. Neurol.*, 34:46–75.
6. Banker, B. Q., and Victor, M. (1966): Dermatomyositis (systemic angiopathy) in childhood. *Medicine (Baltimore)*, 45:261–289.
7. Barnes, B. E. (1976): Dermatomyositis and malignancy. A review of the literature. *Ann. Intern. Med.*, 84:68–76.
8. Barwick, D. D., and Walton, J. N. (1963): Polymyositis. *Am J. Med.*, 33:646–660.
9. Bates, D., Stevens, J. C., and Hudgson, P. (1973): Polymyositis with involvement of facial and distal musculature. *J. Neurol. Sci.*, 19:105–108.
10. Ben-Bassat, M., and Machtey, I. (1972): Picornavirus-like structures in acute dermatomyositis. *Am. J. Clin. Pathol.*, 58a:245–249.
11. Benson, M. D., and Aldo, M. A. (1973): Azathioprine therapy in polymyositis. *Arch. Intern. Med.*, 132:547–551.
12. Bettendorf, U., and Neuhaus, R. (1974): Penicillamininduzierte Polymyositis. *Dtsch. Med. Wochenschr.*, 99:2522–2525.
13. Bitnum, S., Daeschner, C. W., Travis, L. B., Dodge, W. F., and Hopps, H. C. (1964): Dermatomyositis. *J. Pediatr.*, 64:101–131.
14. Black, R. L., Yielding, K. L., and Bunim, J. J. (1957): Observations on new synthetic antirheumatoid steroids and critical evaluation of prednisone therapy in rheumatoid arthritis. *J. Chronic Dis.*, 5:751–763.

15. Bohan, A., and Peter, J. B. (1975): Polymyositis and dermatomyositis. *N. Engl. J. Med.,* 292:344–347, 403–407.
16. Bove, K. E., and Shelburne, S. A., Jr. (1972): Subacute inclusion body encephalitis associated with myopathy. *Arch. Neurol.,* 27:42–44.
17. Boylan, R. C., and Sokoloff, L. (1969): Vascular lesions in dermatomyositis. *Arthritis Rheum.,* 3:379–386.
18. Brooke, M. H., and Kaplan, H. (1972): Muscle pathology in rheumatoid arthritis, polymyalgia rheumatica, and polymyositis. *Arch. Pathol.,* 94:101–118.
19. Brundin, A. (1970): Pulmonary fibrosis in scleroderma and dermatomyositis. *Scand. J. Respir. Dis.,* 51:160–170.
20. Burch, G. E., Sohal, R. S., Colcolough, H. L., and Sun, S. C. (1968): Virus-like particles in skeletal muscle of a heat stroke victim. *Arch. Environ. Health,* 17:984–985.
21. Carlisle, J. W., and Good, R. A. (1959): Dermatomyositis in childhood. *Lancet,* 79:266–273.
22. Carpenter, S., Karpati, G., and Wolfe, L. (1970): Virus-like filaments and phospholipid accumulation in skeletal muscle. *Neurology, (Minneap.),* 20:889–903.
23. Case Records of the Massachusetts General Hospital: Case 13 (1964): Primary systemic amyloidosis. *N. Engl. J. Med.,* 374–582.
24. Caspary, E. A., Currie, S., and Field, E. J. (1971): Sensitized lymphocytes in muscular dystrophy; evidence for a neural factor in pathogenesis. *J. Neurol. Neurosurg. Psychiatry,* 34:384–392.
25. Caspary, E. A., Currie, S., Walton, J. N., and Field, E. J. (1971): Lymphocyte sensitization to nervous tissues and muscle in Guillain-Barré syndrome. *J. Neurol. Neurosurg. Psychiatry,* 34:179–181.
26. Caulfield, J. B., Rebeiz, J., and Adams, R. D. (1968): Viral involvement of human muscle. *J. Pathol.,* 96:232–234.
27. Chandar, K., Mair, H. J., and Mair, N. S. (1968): Case of toxoplasma polymyositis. *Br. Med. J.,* 1:158–159.
28. Chou, S. M. (1967): Myxovirus-like structures in a case of human chronic polymyositis. *Science,* 158:1453–1456.
29. Chou, S. M. (1968): Myoxvirus-like structures and accompanying nuclear changes in chronic polymyositis. *Arch. Pathol.,* 86:649–658.
30. Chou, S., and Gutmann, L. (1970): Picornavirus-like crystals in subacute polymyositis. *Neurology (Minneap.),* 20:205–213.
31. Claman, H. N. (1972): Corticosteroids and lymphoid cells. *N. Engl. J. Med.,* 287:388–397.
32. Clinicopathologic Conference (1969): Polymyositis. *Am. J. Med.,* 46:289–296.
33. Coërs, C., Telerman-Topet, N., and Cremer, N. (1971): Regressive vacuolar myopathy in steatorrhea. *Arch. Neurol.,* 24:217–227.
34. Conn, H. O., and Blitzer, B. L. (1976): Nonassociation of adrenocorticosteroid therapy and peptic ulcer. *N. Engl. J. Med.,* 294:473–479.
35. Cram, R. L., Barmada, R., Gebo, W. B., and Ray, R. D. (1971): Diphosphonate treatment of calcinosis universalis. *N. Engl. J. Med.,* 285:1012–1013.
36. Currie, S., Saunders, M., Nowles, M., and Brown, A. E. (1971): Immunological aspects of polymyositis. The *in vitro* activity of lymphocytes on incubation of muscle antigen and with muscle cultures. *Q. J. Med.,* 157:63–84.
37. Currie, S., and Walton, J. N. (1971): Immunosuppressive therapy in polymyositis. *J. Neurol. Neurosurg. Psychiatry,* 34:447–451.
38. Davis, M. J., Cilo, M., Plaitakis, A., and Yahr, M. D. (1976): Trichinosis: severe myopathic involvement with recovery. *Neurology (Minneap.),* 26:37–40.
39. Dawkins, R. L. (1975): Experimental autoallergic myositis, polymyositis and myasthenia gravis. Autoimmune muscle disease associated with immunodeficiency and neoplasia. *Clin. Exp. Immunol.,* 21:185–210.
40. Dawkins, R. L., and Mastaglia, F. L. (1973): Cell-mediated cytotoxicity to muscle in polymyositis. Effects of immunosuppression. *N. Engl. J. Med.,* 288:434–438.
41. Degos, R., Civatte, J., Balisch, S., and DeLaure, F. (1971): The prognosis of adult dermatomyositis. *Trans. St. Johns Hosp. Dermatol. Soc.,* 57:98–104.
42. Devere, R., and Bradley, W. G. (1975): Polymyositis. Its presentation, morbidity and mortality. *Brain,* 98:637–666.

43. Dietzman, D. E., Schaller, J. G., Ray, C. G., and Reed, M. E. (1976): Acute myositis associated with influenza B infection. *Pediatrics,* 57:255–258.
44. Duncan, P. E., Griffin, J. P., Garcia, A., and Kaplan, S. B. (1974): Fibrosing alveolitis in polymyositis. A review of histologically confirmed cases. *Am. J. Med.,* 57:621–626.
45. Dubowitz, V., and Brooke, M. H. (1973): *Muscle Biopsy: A Modern Approach.* W. B. Saunders, London.
46. Eaton, L. M. (1954): Perspective of neurology in regard to polymyositis. *Neurology (Minneap.),* 4:245–263.
47. Ekbom, K., Hed, R., Kirstein, L., and Astrom, K. E. (1964): Muscular affections in chronic alcoholism. *Arch. Neurol.,* 10:449–458.
47a. Engel, A. G., and Angelini, C. (1973): Carnitine deficiency of human skeletal muscle with associated lipid storage myopathy: a new syndrome. *Science,* 179:899–902.
47b. Engel, A. G., and Siekert, R. G. (1972): Lipid storage myopathy responsive to prednisone. *Arch. Neurol.,* 27:174–181.
48. Epstein, W. V., and Engelman, E. P. (1959): The relation of the rheumatoid factor content of serum to clinical neurovascular manifestations of rheumatoid arthritis. *Arthritis Rheum.,* 2:250–258.
49. Esiri, M. M., Maclennan, I. C. M., and Hazleman, B. L. (1973): Lymphocyte sensitivity to skeletal muscle in patients with polymyositis and other disorders. *Clin. Exp. Immunol.,* 14:25–35.
50. Everett, M. A., and Curtis, A. C. (1957): Dermatomyositis. A review of 19 cases in adolescents and children. *Arch. Intern. Med.,* 100:70–76.
50a. Fidzianska, A. (1973): Virus-like structures in muscle in chronic polymyositis. *Acta Neuropath.* 23: 23–31.
50b. Floyd, M., Ayyar, D. R., Barwick, D. D., Hudgson, P. and Weightman, D. (1974): Myopathy in chronic renal failure. *Quart. J. Med.* 43: 509–524.
51. Fries, J. F., Sharp, G. C., McDevitt, H. O., and Holman, H. R. (1973): Cyclophosphamide therapy in systemic lupus erythematosus and polymyositis. *Arthritis Rheum.,* 16:154–162.
52. Gardner-Thorpe, C. (1972): Muscle weakness due to sarcoid myopathy. Six case reports and an evaluation of steroid therapy. *Neurology (Minneap.),* 22:917–928.
53. Gelderman, A. H., Levine, R. A., and Arndt, K. A. (1962): Dermatomyositis complicated by generalized amyloidosis. *N. Engl. J. Med.,* 267:858–861.
54. Giuliano, V. J. (1974): Polymyositis in a patient with acquired hypogammaglobulinemia. *Am. J. Med. Sci.,* 268:53–56.
55. Goethe, G. (1964): Dermatomyositis treated by triamcinolone. *South. Med. J.,* 57:567–570.
56. Goldenberg, D. L., and Stoz, R. A. (1975): Azathioprine hypersensitivity mimicking an acute exacerbation of dermatomyositis. *J. Rheum.,* 2:346–349.
57. Gonzales-Angulo, A., Fraga, A., and Mintz, G. (1968): Submicroscopic alterations in capillaries of skeletal muscle in polymyositis. *Am. J. Med.,* 45:873–879.
58. Gotoff, S. P., Smith, R. D., and Sugar, O. (1972): Dermatomyositis with cerebral vasculitis in a patient with agammaglobulinemia. *Am. J. Dis. Child.,* 123:53–55.
59. Grace, W. J., Kennedy, R. J., and Formato, A. (1963): Therapy of scleroderma and dermatomyositis. *N. Y. State J. Med.,* 63:140–144.
60. Haas, D. C. (1973): Treatment of polymyositis with immunosuppressive drugs. *Neurology (Minneap.),* 23:55–62.
61. Haas, C. C., and Arnason, B. G. W. (1974): Cell-mediated sensitivity in polymyositis: creatine phosphokinase release from muscle culture. *Arch. Neurol.,* 31:192–196.
62. Hanissian, A. S., Martinez, A. J., Jabbour, J. T., and Duenas, D. A. (1973): Vasculitis and myositis secondary to rubella vaccination. *Arch. Neurol.,* 28:202–204.
63. Hart, F. D., Golding, J. R., and Mackenzie, D. H. (1957): Neuropathy in rheumatoid disease. *Ann. Rheum. Dis.,* 16:471–480.
64. Hashimoto, K., Robison, L., Velayos, E., and Niizuma, K. (1971): Dermatomyositis. Electron microscopic, immunologic and tissue culture studies of paramyxovirus-like inclusions. *Arch. Dermatol.,* 103:120–135.
65. Haslock, D. I., Wright, V., and Harriman, D. G. F. (1970): Neuromuscular disorders in rheumatoid arthritis. *Q. J. Med.,* 39:335–358.

65a. Hewlett, R. H., and Brownell, B. (1975): Granulomatous myopathy: its relationship to sarcoidosis and polymyositis. *J. Neurol. Neurosurg. Psychiatry*, 38:1090–1099.
66. Hill, D. L., and Barrows, H. D. (1968): Identical skeletal and cardiac muscle involvement in a case of fatal polymyositis. *Arch. Neurol.*, 19:545–551.
67. Hill, R. H., and Wood, W. S. (1970): Juvenile dermatomyositis. *Can. Med. Assoc. J.*, 21:1152–1156.
68. Hollindrake, K. (1969): Polymyositis presenting as distal muscle weakness: a case report. *J. Neurol. Sci.*, 8:479–484.
69. Holzmann, H., and Hirz, E. (1969): Über die beziehungen zwischen dermatomyositis und malignenen tumoren. *Arzneim. Forsch.*, 23:335–348.
70. Holzmann, H., Solberg, G., and Elgamili, I. (1967): Zur Kenntnis der psoriatischen Myopathie. *Arch. Dermatol. Forsch.*, 230:329–335.
71. Irby, R., Adams, R. A., and Taone, E. C. (1958): Peripheral neuritis associated with rheumatoid arthritis. *Arthritis Rheum.*, 1:44–53.
72. Jerusalem, F. (1967): Die bioptisch-histologische Differentialdiagnose der Polymyositis und der progressiven Muskeldystrophie. *Dtsch. Z. Nervenheilk*, 191:125–141.
73. Jerusalem, F., Rakusa, M., Engel, A. G., and Macdonald, R. D. (1974): Morphometric analysis of skeletal muscle capillary ultrastructure in inflammatory myopathies. *J. Neurol. Sci.*, 23:391–402.
73a. Johnson, M. A., Fulthorpe, J. J., and Hudgson, P. (1973): Lipid storage myopathy: A recognizable clinicopathological entity? *Acta Neuropathol.*, 24:97–106.
74. Johnson, R. L., Fink, C. W., and Ziff, M. (1972): Lymphotoxin formation by lymphocytes and muscle in polymyositis. *J. Clin. Invest.*, 51:2435–2449.
75. Johnson, R. L., Symth, C. J., Hold, G. W., Lubshenco, A., and Velentin, E. (1959): Steroid therapy and vascular lesions in rheumatoid arthritis. *Arthritis Rheum.*, 2:224–229.
76. Kagen, L. J., Kimball, A. C., and Christian, C. L. (1974): Serologic evidence of toxoplasmosis among patients with polymyositis. *Am. J. Med.*, 56:186–190.
77. Kemper, J. W., Bagenstoss, A. H., and Slocumb, C. H. (1957): The relationship of therapy with cortisone to the incidence of vascular lesions in rheumatoid arthritis. *Ann. Intern. Med.*, 46:831–851.
78. Klug, H., and Sonnichsen, N. (1973): Elektronoptische Untersuchungen über den Nachweis virusartiger Partikeln bei der Dermatomyositis. *Dermatol. Monatsschr.*, 159:97–102.
79. Landry, M., and Winkelmann, R. K. (1972): Tubular cytoplasmic inclusion in dermatomyositis. *Mayo Clin. Proc.*, 47:479–492.
80. Lange, R. K. (1970): Primary amyloidosis of muscle. *South. Med. J.*, 63:321–323.
81. Leddy, J. P., Griggs, R. C., Klemperer, M. R., and Frank, M. M. (1975): Hereditary complement (C2) deficiency with dermatomyositis. *Am. J. Med.*, 58:83–91.
82. Leonhardt, T. (1961): The familial occurrence of collagen diseases. II. Progressive systemic sclerosis and dermatomyositis. *Acta Med. Scand.*, 169:735.
83. Logan, R. G., Bandera, J. M., Mikkelsen, W. M., and Duff, I. F. (1966): Polymyositis: a clinical study. *Ann. Intern. Med.*, 65:996–1007.
84. Lisak, R. P., and Zweiman, B. (1975): Mitogen and muscle extract-induced *in vitro* proliferative responses in myasthenia gravis, dermatomyositis and polymyositis. *J. Neurol. Neurosurg. Psychiatry*, 38:521–524.
85. Lynch, P. G. (1971): Cardiac involvement in chronic polymyositis. *Br. Heart J.*, 33:416–419.
86. Malaviya, A. N., Many, A., and Schwartz, R. S. (1968): Treatment of dermatomyositis with methotrexate. *Lancet*, 2:485–488.
87. Malkinson, F. D., and Rothman, S. (1956): Changes in the gastrointestinal tract in scleroderma and other diffuse connective tissue diseases. *Am. J. Gastroenterol.*, 26:414–431.
88. Manson, S. E. D., and Reese, H. H. (1964): A previously unreported myopathy in patients with schistosomiasis. *Neurology (Minneap.)*, 14:355–361.
89. Martin, J. J., Van Bogaert, L., Van Damme, J., and Peremans, J. (1970): Sur une pseudomyopathie ligneuse généralisée par amyloidose primaire endomysiovasculaire. *J. Neurol. Sci.*, 11:147–166.

90. Martinez, A. J., Hooshmand, H., Mendoza, G. I., and Winston, Y. E. (1974): Fatal polymyositis: morphogenesis and ultrastructural features. *Acta Neuropathol.*, 29:251–262.
91. Mason, W., and Keller, E. (1975): Acute transient myositis with influenza-like illness. *J. Pediatr.*, 86:813–814.
91a. Mastaglia, F. L., McCollum, J. P. K., Larson, P. F., and Hudgson, P. (1970): Steroid myopathy complicating McArdle's disease. *J. Neurol. Neurosurg. Psychiatry*, 33:111–120.
92. Mastaglia, F. L., and Walton, J. N. (1970): Coxsackie virsus-like particles in skeletal muscle from a case of polymyositis. *J. Neurol. Sci.*, 11:593–599.
93. McNicholl, B., and Underhill, D. (1970): Toxoplasmic polymyositis. *Ir. J. Med. Sci.*, 3:525–527.
94. McFarlin, D. E., and Griggs, R. E. (1968): Treatment of inflammatory myopathies with azathioprine. *Trans. Am. Neurol. Assoc.*, 93:244–246.
94a. McKinley, I. A., and Mitchell, I. (1976): Transient acute myositis in childhood. *Arch. Dis. Child*, 51:135–137.
95. Medsger, T. A., Jr., Dawson, W. N., Jr., and Masi, A. T. (1970): The epidemiology of polymyositis. *Am. J. Med.*, 48:715–723.
96. Medsger, T. A., Jr., Robinson, H., and Masi, A. T. (1971): Factors affecting survivorship in polymyositis. A life-table study of 124 patients. *Arthritis Rheum.*, 14:249–258.
97. Metzger, A. L., Bohan, A., Goldberg, L. S., Bluestone, R., and Pearson, C. M. (1974): Polymyositis and dermatomyositis; combined methotrexate and corticosteroid therapy. *Ann. Intern. Med.*, 81:182–189.
98. Metzger, A. L., Singer, F. R., Bluestone, R., and Pearson, C. M. (1974): Failure of disodium etidronate in calcinosis due to dermatomyositis and scleroderma. *N. Engl. J. Med.*, 291:1284–1296.
99. Middleton, P. J., Alexander, R. M., and Szymanski, M. T. (1970): Severe myositis during recovery from influenza. *Lancet*, 2:533–535.
100. Miller, J. J. (1973): Late progression in dermatomyositis in childhood. *J. Pediatr.*, 83:543–548.
101. Mintz, G., Gonzalez-Angulo, A., Fraga, A., and Zavala, B. (1968): The ultrastructure of muscle in polymyositis. *Am. J. Med.*, 44:216.
102. Mollaret, P., Goulon, M., Lissac, J., Margairay, A., and Kochnevis, A. (1960): Un cas de polymyosite survenu au cours d'un traitement par triamcinolone chez un malade atteint de rheumatisme psoriasique. *Bull. Mem. Soc. Med. Hop. Paris*, 76:796–802.
103. Mom, A. M., Polak, M., Febeiro, J. L., and Garibaldi, I. B. (1970): The psoriatic myopathy. *Dermatologica*, 140:214–218.
104. Monif, G. R. G., and Ragan, C. (1962): Anti-inflammatory effect of salicylates in polymyositis. *Arthritis Rheum.*, 5:513–516.
105. Mulder, D. W., Winkelmann, R. K., Lambert, E. H., Diessner, G. R., and Howard, F. M. (1963): Steroid therapy in patients with polymyositis and dermatomyositis. *Ann. Intern. Med.*, 58:969–976.
106. Munsat, T. L., and Cancilla, P. (1974): Polymyositis without inflammation. *Bull. Los Angeles Neurol. Soc.*, 39:113–120.
107. Munsat, T. L., Piper, D., Cancilla, P., and Mendell, J. (1972): Inflammatory myopathy with facioscapulohumeral distribution. *Neurology (Minneap.)*, 22:336–347.
108. Nakashima, N., Tamura, Z., Okamoto, S., and Goto, H. (1970): Inclusion bodies in human neuromuscular disorder. *Arch. Neurol.*, 22:270–278.
109. Nassim, J. R., and Connoly, C. K. (1970): Treatment of calcinosis universalis with aluminum hydroxide. *Arch. Dis. Child.*, 45:118–121.
109a. Nattrass, F. J. (1954): Recovery from "muscular dystrophy." *Brain*, 77:549–570.
110. Nick, J., Prunieras, M., Bakouche, P., Reignier, A., and Nicolle, M. H. (1971): Inclusions dans les cellules endotheliales et les lymphocytes au cours d'un cas de dermatomyosite. *Rev. Neurol. (Paris)*, 125:329–338.
111. Nishikai, M., Fumatsu, Y., and Homma, M. (1974): Monoclonal gammopathy, penicillamine-induced polymyositis and systemic sclerosis. *Arch. Dermatol.*, 110:253–255.
112. Norris, F. H., Jr., Dranow, B., Calder, C. D., and Johnson, S. G. (1969): Virus-like particles in myositis accompanying herpes zoster. *Arch. Neurol.*, 21:25–31.

113. Norton, W. L., Velayos, E., and Robison, L. (1970): Endothelial inclusions in dermato-myositis. *Ann. Rheum. Dis.,* 29:67–72.
114. O'Leary, P. A., and Waisman, M. (1940): Dermatomyositis. A study of 40 cases. *Arch. Dermatol. Syph.,* 41:1001–1019.
115. Park, S., and Nyhan, W. L. (1975): Fatal pulmonary involvement in dermatomyositis. *Am. J. Dis. Child.,* 129:723–726.
116. Pearson, C. M. (1963): Patterns of polymyositis and their responses to treatment. *Ann. Intern. Med.,* 59:827–838.
117. Pearson, C. M. (1966): Polymyositis. *Annu. Rev. Med.,* 17:63–84.
118. Pearson, C. M., and Currie, S. (1974): Polymyositis and related disorders. In: *Disorders of Voluntary Muscle, 3rd Ed.,* edited by J. N. Walton, pp. 614–652. Churchill-Living-stone, Edinburgh and London.
119. Penn, A. S., Schotland, D. L., and Rowland, L. P. (1971): Immunological aspects of muscle disease. *Res. Publ. Assoc. Res. Nerv. Ment. Dis.,* 69:215–240.
120. Perkoff, G. T. (1971): Alcoholic myopathy. *Ann. Rev. Med.,* 22:125–132.
120a. Pinelli, P., Poloni, M., Nappi, G., and Scelsi, R. (1975): A case of late-onset lipid storage myopathy. *Eur. Neurol.,* 13:273–284.
121. Prineas, J. W., Mason, A. S., and Henson, R. A. (1965): Myopathy in metabolic bone disease. *Br. Med. J.,* 1:1034–1036.
122. Prunieras, M., Grupper, C., Durepaire, R., Pourgeois-Spinasse, J., and Edelson, Y. (1971): Inclusions dans la dermatomyosite aigue et chronique. *Nouv. Presse Med.,* 79:1463–1465.
123. Riddoch, D., and Morgan-Hughes, J. A. (1975): Prognosis in adult polymyositis. *J. Neurol. Sci.,* 26:71–80.
124. Rose, A., and Walton, J. N. (1966): Polymyositis. A survey of 89 cases with particular reference to treatment and prognosis. *Brain,* 89:747–768.
125. Rothstein, T. L., Carlson, C. B., and Sumi, S. M. (1971): Polymyositis with facioscapulo-humeral distribution. *Arch. Neurol.,* 25:313–319.
126. Rowland, L. P., and Greer, M. (1961): Toxoplasmic polymyositis. *Neurology (Min-neap.),* 11:367–370.
127. Rowland, L. P., Lisak, R. P., Schotland, D. L., DeJesus, P. V., and Berg, B. (1973): Myasthenic myopathy and thymoma. *Neurology (Minneap.),* 23:282–288.
127a. Rowland, L. P., and Penn, A. S. (1972): Myoglobinuria. *Med. Clin. North Am.,* 56:1233–1256.
128. Rowland, L. P., Sagman, D., and Schotland, D. L. (1966): Polymyositis: a conceptual problem. *Trans. Am. Neurol. Assoc.,* 91:332–334.
129. Rowland, L. P., and Schotland, D. L. (1965): Neoplasms and Muscle Disease. In: *The Remote Effects of Cancer on the Nervous System,* edited by W. R. Brain and F. Norris, p. 83. Grune & Stratton, New York.
130. Samuels, B. S., and Rietschel, R. L. (1976): Polymyositis and toxoplasmosis. *J.A.M.A.,* 235:60–61.
131. Sato, T., Walker, D. L., Peters, H. A., Reese, H. H., and Chou, S. M. (1971): Chronic polymyositis and myxovirus-like inclusions. *Arch. Neurol.,* 24:409–418.
132. Sawhney, B. B., Chopra, J. S., Banerji, A. K., and Wahi, P. L. (1976): Pseudohyper-trophic myopathy in cysticercosis. *Neurology (Minneap.),* 26:270–272.
133. Schaumberg, H. H., Nielsen, S. L., and Yurchak, P. M. (1971): Heart-block in poly-myositis. *N. Engl. J. Med.,* 284:480–481.
134. Schiller, H. H. (1975): Chronic viral myopathy and malignant hyperthermia. *N. Engl. J. Med.,* 292:1409.
135. Schiller, H. H., and Mair, W. G. P. (1974): Ultrastructural changes of muscle in malig-nant hyperthermia. *J. Neurol. Sci.,* 25:93–100.
136. Schirren, C. G. (1966): Antimetaboliten in der Behandlung der Dermatomyositis. *Arch. Dermatol. Forsch.,* 227:371–376.
137. Schmid, F. R., Cooper, N. S., Ziff, M., and McEwen, C. (1961): Arteritis in rheumatoid arthritis. *Am. J. Med.,* 30:56–83.
138. Schochet, S. S., Jr., and McCormick, W. F. (1973): Polymyositis with intranuclear inclusions. *Arch. Neurol.,* 28:280–283.
139. Schott, G. D., and Wills, M. R. (1976): Muscle weakness in osteomalacia. *Lancet,* 1:626–629.

140. Schraeder, P. L., Peters, H. A., and Dahl, D. S. (1972): Polymyositis and penicillamine. *Arch. Neurol.,* 27:456–458.
141. Schrago, R., and Miescher, P. A. (1974): Le traitement de la dermatomyosite. *Schweiz. Med. Wochenschr.,* 104:1311–1316.
141a. Schwarz, M. I., Matthay, R. A., Sahn, S. A., Stanford, R. E., Marmorstein, B. L., and Scheinhorn, D. S. (1976): Interstitial lung disease in polymyositis and dermatomyositis: Analysis of six cases and review of the literature. *Medicine (Baltimore),* 55:89–104.
142. Schuermann, H. (1958): Dermatomyositis. *Ergeb. Inn. Med. Kinderheilkd.,* 10:428–480.
143. Segura, R., and Ziegler, D. K. (1973): Dermatomyositis. A recurrence of symptoms following treatment of neoplasm. *Dis. Nerv. Syst.,* 34:284–286.
144. Sharp, G. C., Irvin, W. S., Tan, E. M., Gould, R. G., and Holman, H. R. (1972): Mixed connective tissue disease; an apparently distinct rheumatic disease syndrome associated with a specific antibody to extractable nuclear antigen. *Am. J. Med.,* 52:148–159.
145. Shy, G. M., and Silverstein, I. (1965): A study of the effects on the motor unit by remote malignancy. *Brain,* 86:515–518.
146. Silverstein, A., and Siltzbach, I. I. (1969): Muscle involvement in sarcoidosis. Asymptomatic, myositis, and myopathy. *Arch. Neurol.,* 21:235–241.
146a. Singsen, B., Goldreyer, B., Stanton, R., and Hanson, V. (1976): Childhood polymyositis with cardiac conduction defects. *Am. J. Dis. Child.,* 130:72–74.
147. Smith, B. (1969): Skeletal muscle necrosis associated with carcinoma. *J. Pathol.,* 97:207–210.
148. Smith, R., and Stern, G. R. (1967): Myopathy, osteomalacia, and hyperparathyroidism. *Brain,* 90:593–602.
149. Smith, R., and Stern, G. R. (1971): Muscular weakness in osteomalacia and hyperparathyroidism. *J. Neurol. Sci.,* 8:511–520.
150. Sokoloff, M. C., Goldberg, L. S., and Pearson, C. M. (1971): Treatment of corticosteroid-resistant polymyositis with methotrexate. *Lancet,* 1:14–16.
151. Sullivan, D. B., Cassidy, J. T., Petty, R. E., and Burt, A. (1972): Prognosis in childhood dermatomyositis. *J. Pediatr.,* 80:555–563.
152. Susac, J. O., Carcia-Mullin, R., and Glaser, J. S. (1973): Ophthalmoplegia in dermatomyositis. *Neurology (Minneap.),* 23:305–310.
153. Talbott, J. H. (1974): *Collagen-Vascular Diseases.* Grune & Stratton, New York.
154. Tang, T. T., Sedmak, G. V., Siegesmand, K. A., and McCreadie, S. R. (1975): Chronic myopathy associated with Coxsackie virus type A9. *N. Engl. J. Med.,* 292:608–611.
154a. Terplank, L., Constantine, A. B., Koepf, G. F., and Dayton, G. O. (1951): Malignant exophthalmos with subacute myocarditis and generalized myositis. *N.Y. State J. Med.,* 51:2750–2752.
155. Vick, N. A. (1970): The fine structure of polymyositis with consideration of capillaries and subcellular organelles. *Neurology (Minneap.),* 20:1062–1068.
156. Vignos, P. J., Jr., Bowling, G. E., and Watkins, M. P. (1964): Polymyositis. Effect of corticosteroids on final result. *Arch. Intern. Med.,* 114:263–277.
157. Vignos, P. J., and Goldwyn, J. (1972): Evaluation of laboratory tests in diagnosis and management of polymyositis. *Am. J. Med. Sci.,* 263:291–308.
158. Vilppula, A. (1972): Muscular disorders in some collagen diseases. A clinical, electromyographic and biopsy study. *Acta Med. Scand. (Suppl.)* 540:1–7.
159. Walton, J. N., and Adams, R. D. (1958): *Polymyositis.* Williams & Wilkins, Baltimore.
160. Webb, D. R., and Currie, G. D. (1972): Pulmonary fibrosis masking polymyositis. Remission with corticosteroid therapy. *J.A.M.A.,* 222:1146–1149.
161. Wedgewood, R. J. P., Cook, C. D., and Cohen, J. (1953): Dermatomyositis; report of 26 cases in children with discussion of endocrine therapy in 13. *Pediatrics,* 12:447–466.
162. Whitaker, J. N., and Engel, W. K. (1972): Vascular deposits of immunoglobulin and complement in idiopathic inflammatory myopathy. *N. Engl. J. Med.,* 286:333–338.
163. Wilner, E. C., and Brody, J. A. (1968): An evaluation of the remote effects of cancer on the nervous system. *Neurology (Minneap.),* 18:1120–1124.
164. Winkelmann, R. K., Mulder, D. W., Diessner, G. R., Howard, F. M., Jr., and Lambert, E. H. (1965): Cyclic myositis, a cortisone-related variety of dermatomyosistis-polymyositis. *Minn. Med.,* 48:164–169.
165. Winkelmann, R. D., Mulder, D. W., Lambert, E. H., Howard, F. M., and Diesner, G. R.

(1968): Course of dermatomyositis-polymyositis: comparison of untreated and cortisone-treated patients. *Mayo Clin. Proc.,* 43:545–556.

166. Yunis, E. J., and Samaha, F. J. (1971): Inclusion body myositis. *Lab. Invest.,* 25:240–248.

167. Ziegler, D. K., and Hamilton, T. R. (1966): Polymyositis: A review of 17 cases. *J. Kans. Med. Soc.,* 67:119–124.

168. Zilko, P. J., and Dawkins, R. L. (1975): Amyloidosis associated with dermatomyositis and features of multiple myeloma. Progression of amyloidosis associated with corticosteroid and cytotoxic drug therapy. *Am. J. Med.,* 59:448–451.

169. Zweymiller, E. (1953): Schwere Haut-muskelerkrankung unter dem klinischen Erscheinungsbild einer Dermatomyositis mit Coxsackievirusbefund. *Dtsch. Med. Wochenschr.,* 78:190–192.

Advances in Neurology, Vol. 17, edited by
R. C. Griggs and R. T. Moxley, III. Raven Press,
New York © 1977.

Treatment of Myasthenia Gravis: Long-Term Administration of Corticosteroids with Remarks on Thymectomy

T. R. Johns

Department of Neurology, University of Virginia Jerry Lewis Neuromuscular Center, University of Virginia, Charlottesville, Virginia 22904

The value of corticotropins in the treatment of myasthenia gravis was demonstrated as early as 1935 by Simon (1). Numerous reports 15 years later evaluated the effectiveness of ACTH and cortisone. Shy et al. (2), Millikan and Eaton (3), and Grob and Harvey (4) observed early deterioration in 14 of their 18 patients treated with short courses of corticotropins or corticosteroids, with little or no subsequent improvement in 16 of those patients. Torda and Wolff (5) and Schlezinger (6), however, observed favorable clinical responses in 20 of their 26 patients treated with steroids.

That short courses of high-dose ACTH were of value in advanced myasthenia gravis was substantiated by Freydberg in 1960 (7) and by Von Reis and co-workers (8), Grob and Namba (9), Osserman and Genkins (10), and Grashchenkov and Perelman (11). ACTH, 100 units daily, was usually given over 8 to 14 days. Clinical improvement, when it occurred, was highly variable in duration, lasting from 2 weeks to over a year (in very few cases), with a mean duration of improvement of approximately 3 months. Therapy consisted of multiple courses of ACTH, and the incidence of exacerbation of myasthenic weakness during early steroid therapy was high. During the same period, Genkins (12) suggested that short courses of corticosteroids (prednisone) could be beneficial in the treatment of myasthenia gravis.

Von Reis (8), Osserman and Genkins (10), and Griggs, McFarlin, and Engel (13) alluded to the potential benefit of chronic ACTH/corticosteroid therapy in myasthenia. Cape and Utterback (14,15) demonstrated the value of using long-term maintenance ACTH in myasthenia. Improvement was achieved in five of their six patients for 16 to 52 months.

In 1971 Kjaer (16) reported seven cases, aged 50 to 73, in which 10 of 13 incidents of maintenance therapy with oral prednisone resulted in "complete" or "almost complete" remission (77%). Warmolts and Engel (17) reported five cases treated with alternate-day high-dose prednisone with "favorable" results (100%), and Jenkins (18) reported nine cases managed in similar fashion with "complete" or "almost complete" recovery in six (67%). Brunner, Namba, and Grob (19) reported nine patients with myasthenia gravis treated with multiple short courses of intramuscular methylprednisolone in doses of 60 mg daily. Some of those courses were followed by maintenance prednisone therapy in the range of 5 to 15 mg daily. The best results were achieved in courses of combined therapy, methylprednisolone followed by oral prednisone, with improvement being maintained for a mean duration of 4 months (range 2 weeks to 13 months).

In 1971 Johns et al. (20) reported 19 patients with myasthenia gravis and polymyositis or atrophy. Corticosteroids (prednisone) in high doses, subsequently maintained at lower doses for many months, led to moderate or marked improvement in both myasthenia and myopathy in all cases. Those observations, along with the lack of good evidence to support the superiority of ACTH over corticosteroids for immunosuppression (21), led the authors to propose therapy with prednisone for myasthenia gravis, with or without myopathy or atrophy.

In 1972 (22) we presented a preliminary report of our results in treating 16 patients with myasthenia gravis with high-dose daily prednisone followed by long-term maintenance therapy with low-dose alternate-day prednisone after initial improvement was sustained. In 26 incidents of treatment, there was complete remission in 46%, marked improvement in 38%, and moderate improvement in 8%.

The following is a report of our experience with 47 consecutive myasthenic patients who were treated initially with high doses of corticosteroids (prednisone) and maintained subsequently for long-term on lower doses. Mann et al. (23) and Jones and co-workers (24) at our institution have reported these results in 1975 and 1976. All patients were treated at the University of Virginia Medical Center. Series A included 30 patients who were treated over a period longer than 5 years ending January 1975 (23,25). Series B included 22 patients who were treated over a subsequent 2-year period ending January 1976 (24). The two series will be discussed separately in order to demonstrate the consistency of results. There was no attempt to have matched controls. No new patients entered these studies after January 1976.

METHODOLOGY

Patient Profile and Classification

SERIES A

A total of 30 patients, 14 male and 16 female, aged 13 to 81 years, underwent 45 incidents of therapy with prednisone for myasthenia gravis (Table 1A). Twenty patients were white and ten were black. That compares with a

TABLE 1A. *Patient profile — series A*

	Male	Female	Total
No. of patients	14	16	30
White	9	11	20
Black	5	5	10
Age range	26–81	13–72	13–81
Mean age	57	34	45
Incidents of treatment	20	25	45

discharge rate from the University of Virginia Hospital of 77% white versus 23% non-white from March 1974 to February 1975. The age of onset of myasthenia was from 10 to 78 years. The mean duration of illness before the first treatment with prednisone was 4 years (range 1 month to 30 years). Three patients had associated polymyositis; two had benign thymomas; one had a malignant thymoma; and one each had thymic vein thrombosis, rheumatoid arthritis, hepatic dysfunction, and scleroderma (see Table 4 for other associated illnesses).

Criteria for the diagnosis of myasthenia gravis included: (a) fluctuating skeletal muscle weakness that was worse after effort, exhibiting some improvement with rest; the extremity weakness was usually proximal and symmetrical, but often distal, and frequently associated with late atrophy; (b) a decrement in the amplitude of the evoked potential electromyogram with a low-frequency stimulation decrement and restoration following edrophonium, neostigmine, or a maximal voluntary contraction; (c) positive pharmacologic testing with edrophonium or neostigmine, usually in a controlled or double-blind procedure; and (d) no evidence of other neuromuscular disease as determined by muscle biopsy, electromyography, serum enzymes, and other diagnostic studies.

The incidents of therapy are displayed in Tables 2A and B, distributed according to the severity of illness at the time of beginning prednisone. We have used a modification of Osserman's classification (26). Generally,

TABLE 2A. *Patient classification — series A (30 patients)*

Classification at initiation of treatment	Incidents of treatment	Duration of myasthenia gravis (MYG) before treatment
1. Ocular	3	6 mo–22 yr
2. Predominantly ocular and mild limb girdle	6	4 mo–30 yr
3. Predominantly faciopharyngeal plus mild limb girdle and/or ocular	7	2.5 mo–8.5 yr
4. Moderate generalized	14	1 mo–28 yr
5. Severe generalized	15	2.5 mo–8 yr
Total	45	1 mo–30 yr

TABLE 2B. *Patient classification — series B*

Classification at initiation of treatment	Incidents of treatment	Duration of MYG before treatment
1. Ocular	2	17 mo–17 yr
2. Predominantly ocular and mild limb girdle	3	7 mo–13 mo
3. Predominantly faciopharyngeal plus mild limb girdle and/or ocular	4	4 mo–5 yr 1 mo
4. Moderate generalized	12	1 mo–12 yr
5. Severe generalized	1	4 mo
Total	22	1 mo–17 yr

class 1 and 2 patients were considered to have mild-to-moderate disease that did not markedly interfere with activities of daily living. However, one class 1 patient initially lost his job as a foreman–truck driver before prednisone therapy, and one class 2 patient, a dentist, was unable to practice because of ocular symptoms. Class 3, 4, and 5 patients were considered to have more severe disease, significantly interfering with activities of daily living and work. Class 3 patients generally had problems with phonation, deglutition, and respiration, even though limb-girdle and ocular involve-

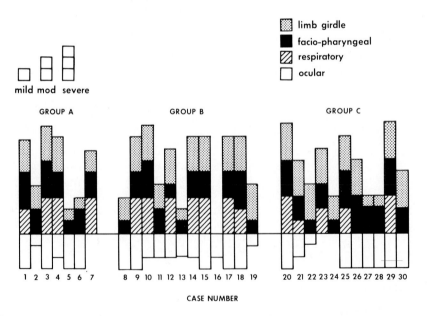

FIG. 1. Degree and distribution of muscle weakness in 30 patients before treatment with corticosteroids. Patients are grouped according to duration of myasthenia before first exposure to prednisone: Group A, less than 6 months, group B, 6 to 24 months, group C, longer than 24 months.

ment was mild. Thus, in series A, 20% of the patients had mild-to-moderate disease with 7% being purely ocular, whereas 80% of the patients had more severe and extensive disease. The duration of disease was over 6 months in 77% of patients. Further characterization of the patient group in terms of distribution and severity of myasthenia before prednisone therapy is shown in Fig. 1.

SERIES B

In the second series, there were 22 patients, 4 male and 18 female, aged 14 to 81 years, and each was treated only once; thus there were 22 incidents of treatment (Table 1B). The mean duration of myasthenia before treatment ranged from 1 month to 17 years. Thus the patient sample was smaller yet comparable to that in series A, but with fewer incidents of treatment because our experience had led us not to discontinue therapy in less than 1 year or after thymectomy.

TABLE 1B. *Patient profile—series B*

	Male	Female	Total
No. of patients	4	18	22
Age range	50–78	14–81	14–81
Mean age	63.5	39.1	43.5
Incidents of treatment	4	18	22

Electrophysiological Studies

Needle electromyography, nerve conductions, and evoked potential studies were performed in all patients. Motor and sensory conductions were normal except for rare instances of seemingly unrelated neuropathy. Evoked potential studies and needle electromyography (EP-EMG) revealed abnormalities in all but two patients (case 24, RBN, and case 5, PGM). Those patients had predominantly laryngeal and ocular myasthenia, respectively. Needle electromyography was performed in proximal muscles, mostly deltoid and biceps, to compare with morphological studies of contralateral muscles. The electromyographic abnormalities ranged from minimal changes of irregularly shaped potentials (13 cases), to a full "myopathic" EMG pattern with short duration, low-amplitude muscle potentials, increased incidence of polyphasic waves, and an interference pattern of reduced amplitude with maximum effort (14 cases). Denervation activity at rest was conspicuously absent in all but one case. The frequent "myopathic" features and lack of denervation on electromyography were in contrast to the scarcity of myopathic findings and frequency of denervation atrophy in the morphologic studies. The evoked potential studies were performed on the ulnar nerve–abductor digiti quinti muscle and/or the facial nerve–orbicularis oculi muscle.

All of the patients, except the two with localized myasthenia, had a significant decrement of the evoked-potential amplitude (more than 7% at 3 c/s stimulation). The decrement occurred 2 to 4 min after brief maximal voluntary effort or tetanic stimulation. In most instances, the administration of edrophonium or neostigmine corrected or ameliorated the evoked potential decrement. A moderate post-tetanic facilitation of no more than 50% was observed in most of the patients.

Muscle Biopsies

The biopsies were obtained from proximal arm muscles, usually deltoid and biceps, and were frozen for histological and histochemical studies.

TABLE 3. *Muscle morphology—series A (30 biopsies)*

Normal	Type II atrophy	Necrosis	Denervation	Cellular reaction
11 (37%)	8 (27%)	8 (27%)	7 (23%)	6 (20%)

Staining reactions were for hematoxylin and eosin, Gomori's trichrome, PAS, Oil Red 0, phosphorylase, myofibrillar ATPase (pH 4.3, 4.7, and 10), diphosphopyridine nucleotide hydrogenase (DPNH), and succinate dehydrogenase. The muscle biopsies were normal in 11 patients. Nineteen patients exhibited one or more of the following abnormalities (Table 3):

A. Atrophy of the histochemical type II fibers was the most common abnormality and was usually associated with one of the others; the atrophic fibers were regularly scattered throughout the sections except in two cases.

B. Denervation atrophy was usually minimal, except for two cases, and consisted of few angular fibers of both histochemical types with dark DPNH staining. Type grouping was never found.

C. Cellular reaction was seen with interstitial and perivascular patterns: the cells were usually round and mononuclear and, for the most part, unrelated to muscle fiber necrosis. Some of those cellular reactions could be called "lymphorrhages."

D. Single-fiber necrosis, with loss of staining features and phagocytosis, when present, affected only a few fibers.

The pathologic findings were frequently mixed in each biopsy. Their incidence in the present series is similar to the findings of Fenichel (27). Normal biopsies were found in patients with a mean duration of myasthenia of 20 months, and abnormal biopsies were found in patients with a mean duration of illness of 70 months.

RESULTS

**Initial Prednisone Therapy and Establishment
of Effective Maintenance Dose**

SERIES A

All patients were hospitalized during the initial phases of treatment with prednisone (Table 4A). Oral prednisone was begun with a mean initial dose of 59 mg daily (range 10 to 100 mg) and continued until there was sustained improvement over a 4- to 5-day period, or, in rare incidents, until untoward side effects led to reduction of the dose. The duration of the initial dose was from 3 days to 5.5 months (mean 29.3 days). Steroids were then gradually decreased, and in most patients an alternate-day (AD) schedule of steroid administration was achieved simultaneously.

TABLE 4A. *Prednisone dosage—series A*

	Range	Mean (SEM)
Initial dose (45 incidents)	10–100 mg daily	59.0 mg daily ($\pm$2)
Duration	3 days–5.5 mo	29.3 days ($\pm$4)
Period to achieve sustained improvement (43 incidents)	3–31 days	13.0 days ($\pm$1)
Maintenance dose		
Alternate day (27 incidents)	10–150 mg	34.8 mg ($\pm$6)
Daily (12 incidents)	5–40 mg	16.7 mg ($\pm$3)
Duration	15 days–5 yr[a]	22.1 mo
Period to achieve maximal response (43 incidents)	3 days–16 mo	3 mo ($\pm$0.5)

[a] Includes 2 patients with polymyositis.

Reduction in corticosteroid dosage from initial high levels was begun when the patient showed sustained improvement over base-line, pre-prednisone strength for at least 4 days. That did not include recovery from weakness during an exacerbation when strength was still below base-line or pretreatment strength. Sustained improvement began between 3 and 31 days after the start of prednisone therapy, with a mean of 13 days. Most of our patients were markedly improved within 6 to 8 weeks after sustained improvement on prednisone was well established. With reduction of steroids during that time, they soon achieved a dose of 60 mg AD. Thereafter, reductions to maintenance levels were made somewhat more slowly, frequently with an 8-week period of observation being allowed before each subsequent reduction of 5 mg in prednisone dosage. The effective maintenance dose (EMD) was determined as the smallest dose of prednisone sufficient to maintain a patient in remission or at maximal improvement. Reduction to EMD required an average of 4.1 months. Early in our experience, we found that rapid or "programmed" reductions in prednisone were often associated with marked fluctuations in the clinical course, occasionally including pronounced episodes of increased weakness, requiring an increase or reinstitution of cholinesterase inhibitors.

The duration of treatment necessary to achieve a maximal response was 3 days to 16 months (mean 3 months). It should be emphasized that it was not necessary to sustain the high initial dose of prednisone until the occurrence of maximal improvement, in that the latter often occurred as steroids were being reduced or even after EMD had been achieved.

Reduction of steroid dosage below maintenance levels resulted in clinical worsening. However, maximal improvement was often reestablished by increasing the prednisone to the last dose on which improvement had been sustained. We also found that sudden large increases over existing dosage had deleterious effects, including a major exacerbation of myasthenic weakness in one case. Dosage adjustments required careful observation for evidence of worsening of myasthenia, as well as for complications of therapy.

In 28 incidents of therapy (62%), patients achieved an AD regimen with a mean maintenance dose of approximately 35 mg AD (Table 4A). In 14 incidents (31%), many of them early in our experience, a daily dosage schedule was adhered to, with a mean maintenance dose of approximately 15 mg daily. In three incidents (7%) EMD was not achieved because steroids were discontinued early in therapy. The duration of EMD was from 15 days to 5 years (mean 22.1 months). The most delayed achievement of maximal response (16 months) and the longest duration of both initial dose (5.5 months) and maintenance dose (5 years) were in one patient who had both myasthenia and polymyositis.

EMD was achieved equally well with an AD or daily regimen, although fewer complications occurred with the former schedule. Some patients on AD steroids complained of mild weakness on days when they were not receiving prednisone, exhibiting some evidence that they were in a 48-hr response cycle to steroids. Four patients showed a return of EP-EMG to normal after remission on prednisone had been achieved.

SERIES B

Patients in series B were more consistently treated with initial doses of prednisone of 60 mg daily (Table 4B), required approximately the same period to achieve sustained improvement, but required a longer period

TABLE 4B. *Prednisone dosage — series B*

(22 incidents)	
Initial dose (daily)	60 mg
Period to achieve sustained improvement	12.5 days
Initial dose (alternate day)	120 mg
Duration	1–2 mo
Period to achieve maximal response	5 mo

to achieve a maximal response (mean 5 months, compared to a mean of 3 months for series A patients).

Cholinesterase Inhibitors

Cholinesterase inhibitors were used as long as they were found to be beneficial early in treatment with prednisone, particularly when they produced a favorable response in oropharyngeal and/or respiratory musculature. However, marked reduction in cholinesterase inhibitor requirements was commonly apparent during the early days or weeks of therapy. Consequently, those drugs were reduced as rapidly as could be tolerated by the patient once prednisone was begun in order to avoid cholinergic weakness. Cholinesterase inhibitors were eventually discontinued in 34 of 43 incidents (79%) of treatment with prednisone, and in 24 incidents of therapy (56%) they were discontinued within the first month. In the entire series, cholinesterase inhibitors were used at low doses and infrequent administrations for a mean of 5.4 months (range 3 days to 31 months) after corticosteroids had been started. In general, requirements for cholinesterase inhibitors were markedly reduced when they were continued with prednisone for prolonged periods. It appeared that many of our patients on prednisone first developed an increased responsiveness to cholinesterase inhibitors; shortly thereafter, muscle power improved independent of the influence of these drugs.

Incidence of Exacerbation

SERIES A

Myasthenic weakness was exacerbated in 20 of 45 incidents of therapy (44%) with prednisone (Table 5A). Exacerbations began between the 1st and 21st days of therapy with a mean of 5 days. The duration of increased muscle weakness was from 1 hr to 20 days with a mean of 6 days. A total of 75% of the exacerbations were mild to moderate in severity, although in 25% of exacerbations (five patients) there was a marked increase in

TABLE 5A. *Exacerbations — series A*

No. 20 (44%)			
	Range		Mean
Onset	1st–21st day		5th day
Duration	1 hr–20 days		6 days
Degree	Mild	Moderate	Severe
No.	10	5	5
Total incidents (%)	22	11	11

muscle weakness, requiring brief periods of respiratory support. Of the patients who experienced exacerbation in the first several weeks of therapy, none improved significantly before the onset of exacerbation while on a constant dose of prednisone. That was true even in those cases in which increased muscle weakness occurred relatively late. Neither the degree nor the duration of exacerbation was a predictor of ultimate therapeutic response to prednisone. Also, the degree of increased muscle weakness was not related to the interval between the beginning of therapy and the onset of exacerbation.

It appeared that more severely involved patients were more likely to experience exacerbation than less severely involved patients: only three patients in that group were in classes 1, 2, or 3. Age, sex, and duration of illness before treatment with prednisone were not significantly related to the probability of worsening during the initial phases of treatment. None of our patients with primarily ocular myasthenia experienced exacerbation. Men who experienced exacerbation tended to be somewhat younger than men who did not (mean age 42.1 versus 63.0 years), whereas women who experienced exacerbation tended to be older than those who did not (mean age 42.1 versus 30.0 years). However, those data represented trends and were not statistically significant. All three patients with thymoma had exacerbation of their muscle weakness, but in one of those patients thymectomy actually preceded the onset of prednisone therapy by 5 years. There was otherwise no relationship between thymus histology and exacerbation.

The concurrent use of cholinesterase inhibitors and prednisone during the first weeks of therapy did not influence the development of increased weakness of a noncholinergic type. Patients who became weaker on prednisone usually had an incomplete response to cholinesterase inhibitors during the period of increased weakness. They were observed closely for any evidence of even slight deterioration in strength, and many of those considered to have "mild" exacerbations experienced increased weakness of only a few hours' duration. In those cases it was frequently difficult to determine whether the increased weakness represented an exacerbation secondary to steroid therapy, or whether the patient was actually undermedicated with cholinesterase inhibitors. Our oldest female myasthenic, aged 74, had an exacerbation with each of three incidents of prednisone therapy. It is also probable that she had two exacerbations during her second incident of therapy. Another patient experienced an exacerbation during the initial part of both incidents of therapy with prednisone, in addition to an exacerbation of her myasthenic weakness after a large increase in her maintenance prednisone. She subsequently achieved moderate improvement. The remaining 14 patients had only one exacerbation each, occurring with the first exposure to prednisone.

SERIES B

Patients in series B had the same percentage of exacerbations but none were severe (Table 5B). The onset of exacerbation remained at a mean of the 5th day, but the range was from 12 hr to 12 days, the duration being approximately the same. This suggests the possibility that hospitalization could be shortened, at least in regard to concern for exacerbation.

TABLE 5B. *Exacerbations — series B*

No. 10 (45%)			
	Range		Mean
Onset	12 hr–12 days		5th day
Duration	1–17 days		4.6 days
Degree	Mild	Moderate	Severe
No.	7	3	0

We do not wish to underemphasize the inherent dangers of exacerbation of myasthenic weakness. There is a definite need for hospitalization and careful observation of patients during the first 2 to 3 weeks of therapy. If exacerbation occurs and is well documented, the patient could be considered eligible for outpatient follow-up, provided he has sufficiently recovered from the episode and is not otherwise at risk. Frequent outpatient contacts have been essential during the ensuing 3 to 6 weeks. Problems of increased myasthenic weakness at other times can be largely avoided if care is taken to make gradual adjustments in the patient's corticosteroid dosage schedule.

Side Effects

SERIES A

The side effects from corticosteroids, aside from exacerbation, were not a major problem in most cases (Table 6A). In 17 patients, mild-to-moderate Cushingoid features developed during the initial period of high-

TABLE 6A. *Complications and side effects — series A*

Defect	No. affected
Cushingoid appearance	17
Diastolic hypertension	3
Cataracts	3
Focal infection	2
Osteoporosis with vertebral collapse	1
Angina	1
Thrombocytopenia	1
Thrombophlebitis	1
Pulmonary emboli	1
Aseptic necrosis of femoral heads	1

dose prednisone. Those signs usually resolved completely as the dosage was reduced and an AD schedule was established.

Major complications occurred in nine patients (aged 28 to 81, mean 61 years), five of whom had predisposing associated illnesses. Osteoporosis with vertebral collapse occurred in our oldest female patient after 15 months of treatment with prednisone. She had had myasthenia gravis 84 months before beginning steroids, and her course during that time was characterized by major fluctuations in muscle strength, difficulty of control with cholinesterase inhibitors, and prolonged periods of hospitalization and inactivity.

Thrombocytopenia, thrombophlebitis, and pulmonary emboli all occurred in one patient, a 69-year-old man with arteriosclerotic cardiovascular disease and multifocal preventricular contractions. The entire episode was of short duration, with improvement coinciding with reduction of prednisone to 5 mg daily. He subsequently achieved and maintained complete remission on 25 mg AD. Aseptic necrosis of the femoral heads occurred in our patient on steroids for the longest period, a patient with both polymyositis and myasthenia gravis. He had relapses when steroids were discontinued or reduced below maintenance levels. Eight patients had significant hypertension before beginning therapy with prednisone. Five of them exhibited no worsening, even when taking high daily doses of corticosteroids. Diastolic hypertension became worse in three patients, responding in all three to antihypertensive medications, and eventually to reduction of prednisone dosage. Three patients developed cataracts after 15, 18, and 20 months of therapy. Two other patients had mild transient infections of the urinary tract and skin.

SERIES B

Patients in series B had complications and side effects similar in incidence, type, and severity to those in series A patients (Table 6B).

TABLE 6B. *Complications and side effects — series B*

Defect	No. affected	Percent
Cushingoid appearance	14	63.6
Diastolic hypertension	3	13.6
Cataracts	5	22.7
Osteoporosis with vertebral collapse	1	4.5
Aseptic necrosis of femoral head	1	4.5
Ruptured diverticuli	1	4.5

Improvement of Muscle Strength

SERIES A

There were 45 incidents of long-term prednisone therapy in 30 patients (Table 7A). In nine incidents (20%) patients had mild-to-moderate myasthenia at the beginning of prednisone therapy (classes 1 and 2); and in 36 incidents (80%) patients had more severe involvement (classes 3, 4, and 5).

In those with moderate involvement, there were two incidents of marked improvement and seven of complete remission, all without continued use of cholinesterase inhibitors. Although the number of incidents is small, it is important to observe that of the nine incidents of therapy in classes 1 and 2, 100% achieved marked improvement or complete remission, and all those with mainly ocular involvement sustained a complete remission on prednisone. In the 36 incidents involving patients with more severe myasthenia, there were 3 incidents of moderate improvement, 7 incidents of marked improvement, and 24 incidents of complete remission, with ultimate discontinuation of cholinesterase inhibitors.

TABLE 7A. *Results — series A*

Classifi-cation	Incidents	Unimproved	Moderate improve-ment	Marked improve-ment	Remission	Total remission and marked improve-ment (%)
1	3	0	0	0	3	100
2	6	0	0	2	4	100
3	7	0	1	2	4	86
4	14	0	0	4	10	100
5	15	2[a]	2	1	10	73
Total	45	2[a]	3	9	31	
	(100%)	(4%)	(7%)	(20%)	(69%)	(89%)

[a] Two patients treated with low dose or short duration: both had thymic recurrence.

Two patients in class 5 failed to improve in two incidents of therapy. Both were young women who were treated early in our experience with prednisone and late in the course of their illnesses, for only 3 and 5 weeks, at daily doses of 60 and 40 mg, respectively. Prior thymectomy and several courses of ACTH had produced only mild unsustained improvement. Each died in the 4th year of illness, and both were found to have recurrence of the thymus gland without neoplasia.

Thus, in series A, 20% of incidents of therapy with prednisone led to marked improvement and 69% to complete remission, so that in 89% there was essentially complete loss of disability. Another 7% experienced moderate improvement.

SERIES B

In the more recent series B (Table 7B), 22 patients were treated with long-term prednisone. Five patients (23%) had mild-to-moderate myasthenia at the beginning of prednisone therapy, and 17 patients (77%) had more severe involvement. However, in this series only one patient was in class 5.

In those with moderate involvement, there were four incidents of marked improvement and one of complete remission—confirming the results of series A. In the 17 patients with more severe myasthenia, there were three incidents of moderate improvement (18%), nine incidents of marked improvement (53%), and five incidents of complete remission (29%).

Therefore, in the entire series B, 59.1% of patients experienced marked improvement and 27.3% experienced complete remission, so that 86.4% of patients achieved essentially a complete loss of disability. Another 13.6% experienced moderate improvement.

However, even with this confirmatory data of significant improvement, it should be noted that in series A 60% of patients achieved complete remission, whereas in series B only 27.3% did. Conversely, in series A 20% achieved marked improvement, and in series B 59.1% did.

TABLE 7B. Results — series B

Classification	Patients	Unimproved	Moderate improvement	Marked improvement	Remission	Remission and marked improvement (%)
1	2	0	0	2	0	100.0
2	3	0	0	2	1	100.0
3	4	0	1	0	3	75.0
4	12	0	1	9	2	91.6
5	1	0	1	0	0	———
Total	22	0	3	13	6	
		(0%)	(13.6%)	(59.1%)	(27.3%)	(86.4%)

Thymectomy

SERIES A

Thymectomy was performed in twenty-three patients, in four before the institution of prednisone and in nineteen after achievement of marked improvement or remission on steroids. (These figures represent a period of follow-up through May 1975.) In the first group, the two young women with recurrent thymus referred to above (Table 7A) had mild, unsustained improvement 18 and 24 months after thymectomy. Their response to prednisone was negligible. Two other patients were unimproved 5 and 8 years after thymectomy and had evidence of moderate muscle atrophy. Both responded to long-term prednisone with marked improvement.

In the second group of nineteen patients treated with prednisone before thymectomy (Table 8A), there were fifteen females and four males, with a duration of myasthenia before prednisone of 3 to 96 months. Eleven of those patients achieved complete remission and eight showed marked improvement before surgery. The duration of prednisone treatment before thymectomy was from 1 to 30 months with a mean of 10.5 months.

All of our thymectomy patients underwent a sternum-splitting procedure, usually with only the upper one-half, or less, of the sternum being divided. With a single exception, the morbidity associated with surgery was insignificant and the postoperative period uneventful. Marked postoperative morbidity was experienced by our oldest thymectomy patient, a 65-year-old woman with a large malignant thymoma requiring extensive surgical resection. She received prednisone for only 1 month before surgery. The relative lack of morbidity associated with thymectomy in our patients contrasts with

TABLE 8A. *Thymectomy after prednisone—series A*

Characteristic	No.	
Sex		
Male	4	
Female	15	
Classification		
1, 2, and 3	7	
4 and 5	12	
Morbidity		
None	14	
Mild	4	
Marked	1	
	Range	Mean
Age (yr)	13–65	31.2
Months of prednisone prethymectomy	1–30	10.5

the frequently stormy postoperative courses experienced by myasthenics not on prednisone.

No patient with normal or involuted thymus failed to achieve remission on prednisone. Hyperplastic thymus was found in only five of our younger female patients. Of that group, two patients failed to respond to prednisone, which was begun after thymectomy. Our youngest patient, aged 13, exhibited marked improvement on prednisone, and two other patients with hyperplastic thymus responded to corticosteroids with sustained remission before thymectomy. All of our patients with thymoma experienced either remission or marked improvement with prednisone.

SERIES B

Of the twenty-two patients in series B, ten — one male and nine females — proceeded to thymectomy (Table 8B). They had been treated with prednisone for from 4 to 17 months (mean 19.8 months). Four of them (40%) had achieved complete remission, and six (60%) marked improvement. At subsequent thymectomy there was essentially no morbidity in nine (90%) and severe morbidity in one (10%), a 30-year-old woman whose phrenic nerve was resected at removal of a malignant thymoma, leading to assisted ventilation for 48 hr. All of the patients maintained their prethymectomy improvement after the operative procedure.

Although the number of cases is small, series B does confirm series A in that there was little morbidity at thymectomy and the patients maintained their prethymectomy improvement post-thymectomy. The fewer complete remissions in series B are reflected in the pre- and post-thymectomy status.

TABLE 8B. *Thymectomy after prednisone — series B*

Characteristic	No.	
Sex		
Male	1	
Female	9	
Total	10	
Results in thymectomized patients		
Remission	4 (40%)	
Marked improvement	6 (60%)	
Morbidity		
None	9	
Severe	1	

	Range	Mean
Age (yr)	14–50	26.5
Months of prednisone prethymectomy	4–17	9.8

Discontinuation of Corticosteroids After Thymectomy

Our patients have been continued on maintenance prednisone after surgery for an arbitrary period of time. Currently available evidence indicates that improvement induced by thymectomy may not occur for as long as 10 years, and the best prediction is that approximately 50% of patients who improve achieve their maximum improvement within 2.5 years after surgery (41). We have therefore attempted to discontinue steroids approximately 1 year after thymectomy, and thus far four of our thirty patients in series A have been tapered off steroids completely after thymectomy and have sustained prolonged remission. The few patients in whom steroids were discontinued completely and who eventually relapsed did so at a mean of 4.1 months after discontinuation of prednisone. In most cases, when patients had relapsed off steroids, prednisone was reinstituted in an inpatient setting using the high-dose daily regimen described above. We found that with repeated courses of prednisone, higher maintenance doses were often required to sustain significant improvement.

Of the original 30 patients in series A, 25 were available for additional 2 years' follow-up between January 1974 and January 1976 (Table 9A). The percentage of patients maintaining marked improvement or complete remission remained the same (89 versus 88%). However, whereas 69% had been in complete remission in January 1974, only 32% had maintained that improvement permanently. Conversely, in January 1974, 20% exhibited marked improvement, but that group had enlarged to 56% 2 years later. The other categories had not changed.

In some cases there had been a transient worsening, with return to complete remission with slight increases in doses of prednisone.

In combining the results of the current status of series A and series B (Table 10), we found that patients continue to have an excellent result in marked improvement and complete remission (87.3%). However, we observed that the percentage of patients achieving and maintaining complete

TABLE 9. *Original classification and current status—series A (review 1/74)*

Classification	Patients	Unimproved	Moderate improvement	Marked improvement	Remission
1	1	0	0	0	1
2	5	0	0	4	1
3	5	0	1	2	2
4	8	0	0	5	3
5	6	1	1	3	1
Total	25	1	2	14	8
		(4%)	(8%)	(56%)	(32%)

Marked improvement/remission = 88%.

TABLE 10. *Combined series (1/76 and review 1/74)*

Classification	Patients	Unimproved	Moderate improvement	Marked improvement	Remission
1	3	0	0	2	1
2	8	0	0	6	2
3	9	0	2	2	5
4	20	0	1	14	5
5	7	1	2	3	1
Total	47	1	5	27	14
		(2.1%)	(10.6%)	(57.5%)	(29.8%)

Marked improvement/remission = 87.3%.

remission had decreased from the January 1974 series A figure of 69% to the January 1976 combined figure of 29.8%.

DISCUSSION

Administration of Corticosteroids

As our experience with oral corticosteroids in the treatment of myasthenia gravis has increased, we have identified several advantages in treating patients with high daily doses of prednisone early in therapy, and subsequently reducing dosage to much lower alternate-day maintenance levels: (a) rapid induction of remission or marked improvement in a high percentage of myasthenic patients within a predictable period of time; (b) rapid reduction of cholinesterase inhibitor requirements and simplification of medical regimens; (c) generally mild exacerbations occurring early in therapy when patients are closely supervised in a hospital setting; (d) early return to normal activities of daily living with outpatient management; and (e) reduced morbidity at thymectomy, usually performed 3 to 5 months after prednisone is begun, when the patient is in a state of maximal improvement.

Most of our patients experienced sustained improvement in the first 2 weeks of therapy and reached a state of maximal improvement within 5 months. During the early part of therapy, cholinesterase inhibitor requirements dropped dramatically so that simultaneous regulation of two antimyasthenic agents was, in most cases, obviated. That was particularly useful in those few patients whose poor cooperation complicated treatment. Those patients were best managed by rapid induction of remission or marked improvement while under our care in a hospital setting, with consequent simplification of drug administration for outpatient management.

Several investigators (16,17) have urged the use of high-dose AD prednisone at the beginning of steroid therapy. Some of the patients in those series experienced a significant increase in weakness on days when prednisone was omitted, requiring further dosage adjustments by the addition of significant amounts of prednisone on the "off" days. In one study in which cholinesterase inhibitors were withheld entirely and patients were treated with high-dose AD prednisone, pulmonary function studies revealed significant deterioration on the days when steroid was not administered (30). We have avoided those problems by giving prednisone on a daily basis from the beginning of therapy, later tapering to an individualized AD or low daily maintenance dose. Brunner et al. (31) and Jenkins (18) have reached similar conclusions concerning the initiation of steroids in myasthenia.

Comparison of exacerbation rates does not provide evidence supporting the use of high-dose AD over high-dose daily steroids. In a recent study evaluating many methods of steroid administration in a large number of myasthenic patients, Brunner et al. (31) reported an overall exacerbation rate of 80%, with the longest exacerbations occurring in patients beginning prednisone on a high-dose AD schedule. Comparisons with other series are difficult, considering the small numbers of patients in some reports and the failure to report incidence of exacerbations in others (30). Nevertheless, the rate for moderate and severe exacerbation in our series was 19%, similar to the rate observed by Jenkins (18) in patients begun on prednisone. Other major complications of prednisone therapy were infrequent during the early part of therapy and probably would not have been avoided by using high-dose AD steroids.

Seybold and Drachman (32) have advocated a regimen of low-dose AD steroids at the beginning of therapy, followed by a gradual increase in dosage over a period of months, in order to reduce the incidence of exacerbation and related complications. It is evident from the observations of McQuillen (33) and others (31) that the risk of exacerbation is not eliminated for patients treated in that fashion. In addition to the off-day phenomenon referred to above, the low-dose AD schedule leads to other problems in patient management. These arise from the need to continue adjustment of prednisone and significant doses of cholinesterase inhibitors over longer periods of time because of the delayed achievement of rapid resolution of the myasthenic weakness and the associated reduction of cholinesterase inhibitor requirements. In contrast, our current approach of rapid induction of clinical improvement with high-dose daily prednisone allows us to bring the patient to thymectomy in remission or marked improvement within a relatively short time after beginning steroid treatment.

Use of Cholinesterase Inhibitors

In some of our patients, clinical improvement took place early and very rapidly, sometimes within 1 or 2 days of beginning prednisone. This may reflect, in part, prednisone-facilitated release of acetylcholine at the neuromuscular junction, as demonstrated by Wilson et al. (34) in intracellular recordings from rat diaphragm. The hazard of cholinergic weakness in rapid responders was real, and close monitoring was required during the early phases of prednisone therapy when cholinesterase inhibitor requirements were decreasing. Although that represented a problem to physician and nursing staffs, the duration of intensive monitoring required was relatively brief, and evidence of cholinergic weakness appeared transiently in only two patients. We consider close, short-term monitoring of cholinesterase inhibitor requirements in patients beginning high-dose daily prednisone preferable to dealing with the acute decompensation that might have taken place in some of our patients had cholinesterase inhibitors been abruptly withdrawn before administration of steroids (30,35).

On the basis of twitch-tension studies of the rat diaphragm, Patten et al. (36) have shown that there may be an antagonistic effect between prednisone and cholinesterase inhibitors at the neuromuscular junction. The magnitude of that effect in humans is uncertain, and there was no evidence for it in our patient series. Nevertheless, the ever-present threat of cholinergic weakness supports the practical clinical concept of reducing cholinesterase inhibitors as much as possible in myasthenic patients on prednisone, particularly during the early part of therapy. Reduction of cholinesterase inhibitors is also important in terms of evaluating the effects of steroid therapy alone.

Exacerbation of myasthenic weakness may reflect, in part, an adverse interaction between cholinesterase inhibitors and prednisone. However, based on our experience as well as that of Engel et al. (30), we feel that complete discontinuation of cholinesterase inhibitors early in prednisone therapy is more hazardous than exacerbation itself. The 79% rate of cholinesterase inhibitor discontinuation in our group is comparable to the 84% reported by Engel et al. (30) in patients whose medications were initially withheld and then added as needed after prednisone had been started.

Thymectomy and Steroid Therapy

Thymectomy has been shown to be an effective mode of therapy in myasthenia gravis (26,37,38). Remission or significant improvement has been reported in a high percentage of nonthymomatous patients undergoing thymectomy, with all age groups in both sexes showing improved strength. Of patients exhibiting improvement after thymectomy, 50% achieve that improvement during the first 2.5 years (41), and 50% of all patients undergoing thymectomy exhibit some improvement within 5 years (28). It has been postulated that the delayed response may be because of the persistence of circulating thymic lymphocytes. The results in those with myasthenia and thymoma, although less impressive, are significant. Thymectomy, then, seems to be the form of therapy for myasthenia gravis that offers the best chance for sustained improvement with no long-term medication.

It has been proposed that delayed remission after thymectomy is related to the duration and severity of myasthenia before surgery, and that numbers of thymic germinal centers might be directly related to the duration of the illness (37). The incidence of malignant thymoma was higher in patients who underwent thymectomy 1 year or more after the onset of myasthenia. Those findings argue in favor of early thymectomy with related early improvement in myasthenic patients.

However, there are many cases on record of no favorable response to early thymectomy and of development of myasthenia after thymothymectomy. Further, the early use of corticosteroids is probably more effective than delayed treatment; early treatment with any agent is usually more effective than delayed treatment.

Accordingly, our current approach is to use both prednisone and thymectomy, when possible, in order to provide our myasthenic patients an opportunity for early, predictable, sustained clinical improvement with prednisone; low operative morbidity during surgery; gradual reduction or cessation of prednisone; and permanent remission at some time after thymectomy.

Present Concepts of Management – A Summary

The present series of 47 patients has led us to certain conclusions concerning the management and treatment of patients with myasthenia gravis (Table 11). The use of cholinesterase inhibitors alone is reserved for those patients with purely ocular myasthenia whose deficits can be corrected satisfactorily with those agents. Some of those with ocular involvement may be disabled. In light of our excellent results with that small group, as well as similar findings presented by Fischer and Schwartzman (39), patients with disabling or refractory ocular myasthenia should be considered for treatment with prednisone and thymectomy. All other patients with myasthenia are given a course of oral corticosteroids (prednisone) initially

TABLE 11. *Current management of myasthenia gravis at the University of Virginia Medical Center*

A. Cholinesterase inhibitors alone
   (when effective for case with mild, restricted involvement)
B. Long-term corticosteroids
   (in combination with cholinesterase inhibitors as needed)
C. Thymectomy
   (usually after maximal response to prednisone)
D. Attempted corticosteroid discontinuance
   (presently arbitrarily, 1–2 yr after thymectomy)
E. With relapse off steroids
   (corticosteroids reinstituted)
F. With repeated steroid failures consider:
   Thymic recurrence (40)
   Antimetabolites (29,42)
   Antithymocyte serum

at high doses, with subsequent tapering to maintenance, AD low dose therapy. Cholinesterase inhibitors are used as needed while the patient is receiving corticosteroids. We now anticipate that most patients will exhibit sustained improvement within the first 2 weeks, reaching maximal improvement at approximately 3 to 5 months. Myasthenic weakness may be exacerbated in the early phases of treatment. Such exacerbations commonly are mild, occur with a mean onset at 5 days, and have a mean duration of 5 days. Most patients have been able to tolerate an AD schedule of prednisone therapy when maintenance levels were achieved.

After the establishment of maximal improvement, patients have been considered for thymectomy. In our experience, the sternum-splitting procedure has been tolerated extremely well by patients exhibiting marked improvement or remission while on corticosteroids. Patients are continued on maintenance steroid therapy after surgery for an arbitrary period of time. On the basis of data relating to anticipated time of improvement after thymectomy, we have considered an attempt to discontinue steroids at approximately 1 year reasonable. Reduction of dosage during attempted steroid discontinuation should be safe if several months is allowed for observation of patient response after each reduction. Large rapid increases in steroids must be avoided.

Should the patient relapse after the medication has been discontinued, oral corticosteroids are reinstituted. Consideration may be given to the possibility of recurrent thymus (40) in patients who repeatedly fail to maintain a remission when steroids have been stopped. Tomography of the anterior mediastinum and mediastinoscopy may be the most useful means of searching for a recurrent thymus. Our experience has not permitted us to draw firm conclusions concerning how long high-dose daily steroids should be continued in patients who do not show a favorable response to therapy. Thymectomy remains the choice of treatment in that group. Finally, we have not had to resort to the use of antimetabolites or antithymocyte serum in myasthenics refractory to corticosteroids (29,42).

ACKNOWLEDGMENT

William H. Muller, M.D., Professor and Chairman, Department of Surgery, University of Virginia Medical Center, has performed all the postprednisone thymectomies in these series. His diligence and skill have undoubtedly contributed to the minor postoperative morbidity, and to what we hope will be favorable results. I wish to thank Ms. Page O'Neill for her editorial assistance.

REFERENCES

1. Simon, H. E. (1935): Myasthenia gravis: Effect of treatment with anterior pituitary extract. *J.A.M.A.*, 104 (23):2065–2066.

2. Shy, G. M., Brendler, S., Rabinovitch, R., et al., (1950): Effects of cortisone in certain neuromuscular disorders. *J.A.M.A.*, 155 (16): 1353–1358.
3. Millikan, C. H., and Eaton, L. M. (1951): Clinical evaluation of ACTH in myasthenia gravis. *Neurology (Minneap.)*, 1:145–152.
4. Grob, D., and Harvey, A. M. (1952): Effect of adrenocorticotrophic hormone (ACTH) and cortisone administration in patients with myasthenia gravis. *Johns Hopkins Med. J.*, 91:124–136.
5. Torda, C., and Wolff, H. G. (1951): Effects of administration of ACTH on patients with myasthenia gravis. *Arch. Neurol. Psychiatry*, 66:163–170.
6. Schlezinger, N. S. (1952): Present status of therapy in myasthenia gravis. *J.A.M.A.*, 148:508–513.
7. Freydberg, L. D. (1960): The place of corticotrophin in the treatment of myasthenia gravis. *Ann. Intern. Med.*, 52:108–118.
8. Von Reis, G., Liljestrand, A., and Matell, G. (1965): Results with ACTH and spironolactone in severe cases of myasthenia gravis. *Acta Neurol. Scand. Suppl. 13*, 41:463–471.
9. Grob, D., and Namba, T. (1966): Corticotropin in generalized myasthenia gravis. *JAMA*, 198:703–707.
10. Osserman, K. E., and Genkins, G. (1966): Studies in myasthenia gravis. *J.A.M.A.*, 198:669–702.
11. Graschenkov, N., and Perelman, L. B. (1966): Some aspects of myasthenia gravis. *Ann. N.Y. Acad. Sci.*, 135:399–408.
12. Genkins, G. (1966): Discussion of G. Glaser: Crisis, precrisis and drug resistance in myasthenia gravis. *Ann. N.Y. Acad. Sci.*, 135:348–349.
13. Griggs, R. C., McFarlin, D. E., and Engel, W. K. (1968): Severe occult juvenile myasthenia gravis responsive to long term corticosteroid therapy. *Trans. Am. Neurol. Assoc.*, 93:216–218.
14. Cape, C. A., and Utterback, R. A. (1969): Treatment of myasthenia gravis with ACTH: massive short term and maintenance treatment. *J. Neurol. Neurosurg. Psychiatry*, 32:290–296.
15. Cape, C. A., and Utterback, R. A. (1971): Long term maintenance ACTH therapy in myasthenia gravis. *Neurology (Minneap.)*, 21:411.
16. Kjaer, M. (1971): Myasthenia gravis and myasthenic syndromes treated with prednisone. *Acta Neurol. Scand.*, 47:464–474.
17. Warmolts, J. R., and Engel, W. K. (1972): Benefit from alternate day prednisone in myasthenia gravis. *N. Engl. J. Med.*, 286:17–20.
18. Jenkins, R. B. (1972): Treatment of myasthenia gravis with prednisone. *Lancet*, 1:765–767.
19. Brunner, N. G., Namba, T., and Grob, D. (1972): Corticosteroids in management of severe, generalized myasthenia gravis. *Neurology (Minneap.)*, 22:603–610.
20. Johns, T. R., Crowley, W. J., Miller, J. Q., et al. (1971): The syndrome of myasthenia and polymyositis with comments on therapy. *Ann N.Y. Acad. Sci.*, 183:64–71.
21. Allander, E. (1969): ACTH or corticosteroids? A critical review of results and possibilities in the treatment of severe chronic disease. *Acta Rheumatol. Scand.*, 15:227–296.
22. Johns, T. R., Mann, J. D., Joseph, B. S., et al. (1972): Long term administration of corticosteroids in myasthenia gravis. *Neurology (Minneap.)*, 22:400 (abs.).
23. Mann, J. D., Johns, T. R., Campa, J. F., and Muller, W. H.: (1976): Long-term prednisone followed by thymectomy in myasthenia gravis. *Ann. N.Y. Acad. Sci.*, 274:608–622.
24. Jones, V. R., Johns, T. R., Sanders, D. B., and Campa, J. F. (1976): Long term administration of corticosteroids in myasthenia gravis: Two years' additional experience. *Neurology (Minneap.)*, 26:372 (Abs.).
25. Mann, J. D., Johns, T. R., and Campa, J. F. (1976): Long-term administration of corticosteroids in myasthenia gravis. *Neurology*, 26:729–740.
26. Perlo, V. P., Arnason, B., Poskanzer, D., et al. (1971): The role of thymectomy in the treatment of myasthenia gravis. *Ann. N.Y. Acad. Sci.*, 183:308–315.
27. Fenichel, G. M. (1966): Muscle lesions in myasthenia gravis. *Ann. N.Y. Acad. Sci.*, 135:60–67.
28. Papatestas, A. E., Alpert, E. I., Osserman, K. E., et al. (1971): Studies in myasthenia gravis: Effects of thymectomy. *Am. J. Med.*, 50:465–474.
29. Mertens, H. G., Balzereit, F., and Leipert, M. (1969): The treatment of severe myasthenia gravis with immunosuppressive agents. *Eur. Neurol.*, 2:321–339.

30. Engel, W. K., Festoff, B. F., Patten, B. M., et al. (1974): N. I. H. Conference: Myasthenia Gravis. *Ann. Intern. Med.,* 81:225–246.
31. Brunner, N. G., Berger, C. L., Namba, T., and Grob, D. (1976): Corticotropin or corticosteroids in generalized myasthenia gravis: Comparative studies and role in management. *Ann. N. Y. Acad. Sci.,* 274:577–595.
32. Seybold, M. E., and Drachman, D. B. (1974): Gradually increasing doses of prednisone in myasthenia gravis. *N. Engl. J. Med.,* 290:81–84.
33. McQuillen, M. P. (1974): Prednisone schedule for myasthenia gravis, Letter to editor. *N. Engl. J. Med.,* 290:631.
34. Wilson, R., Ward, M. D., and Johns, T. R. (1974): Corticosteroids: a direct effect on the neuromuscular junction. *Neurology (Minneap.),* 24:1091–1095.
35. Kinney, A. B., and Blount, M. (1971): Systems approach to myasthenia gravis. *Nurs. Clin. North Am.,* 6:435–453.
36. Patten, B. M., Oliver, K. L., and Engel, W. K. (1974): Adverse interaction between steroid hormones and anticholinesterase drugs. *Neurology (Minneap.),* 24:442–448.
37. Genkins, G., Papatestas, A. E., Horowitz, S. H., et. al. (1975): Studies in myasthenia gravis: early thymectomy. *Am. J. Med.,* 58:517–524.
38. Genkins, G. (1975): For less gravis myasthenia. *Emergency Med.,* 7:173–179.
39. Fischer, K. C., and Schwartzman, R. J. (1974): Oral corticosteroids in the treatment of ocular myasthenia gravis. *Neurology (Minneap.),* 24:795–798.
40. Joseph, B. S., and Johns, T. R. (1973): Recurrence of nonneoplastic thymus after thymectomy for myasthenia gravis. *Neurology (Minneap.),* 23:109–116.
41. Perlo, V. P., Poskanza, D. C., Schwab, R. S., et al. (1966): Myasthenia gravis: Evaluation of treatment in 1355 patients. *Neurology (Minneap.),* 16:431–439.
42. Matell, G., Bergstrom, K., Franksson, C., et al. (1976): Effects of some immunosuppressive procedures on myasthenia gravis. *Ann. N.Y. Acad. Sci.,* 274:659–682.

Advances in Neurology, Vol. 17, edited by
R. C. Griggs and R. T. Moxley, III. Raven Press,
New York © 1977.

Disorders of Glycogen and Lipid Metabolism

Salvatore DiMauro and Abraham B. Eastwood

H. Houston Merritt Clinical Research Center for Muscular Dystrophy and Related Diseases, College of Physicians and Surgeons, Columbia University, and Neurological Institute, Presbyterian Hospital, New York, New York 10032

DISORDERS OF GLYCOGEN METABOLISM

Muscle is involved in five forms of glycogen storage disease: types 2, 3, 4, 5, and 7 (Table 1). In three of these (types 2, 5, and 7), muscle symptoms are the sole or predominant manifestation of the disease; in the other two forms (types 3 and 4) the clinical picture is dominated by liver dysfunction.

Type 5 (McArdle Disease)

McArdle disease is owing to a defect of muscle phosphorylase. The metabolic block was elegantly demonstrated in 1951 by Brian McArdle (1), although the enzyme defect was not recognized until 8 years later (2,3). About 50 cases have been reported, with a definite prevalence in men (approximately 4:1). The clinical picture is characterized by exercise intolerance; soon after starting vigorous exercise, the patients experience muscle stiffness and ache. Most patients learn what their limits are, and, within that framework, they can enjoy a nearly normal life. However, when they exceed their limits, they experience painful cramps. In contrast to the interference pattern generated by volitional movement, the shortening of these cramps is electrically silent and, therefore, fits the physiological definition of "contracture" (4). If exercise is prolonged further, contracture may be followed by muscle necrosis and myoglobinuria. Renal shutdown has been reported as a complication of myoglobinuria in five patients with this disease (5,6). After uncomplicated episodes of myoglobinuria, there is complete functional recovery. Symptoms and signs of McArdle disease are rarely a problem in childhood. Permanent myopathy with weakness was reported as a late consequence in two cases (3,7), and it characterized the clinical picture in a family with late-onset form of the disease (8).

Because of the block of glycogenolysis, venous lactate fails to rise after ischemic exercise as it does in normal individuals (19), and glycogen of normal structure accumulates in the sarcoplasm, particularly under the sarcolemma (9,10).

Most patients with McArdle disease experience a characteristic "second

TABLE 1. *Glycogen storage disease*

Type (eponym)	Affected tissues	Clinical picture	Glycogen structure	Enzyme defect
1. (Von Gierke)	Liver, kidney	Hepatomegaly, growth retardation, hypoglycemia, ketosis, hyperlipemia, hyperlactacidemia	Normal	Glucose-6-phosphatase
2. Infancy (Pompe)	All tissues	Cardiomegaly, extreme weakness; death within first year of life	Normal	Acid (lysosomal) α-1,4- and α-1,6-glucosidase
Childhood	Skel. muscle, liver	Myopathy simulating Duchenne muscular dystrophy	Normal (?)	
Adult	Skel. muscle, liver	Myopathy simulating limbgirdle muscular dystrophy or polymyositis	Normal (?)	
3. (Cori-Forbes)	Liver, muscle, RBC fibroblasts	Hepatomegaly, fasting hypoglycemia. weakness	Phosphorylase-limit dextrin	Debrancher system
4. (Andersen)	Liver, kidney, WBC, heart, skel. muscle, spinal cord, spleen	Hepatosplenomegaly, cirrhosis of liver	Longer peripheral chains, fewer branching points	Branching enzyme
5. (McArdle)	Skel. muscle	Cramps after exertion, myoglobinuria	Normal	Muscle phosphorylase
6. (Hers)	Liver, WBC	Hepatomegaly, hypoglycemia, acidosis	Normal	Liver phosphorylase
7. (Tarui)	Skel. muscle	Cramps after exertion, myoglobinuria	Normal	Muscle phosphofructokinase
8. (Hug)	Liver	Asymptomatic hepatomegaly	Normal	Liver dephosphophosphorylase kinase

wind" phenomenon. If they rest briefly when muscles ache or feel stiff during exercise, they can resume physical activity more vigorously and for a longer period. Two factors apparently contribute to this phenomenon: increased mobilization of free fatty acids, providing muscle with alternative fuel, and increased blood flow to the exercising muscles (11,12).

Both contracture and myoglobinuria in McArdle disease are attributed to a critical shortage of ATP during strenuous exercise, when most of the energy for normal muscle contraction derives from glycogen breakdown and glycolysis. A defect of ATP could impair muscle relaxation by inhibiting the energy-dependent calcium uptake of the sarcoplasmic reticulum: more severe or prolonged depletion of ATP could alter the integrity of cell membranes and cause muscle necrosis. This pathogenetic mechanism, however, has not been verified experimentally, and in one study (13) the concentration of ATP did not change, although creatine phosphate, creatine, and inorganic phosphate were appropriately altered in muscle taken before and during contracture in two patients. Lack of change in ATP content of whole-muscle homogenates in these experiments might have obscured a local defect in the ATP of sarcoplasmic reticulum. A localized defect of ATP may explain the observation that muscle fibers stripped of their sarcolemma ("skinned fibers") develop prolonged contractures after repetitive applications of calcium (14), suggesting functional impairment of sarcoplasmic reticulum calcium uptake. Structural damage of sarcoplasmic reticulum membranes probably does not accompany contractures because no defect of calcium uptake or APTase was found in sarcoplasmic reticulum fractions isolated from contractured muscle in Brody's (15) and in our own laboratory (Fig. 1).

McArdle disease is not a single genetic entity. In most cases the mode of transmission appears to be autosomal recessive, but autosomal dominant inheritance was observed in one family (16), and a genetic basis for the striking prevalence of male patients remains to be explained. A more striking example of genetic heterogeneity is the demonstration in some patients that no enzyme protein is detectable by immunological methods (5,9,17), whereas in others enzyme protein seems to be present, although inactive or only

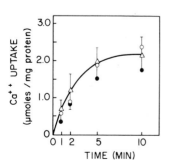

FIG. 1. Calcium uptake by sarcoplasmic reticulum (SR) vesicles isolated from normal muscle biopsies (*triangles; bars* represent SD), and from the gastrocnemius muscle of a patient with McArdle disease, before (*open circles*) and during (*full circles*) contracture induced by ischemic exercise. SR vesicles were isolated between 8,000 and 30,000 g for 60 min and calcium uptake was measured with ^{45}Ca by a Millipore filtration method (106,107).

partially active (5,17,18). Because immunological evaluation has not been carried out in all patients, it is not known which type is more common. Another genetic puzzle was the histochemical demonstration of phosphorylase activity in regenerating and cultured muscle fibers from three patients with McArdle disease (19).

Because symptoms in McArdle disease are intermittent and transitory, there is less need for effective therapy than in other progressively crippling metabolic disorders. However, because of the severe limitation of exercise in otherwise healthy people and the risk of myoglobinuria, several therapeutic measures have been tried. Initial attempts to bypass the metabolic block and provide muscle with glycolytic fuels were based on the observation that the working capacity of patients with McArdle disease could be increased by intravenous infusions of glucose or by the hyperglycemic effect of glucagon (3,20). The demonstration that infusions of fructose (21) were similarly beneficial evoked varying interpretations; some thought that fructose could be used directly by muscle, whereas others favored the view that fructose was converted in the liver to lactate or glucose (22–24). However, frequent ingestion of sugars was not always therapeutically effective (9,25) and might cause undesirable weight gain, whereas repeated injections of glucagon are objectionable for prolonged treatment. As an alternative, Rowland and Layzer (*unpublished observations*) used a hypoglycemic agent (phenformin) believed to promote peripheral utilization of glucose and a hyperglycemic agent (diazoxide) that has complex actions, including inhibition of insulin release. In one patient, phenformin (250 mg daily for 5 days) had no effect on blood sugar and caused no symptomatic relief. Various doses of diazoxide (1,200 mg daily for 5 days; 400 mg daily for a week) were administered to two patients. Blood sugars tended to be higher than normal, but there was no improvement in exercise tolerance and both patients complained of headache and edema (L. P. Rowland and R. B. Layzer, unpublished observations). Other potential therapeutic approaches remain to be evaluated. One, suggested by the studies of the second wind phenomenon, would be to raise the concentration of serum free fatty acids and ketone bodies by diet or drugs (e.g., sublingual isoproterenol).

Type 7 (Tarui Disease)

Tarui disease is owing to a defect of muscle phosphofructokinase (PFK). Six cases have been reported (26–29), and we have recently studied a seventh. In six, the clinical picture — exercise intolerance, contractures, and myoglobinuria — was virtually identical to that of McArdle disease. In glycogenosis type 7, as in McArdle disease, there is a second wind phenomenon and ischemic exercise results in no venous lactate response. Muscle morphology and the degree of glycogen accumulation are also similar in the two diseases. Differential diagnosis may be suggested by erythrocyte studies because a partial defect of the red blood cell enzyme has been found in all cases of muscle PFK deficiency. The erythrocyte abnormality results in a mild hemolytic tendency and is attributed to an alteration of the subunit composition of the erythrocyte enzyme. In normal red blood cells PFK is composed of both muscle-type (M) and red blood cell–type (R) subunits (30–32), and in patients the M subunits are lacking. In PFK-deficient muscle, hexose phosphate intermediates that precede the metabolic block — fructose-6-phosphate, and, particularly, glucose-6-phosphate — accumulate excessively (26,27,33). The genetic transmission of muscle PFK deficiency appears to be autosomal recessive, on the basis of the pedigree of Tarui's original family (26) and because PFK activity was decreased in the red blood cells of both parents of Layzer's patient (27). One of the six reported patients was atypical in many respects (28). Myopathic weakness started in adolescence, but without contracture and pigmenturia, and the muscle biopsy showed degenerative changes without glycogen storage. PFK activity was decreased in both muscle (undetectable in one biopsy, but 19% of normal in another) and erythrocytes, and venous lactate did not increase after ischemic exercise. Similar clinical disorder was present in three other members of the family in three subsequent generations, suggesting autosomal dominant inheritance.

No therapy has been attempted so far in muscle phosphofructokinase deficiency. Because the metabolic block affects glycolysis rather than glycogenolysis, there is no rationale for the administration of glucose or hyperglycemic agents in this condition. However, dietary regimens or drugs causing increased levels of plasma fatty acids and ketone bodies might be beneficial.

Type 3 (Cori-Forbes' Disease)

Cori-Forbes' disease is owing to a defect of debrancher enzyme. The disorder is dominated by liver involvement, with hepatomegaly, growth retardation, hypoglycemia, and seizures. For unknown reasons, all symptoms and signs tend to disappear at puberty. Myopathy is rarely a major problem. In two patients a progressive myopathy of late onset was described (34,35), and in two others (36,37) intolerance to exercise was the main complaint but without contractures or myoglobinuria. It is surprising that exercise intolerance is not more common in these patients since the metabolic block is only one step removed from that of phosphorylase deficiency. One possible explanation for this apparent protection is that some glucose-1-phosphate can be formed from the peripheral chains of glycogen through the action of phosphorylase. However, this source of energy should be limited, because the polysaccharide that accumulates in muscle has abnormally short peripheral chains (38–40). This is reflected functionally by the failure of venous lactate to rise after ischemic exercise in all four

TABLE 2. *Anaerobic glycolysis in muscle homogenates*

Substrate	Controls (8)	Phosphorylase deficiency	Debrancher deficiency	Phosphofructokinase deficiency[a]
None	53 ± 19	10	3	0
0.15% Glycogen	121 ± 29	13	54	0

Anaerobic glycolysis was measured by the method of Layzer et al. (27) and is expressed as μmoles lactate per gram fresh tissue. Control values ± SD.
[a] Data from Layzer et al. (27).

reported patients with myopathy (34–37). Similarly, virtually no lactate was produced from endogenous polysaccharide in anaerobic glycolysis of muscle homogenate from a 10-year-old patient without muscle symptoms (Table 2). The lack of symptomatic exercise intolerance in most patients with type 3 disease may also be due, in part at least, to the chronically increased plasma content of fatty acids and ketones (41,42), a situation similar to that realized during the second wind phenomenon in glycogenosis types 5 and 7.

The debranching of a phosphorylase-limit dextrin requires two sequential enzymatic reactions: transfer of a maltotriosyl unit from a donor to an acceptor chain of the glycogen molecule, followed by the hydrolysis of the α-1,6-glucosidic link. Using appropriate substrates, one can assay the overall debrancher reaction or analyze the transferase and α-1,6-glucosidase activities separately (43). Employing four different assays in liver and muscle biopsies, Van Hoof and Hers (39) studied 45 clinically indistinguishable patients, none with clinical myopathy. They separated these patients into six subgroups, the first example of genetic heterogeneity in glycogen storage disease. The largest group, approximately 75% of the cases, showed very low activity with all four assays and in both tissues. In the other 11 patients, only some of the reactions were negative in one or both tissues. In rabbit muscle and liver both transferase and glucosidase activities seem to be properties of a single protein (44–46). If this is also true for human tissues, the various subgroups of glycogenosis type 3 are likely to be allelic disorders, probably because of different point mutations, as originally suggested by Van Hoof and Hers (39). Inheritance in all forms appears to be autosomal recessive. Therapy is limited to controlling hypoglycemia.

Type 4 (Andersen's Disease)

Caused by a defect of the brancher enzyme, Andersen's disease is a rapidly progressive disease of early childhood (47,48). The clinical picture is dominated by liver disorder, with hepatosplenomegaly, progressive cirrhosis, and, ultimately, fatal hepatic failure. The accumulated polysaccharide has abnormally long outer chains and relatively few branching points (49,50). On the basis of morphological (47,48) and biochemical (51–53) studies, glycogenosis type 4 appears to be a generalized disorder, although the degree of involvement of different tissues varies from case to case. In one patient with severe muscle weakness and atrophy (54) there were characteristic ultrastructural lesions in skeletal muscle: intermyofibrillar, non-membrane-bound deposits of branched filaments and osmiophilic granules, similar to those observed in liver, and presumably representing accumulations of abnormal polysaccharide. In muscle, as in liver, normal glycogen particles were present together with abnormal storage material (54). The presence of some degree of branching in the abnormal polysaccharide has been attributed to a reverse action of the debrancher enzyme (55), but the origin of morphologically normal glycogen particles in both liver and muscle remains unexplained. Transmission is autosomal recessive. No therapy is available.

Type 2 (Pompe Disease)

A different picture is offered by glycogenosis type 2, owing to acid maltase deficiency (Table 1). In the infantile, generalized form, the disease is rapidly progressive and death occurs before age 1 year. There is massive accumulation of glycogen in the heart, skeletal muscle, and the central (56–58) and peripheral (57–59) nervous systems. The clinical disorder is characterized by profound weakness (attributable to both motor neuron and muscle disease), cardiomegaly with heart failure, and, in some cases, macroglossia. It is probably appropriate to restrict the eponym Pompe disease to infantile cases, but recently a more benign form of acid maltase deficiency (AMD) has been recognized. Symptoms begin later, in childhood (60–68) or adult life (67–70), and, with very few exceptions (62,63), they are limited to skeletal muscle, simulating muscle dystrophy or polymyositis, with no cardiac or neuronal disorder. Weakness, generally of trunk and proximal limb muscles, is slowly progressive, but involvement of respiratory muscles in approximately 50% of cases (68,71) may cause severe ventilatory insufficiency. Serum creatine phosphokinase is consistently elevated, and electromyography characteristically shows myotonic discharges in the absence of clinical myotonia, for reasons still not known. The histopathological features are those of a vacuolar myopathy and glycogen is variably increased, but this may escape routine histological observation. It is, therefore, important to consider late-onset AMD in the differential diagnosis of myopathic syndromes. We found that daily urinary excretion of acid maltase is markedly reduced in patients and heterozygotes with late-onset AMD (72). This noninvasive urinary assay represents an alternative to muscle biopsy as a tool in diagnosis and genetic counseling.

In 1963 Hers (73) described the absence of acid maltase in tissues of patients with the generalized form of the disease and formulated the general concept of "inborn lysosomal diseases" (74,75). In glycogenosis type 2, this concept is based on a phenomenon called "autophagy" (74,75), a normal mechanism of cellular renewal, in which portions of the cytoplasm are surrounded by a membrane and physically isolated from the rest of the cell within an "autophagic vacuole" or "autophagosome" (75). When merged with a primary lysosome containing several acid hydrolases, the autophagic vacuole is transformed into a "digestive vacuole" or "autolysosome" (75). Once all the components of the sequestered cytoplasm have been digested by appropriate hydrolases, small molecules pass through the lysosomal membrane and are reused by the cell, while undigested material is retained within "residual" or "dense bodies." In glycogenosis type 2, the absence of acid maltase, which has both α-1,4- and α-1,6-glucosidase activities and is therefore capable of digesting glycogen to glucose (76), results in continuous accumulation of undigested glycogen within lysosomes until the cell is literally engorged with these "glycogenosomes." Although there is little doubt that this is the basic pathogenetic mechanism in type 2 glycogenosis, some observations remain difficult to explain. One question that reflects our ignorance of the functional role of lysosomal glycogen metabolism in normal muscle is why this tissue, which normally appears to have few lysosomes, is so severely affected. A more important question is why such a large proportion of the accumulated glycogen is not intralysosomal, but free in the cytoplasm, a phenomenon particularly apparent in muscle and in the infantile form of the disease (Fig. 2). Further, irrespective of the mechanism by which it accumulates, why is this free glycogen not degraded through the normal glycogenolytic pathways of the cytoplasm?

Another puzzling question regards the biochemical basis for the clinical differences between infantile and late-onset AMD. Angelini and A. G. Engel drew attention to neutral maltase, an enzyme apparently bound to the sarcoplasmic reticulum (77) and whose functional role is obscure. In a comparative study (78), they found decreased neutral maltase activity in several tissues from infantile, but not late-onset AMD, and suggested that the normal complement of neutral enzyme in late-onset AMD may partially compensate for the lack of acid maltase.

Dreyfus et al. (79,80) reported electrophoretic studies suggesting the presence of abnormal isozymes of acid maltase in these conditions. We determined acid maltase activity by a very sensitive fluorometric assay, using the artificial substrate 4-methylumbelliferyl-α-D-glucoside, and found some residual activity (3 to 12% of normal) in muscle from 15 cases with late-onset AMD but no enzyme activity in 3 infantile cases (71). The residual acid maltase in late-onset AMD muscle was electrophoretically and kinetically normal, and neutral maltase activity was decreased only in 1 of the 3 infantile cases (71).

In leukocytes acid maltase activity is either normal (65,81) or only partially reduced (71,78,82) in late-onset AMD cases, but it is undetectable in the infantile form (76).

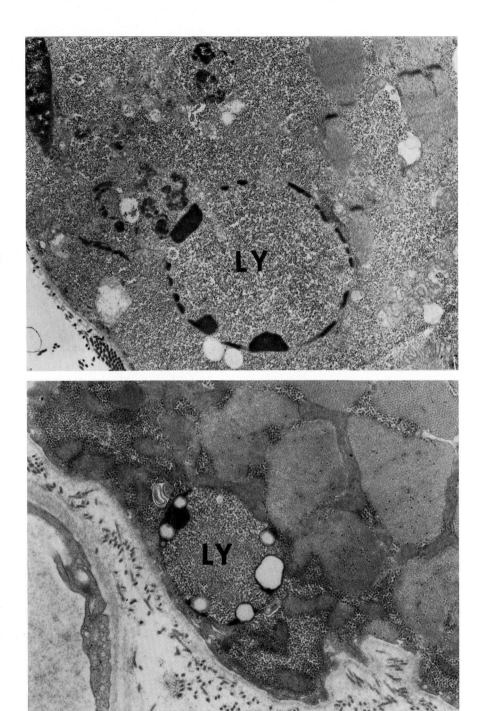

FIG. 2. Top: Acid maltase deficiency, infantile form. In this longitudinal section, a lyso-some (Ly) containing glycogen and electron-opaque material is surrounded by abundant free glycogen. Myofibrils are sparse and distended by glycogen accumulation.

Bottom: Acid maltase deficiency, adult form. In this cross section, a lysosome (Ly) containing glycogen, lipid, and electron-opaque material is present near the sarcolemma. Free glycogen is increased, but myofibrils are not disrupted.

These observations and the fact that there have been no families with both infantile and late-onset forms suggest that these are two different genetic disorders affecting the same enzyme, another example of genetic heterogeneity.

Several different therapeutic strategies have been tried, particularly in the infantile form, including labilization of lysosomes, stimulation of glycogenolysis, and enzyme replacement. Vitamin A, progesterone, and hyperbaric oxygen (83) are among the "lysosome-labilizing" agents used to make the trapped glycogen available to cytoplasmic enzymes. These agents were clinically ineffective, and the rationale of this approach may be questionable in infantile AMD, where there is much free glycogen in addition to the lysosomal accumulation. Stimulation of glycogenolysis by administration of epinephrine resulted in a decrease of cytoplasmic but not intralysosomal glycogen in the liver (83), demonstrating that extralysosomal glycogen breakdown is normal. Administration of α-glucosidase prepared from *Aspergillus niger* (83,84) or human placenta (85) was attempted in a few cases. In one patient administered enzyme could be detected in a liver biopsy, and intralysosomal glycogen decreased significantly in this tissue (83). In no case, however, did the exogenous enzyme enter skeletal or heart muscle, and the clinical course was not changed by this treatment. In patients with late-onset AMD, ketogenic diet with or without administration of epinephrine has been suggested to retard glycogen accumulation in muscle.

DISORDERS OF LIPID METABOLISM

Although a great amount of work has been done in the past 25 years on glycogen metabolism of muscle and its disorders, relatively little clinical attention has been directed to lipid metabolism. Yet lipid is at least as important as glycogen as a source of energy for muscle contraction. Glycogen breakdown is ideally suited for the rapid provision of energy in "fight or flee" situations or other strenuous effort, but muscle glycogenolysis cannot sustain exercise for more than a few minutes (86). The energy for prolonged exercise derives mainly from lipid metabolism, largely an intramitochondrial process. Once free fatty acids, which are the circulating lipid "currency," enter the cell, they are activated to fatty acyl-CoA at the expense of ATP by fatty acyl-CoA synthetase. Long-chain fatty acyl residues are then transferred from coenzyme A to carnitine (γ-trimethylamino-β-hydroxybutyrate) by carnitine palmityltransferase I(CPT I), located on the outer face of the inner mitochondrial membrane (86). Carnitine is the obligatory carrier of long-chain fatty acids across the mitochondrial barrier. Inside the mitochondria, a second carnitine palmityltransferase (CPT II), bound to the inner face of the inner mitochondrial membrane (87), catalyzes the reverse reaction, reconverting fatty acyl carnitine to fatty acyl-CoA. Inside the mitochondria, the fatty acyl-CoA undergoes β-oxidation. In this stepwise process, one acetyl-CoA is formed at each step and is oxidized in the Kreb's cycle.

Two disorders of muscle lipid metabolism have been identified, one characterized clinically by recurrent myoglobinuria, the other by progressive weakness.

In 1973 we studied two brothers, 33 and 29 years old, with recurrent myoglobinuria beginning around puberty (88,89). In contrast to muscle phosphorylase and phosphofructokinase deficiency, there was no history of cramps or intolerance to strenuous exercise of short duration. Myoglobinuria usually followed sustained exercise—mountain hiking, unloading lumber, painting walls—of approximately 2-hr duration. Another distinctive feature was that fasting seemed to precipitate myoglobinuria, and the most severe attacks in both patients were caused by a combination of prolonged exercise and not eating (89). Glycogen storage disease was excluded by the normal content of glycogen and the normal activities of phosphorylase and phosphofructokinase in muscle biopsies. Muscle morphology was normal. The concentration of carnitine was slightly increased, and the activities of palmityl CoA synthetase and carnitine acetyltransferase were normal.

Muscle carnitine palmityltransferase activity, measured by three different methods in both crude extracts and isolated mitochondria, varied from undetectable to 20% of normal in both patients. The enzyme defect was also expressed in leukocytes, and intermediate values were found in white blood cells from the asymptomatic, presumably heterozygote mother (Fig. 3). These findings suggest autosomal recessive inheritance, although in the absence of data from the father, an X-linked mode of transmission cannot be excluded.

Plasma free fatty acids were normal in both patients on a balanced diet,

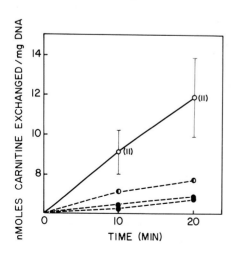

FIG. 3. Carnitine palmityltransferase activity ($\pm$ SD) in leukocytes of 11 adult controls (6 men, 5 women), two brothers with muscle CPT deficiency (*full circles*), and their asymptomatic mother (*half-shaded circles*). CPT activity was measured by the isotope-exchange method (108) in 0.1-ml suspensions of leukocytes. Leukocytes were isolated by the method of Mellman and Tedesco (109) and resuspended in 0.5 to 1.0 ml of 0.15 M KCl–50 mM Tris, pH 7.5, by manual homogenization with a Teflon pestle. DNA was measured by the method of Richards (110).

but cholesterol was slightly increased, and triglycerides were two to three times higher than normal. After a 72-hr fast without exercise, one patient showed a sharp increase of serum creatine phosphokinase, and traces of myoglobin were detected in plasma and urine (89). In contrast to the pattern in normal individuals, ketone bodies did not rise in plasma until the third day of fasting, but ketones appeared promptly after an oral meal of medium-chain triglycerides, suggesting that the enzyme defect may involve the liver as well as muscle and leukocytes.

Impairment of long-chain fatty acid utilization by muscle and perhaps by liver may account for the increased plasma content of free fatty acids and secondary hypertriglyceridemia. During normal activity and on a normal diet, these patients can use muscle glycogen and blood glucose: normal activity and moderate or short exercise are well tolerated. After prolonged exercise, however, especially with some degree of fasting, muscle and liver glycogen stores are probably depleted, and because of the defect of CPT, long-chain fatty acids cannot enter muscle mitochondria. The decreased concentration of plasma ketone bodies may further aggravate this shortage of fuel for muscle contraction. In this disorder, as in glycogenosis types 5 and 7, myoglobinuria is attributed to acute muscle necrosis related to a defect of ATP, due in this case to a block of lipid rather than glycogen metabolism, but this has not been proven.

A similar disorder was described in 1970 by W. K. Engel et al. (90) in identical twin girls, 18 years old, with intermittent "cramps" and myoglobinuria related to exercise but also induced by fasting or high-fat diet. Metabolic studies suggested a defect in the utilization of long-chain fatty acids by skeletal muscle. Long-chain fatty acyl-CoA synthetase activity was normal in muscle biopsies, and a defect of muscle CPT was posulated. However, a few important differences between these patients and the brothers with CPT deficiency suggest that the two disorders may not be owing to the same enzyme defect. There was no hypertriglyceridemia in the twins, fat tolerance was normal, ketone production was totally lacking during fasting, and lipid accumulation was seen in muscle.

In 1972 A. G. Engel and Siekert (91) described a 19-year-old woman with severe, generalized weakness and a muscle biopsy characterized by great accumulation of lipid droplets, particularly in type 1 fibers, a true "lipid storage myopathy." The following year A. G. Engel and Angelini (92) found that *"in vitro"* utilization of long-chain fatty acids by a homogenate of the patient's muscle was defective in the absence of exogenous carnitine, but it became normal after addition of carnitine to the incubation mixture. This led them to measure the concentration of carnitine; values ranging from 8 to 31% of normal were found in five different muscle biopsies. Lipid analysis showed a marked increase of muscle tri- and diglycerides (93). Serum contents of triglycerides, cholesterol, and free fatty acids were normal, and ketone bodies were formed normally during fasting, suggesting that liver lipid metabolism was not impaired.

Therapy with corticosteroids (prednisone, 60 mg/day, gradually tapered to a maintenance dose of 35 mg/day), initiated before the defect of muscle carnitine had been discovered, was followed by dramatic improvement (91–93). Replacement therapy with oral carnitine (4000 mg DL-carnitine daily) was attempted when serum carnitine concentration was found to be slightly lower than normal (93). After a year of carnitine administration (together with prednisone and low-fat diet), the clinical condition of the patient had not further improved, and the concentration of carnitine in skeletal muscle was unchanged.

Carnitine is synthesized exclusively or predominantly in the liver and is "exported" through the blood to other tissues. The much higher concentration of carnitine in muscle than in plasma implies that the uptake of carnitine depends on an active transport mechanism or may be facilitated by specific membrane or intracellular receptors (93).

In Engel and Angelini's case, low muscle carnitine content after 1 year of replacement therapy (which reestablished normal blood levels of carnitine) suggested a defect of the muscle uptake mechanism. Alternatively, the rate of carnitine synthesis in the liver might be sufficient to maintain normal liver concentration, but it is not enough to replenish other tissues, particularly skeletal muscle (93).

Six other cases with carnitine deficiency of muscle have been reported (94–98) (Table 3). In all of these, weakness was prominent, serum enzymes were elevated, and muscle disease was characterized by lipid storage, especially in type-1 fibers. However, there was considerable variability in clinical presentation, age of onset, degree of weakness, and involvement of tissues other than muscle, suggesting that "carnitine deficiency" is a syndrome possibly owing to several different specific biochemical abnormalities. The patient of Karpati et al. (95) had two episodes of acute hepatic encephalopathy at ages 3 and 9, before progressive muscle weakness developed when the child was 11. Carnitine concentration was much decreased in both liver and plasma, suggesting a defect of carnitine synthesis. This hypothesis, however, is difficult to reconcile with the observation that replacement therapy with oral carnitine (DL-form, 2 g/day) for 5 months resulted in normal plasma carnitine levels and was accompanied by dramatic clinical improvement, although liver carnitine remained low. To explain all the findings in this case, investigators postulated a combined defect of carnitine synthesis in the liver and impaired uptake or storage in skeletal muscle (95). Excessive accumulation of lipid droplets was observed in leukocytes and Schwann cells in one patient (94), who also had electromyographic signs of peripheral nerve involvement. Cardiac involvement was suggested in one case (96).

TABLE 3. *The syndrome of carnitine deficiency*

Case No. (ref.)	Sex	Age at onset	Clinical picture	Tissues affected	Serum carnitine	Therapy
1. Engel and Siekert (91)	F	Childhood	Generalized weakness, worsening at age 18; respiratory muscles involved	Muscle	Slightly decreased	Prednisone, carnitine
2. Markesbery et al. (94)	F	38 yr	Generalized weakness	Muscle, nerve, WBC	Normal	—
3. VanDyke et al. (96)	M	18 mo	Progressive weakness (proximal > distal)	Muscle	Normal	Prednisone
4. Angelini et al. (98)	F	7 yr	Weakness of proximal limb and trunk muscles	Muscle	Normal	Carnitine
5. Smyth et al. (97)	M	5 yr	Generalized weakness; growth failure, hearing loss; lactic acidosis	Muscle, WBC	?	—
6. Karpati et al. (95)	M	Infancy	Weakness, worsening at age 11; 2 episodes of acute hepatic encephalopathy (ages 3 and 9)	Muscle, liver	Low	Carnitine

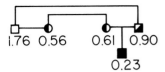

FIG. 4. Pedigree of a patient with muscle carnitine deficiency (96). Numbers represent muscle carnitine concentrations in μmoles/g tissue. Normal values (26 controls): 2.64 $\pm$ 0.69 (range: 1.53 to 4.10).

The patient of Smyth et al. (97), an 11-year-old boy, had a unique clinical picture, characterized by the association of progressive muscle weakness and CNS involvement (calcification of basal ganglia, increased CSF protein concentration, high-tone hearing loss), growth retardation, episodic vomiting, exertional dyspnea, and high serum levels of lactate, pyruvate, and alanine. Liver function was normal and serum carnitine was not measured.

Although the mechanism of action is not clear, replacement therapy with oral carnitine was very effective in two patients (95,98) and should be tried in all cases before resorting to steroids.

Genetic transmission was demonstrated only in the family reported by VanDyke et al. (96). Lower-than-normal concentrations of carnitine were found in muscle biopsies from both parents and a maternal aunt of the propositus (Fig. 4), suggesting autosomal recessive inheritance. However, carnitine deficiency may be acquired in some cases. In experimental animals, decreased concentrations of carnitine were found in the heart after administration of diphtheria toxin (99), in heart and liver after a choline-deficient diet (100), and in heart and skeletal muscle after a lysine-deficient diet (101).

All cases of carnitine deficiency reported so far showed increased lipid droplets in muscle, but not all cases of lipid storage myopathy are owing to carnitine deficiency. Increased numbers of lipid droplets were seen in muscle in a patient with an intermittent movement disorder owing to pyruvate dehydrogenase deficiency (102), in the twin girls with recurrent myoglobinuria and postulated CPT deficiency (90), and in a patient with congenital muscle weakness of unknown etiology (103). Recently, massive lipid storage was seen in several tissues, including muscle, and in cultured skin fibroblasts from a patient with congenital ichthyosis as the sole clinical disorder (104). Carnitine concentration was not measured in muscle but was normal in plasma, and addition of L-carnitine to the fibroblasts in culture did not correct the metabolic defect. We have seen a similar patient with congenital ichthyosis, chronic diarrhea, and proximal myopathic weakness who also had generalized lipid storage, particularly evident in muscle and fibroblasts in culture, but normal muscle carnitine concentration (105).

As far as skeletal muscle is concerned, the area of lipid metabolism and its disorders is largely uncharted territory. As was the case with glycogen storage disease, it is likely that a number of biochemically distinct lipid storage diseases affecting muscle will be recognized in the near future.

ACKNOWLEDGMENTS

We thank Dr. Lewis P. Rowland for reviewing the manuscript. This study was supported by Clinical Center Grants from the National Institute of Neurological and Communicative Disorders and Stroke (NS-117766) and the Muscular Dystrophy Association.

REFERENCES

1. McArdle, B. (1951): Myopathy due to a defect in muscle glycogen breakdown. *Clin. Sci.,* 10:13–33.
2. Mommaerts, W. F. H. M., Illingworth, B., Pearson, C. M., Guillory, R. J., and Seraydarian, K. (1959): A functional disorder of muscle associated with the absence of phosphorylase. *Proc. Natl. Acad. Sci. U.S.A.,* 45:791–797.
3. Schmid, R., and Mahler, R. (1959): Chronic progressive myopathy with myoglobinuria: Demonstration of a glycogenolytic defect in the muscle. *J. Clin. Invest.,* 38:2044–2058.
4. Layzer, R. B., and Rowland, L. P. (1971): Cramps. *N. Engl. J. Med.,* 285:31–30.
5. Grünfeld, J. P., Ganeval, D., Chanard, J., Fardeau, M., and Dreyfus, J. C. (1972): Acute renal failure in McArdle's disease. *N. Engl. J. Med.,* 286:1237–1241.
6. Bank, W. J., DiMauro, S., and Rowland, L. P. (1972): Renal failure in McArdle's disease. *N. Engl. J. Med.,* 287:1102.
7. Schmid, R., and Hammaker, L. (1961): Hereditary absence of muscle phosphorylase (McArdle's syndrome). *N. Engl. J. Med.,* 264:223–225.
8. Engel, W. K., Eyerman, E. L., and Williams, H. E. (1963): Late-onset type of skeletal-muscle phosphorylase deficiency. *N. Engl. J. Med.,* 268:135–137.
9. Rowland, L. P., Fahn, S., and Schotland, D. L. (1963): McArdle's disease. *Arch. Neurol.,* 9:325–342.
10. Schotland, D. L., Spiro, D., Rowland, L. P., and Carmel, P. (1965): Ultrastructural studies of muscle in McArdle's disease. *J. Neuropathol. Exp. Neurol.,* 24:629–644.
11. Porte, D., Crawford, D. W., Jennings, D. B., Aber, C., and McIlroy, M. B. (1966): Cardiovascular and metabolic responses to exercise in a patient with McArdle's syndrome. *N. Engl. J. Med.,* 275:406–412.
12. Pernow, B. B., Havel, R. J., and Jennings, D. B. (1967): The second wind phenomenon in McArdle's syndrome. *Acta Med. Scand.,* 472:294–307.
13. Rowland, L. P., Araki, S., and Carmel, P. (1965): Contracture in McArdle's disease. *Arch. Neurol.,* 13:541–544.
14. Gruener, R., McArdle, B., Ryman, B., and Weller, R. O. (1968): Contracture of phosphorylase deficient muscle. *J. Neurol. Neurosurg. Psychiatry,* 31:268–283.
15. Brody, I. A., Gerber, C. J., and Sidbury, J. B. (1970): Relaxing factor in McArdle's disease. Calcium uptake by sarcoplasmic reticulum. *Neurology (Minneap.),* 20:555–558.
16. Chui, L. A., and Munsat, T. L. (1976): McArdle's syndrome. A third type of myophosphorylase deficiency? *Arch. Neurol. (in press).*
17. Dreyfus, J. C., and Alexandre, Y. (1971): Immunological studies on glycogen storage diseases type III and V. Demonstration of the presence of an immunoreactive protein in one case of muscle phosphorylase deficiency. *Biochem. Biophys. Res. Commun.,* 44:1364–1370.
18. Bank, W. J., DiMauro, S., Rowland, L. P., (1972): Renal failure in McArdle's disease, N. Engl. J. Med., 287:1102.
19. Roelofs, R. I., Engel, W. K., and Chauvin, P. B. (1972): Histochemical phosphorylase activity in regenerating muscle fibers from myophosphorylase-deficient patients. *Science,* 177:795–797.
20. Pearson, C. M., Rimer, D. G., and Mommaerts, W. F. H. M. (1961): A metabolic myopathy due to absence of muscle phosphorylase. *Am. J. Med.,* 30:502–517.
21. Pearson, C. M., and Rimer, D. G. (1959): Evidence for direct utilization of fructose in working muscle in man. *Proc. Soc. Exp. Biol. Med.,* 100:671–672.
22. Steinitz, K. (1962): McArdle's syndrome. *Lancet,* 1:1406.

23. Mahler, R., Mellick, R. S., and Hughes, B. P. (1962): McArdle's syndrome. *Lancet,* 1:1234–1235.
24. Opie, L. H., Evans, J. R., and Renold, A. E. (1962): Fructose in McArdle's syndrome. *Lancet,* 2:358–359.
25. Rowland, L. P., Lovelace, R. E., Schotland, D. L., Araki, S., and Carmel, P. (1966): The clinical diagnosis of McArdle's disease. *Neurology (Minneap.),* 16:93–100.
26. Tarui, S., Okuno, G., Ikura, Y., Tanaka, T., Suda, M., and Nishikawa, M. (1965): Phosphofructokinase deficiency in skeletal muscle. A new type of glycogenosis. *Biochem. Biophys. Res. Commun.,* 19:517–523.
27. Layzer, R. B., Rowland, L. P., and Ranney, H. M. (1967): Muscle phosphofructokinase deficiency. *Arch. Neurol.,* 17:512–523.
28. Serratrice, G., Monges, A., Roux, H., Aquaron, R., and Gambarelli, D. (1969): Forme myopathique du deficit en phosphofructokinase. *Rev. Neurol. (Paris),* 120:271–277.
29. Tobin, W. E., Huijing, F., Porro, R. S., and Salzman, R. T. (1973): Muscle phosphofructokinase deficiency. *Arch. Neurol.,* 28:128–130.
30. Tarui, S., Kono, N., Nasu, T., and Nishikawa, M. (1969): Enzymatic basis for the coexistence of myopathy and hemolytic disease in inherited muscle phosphofructokinase deficiency. *Biochem. Biophys. Res. Commun.,* 34:77–83.
31. Layzer, R. B., and Conway, M. M. (1970): Multiple isoenzymes of human phosphofructokinase. *Biochem. Biophys. Res. Commun.,* 40:1259–1265.
32. Layzer, R. B., and Rasmussen, J. (1974): The molecular basis of muscle phosphofructokinase deficiency. *Arch. Neurol.,* 31:411–417.
33. DiMauro, S., Rowland, L. P., and DiMauro, P. M. (1970): Control of glycogen metabolism in human muscle. Evidence from glycogen storage disease. *Arch. Neurol.,* 23:534–540.
34. Oliner, L., Schulman, M., and Larner, J. (1961): Myopathy associated with glycogen deposition resulting from generalized lack of amylo-1,6 glucosidase. *Clin. Res.,* 9:243.
35. Brunberg, J. A., McCormick, W. F., and Schochet, S. S. (1971): Type III glycogenosis. An adult with diffuse weakness and muscle wasting. *Arch. Neurol.,* 25:171–178.
36. Özand, P., Tokatli, M., and Amiri, S. (1967): Biochemical investigation of an unusual case of glycogenosis. *J. Pediatr.,* 71:225–232.
37. Murase, T., Ikeda, H., Muro, T., Nakao, K., and Sugita, H. (1973): Myopathy associated with type III glycogenosis. *J. Neurol. Sci.,* 20:287–295.
38. Illingworth, B. (1961): Glycogen storage disease. *Am. J. Clin. Nutr.,* 9:683–690.
39. Van Hoof, F., and Hers, H. G. (1967): The subgroups of type III glycogenosis. *Eur. J. Biochem.,* 2:265–270.
40. Garancis, J. C., Panares, R. P., Good, T. A., and Kuzma, J. F. (1970): Type III glycogenosis. A biochemical and electron microscopic study. *Lab. Invest.,* 22:468–477.
41. Fernandes, J., and Pikaar, N. A. (1969): Hyperlipemia in children with liver glycogen disease. *Am. J. Clin. Nutr.,* 22:617–627.
42. Fernandes, J., and Pikaar, N. A. (1972): Ketosis in hepatic glycogenosis. *Arch. Dis. Child.,* 47:41–46.
43. Hers, H. G., Verhue, W., and Van Hoof, F. (1967): The determination of amylo-1,6-glucosidase. *Eur. J. Biochem.,* 2:257–264.
44. Nelson, T. E., Kolb, E., and Larner, J. (1969): Purification and properties of rabbit muscle amylo-1,6-glucosidase-oligo-1,4; 1,4-transferase. *Biochemistry,* 8:1419–1428.
45. Brown, D. H., Gordon, R. B., and Illingworth-Brown, B. (1973): Studies on the structure and mechanism of action of the glycogen debranching enzymes of muscle and liver. *Ann. N.Y. Acad. Sci.,* 210:238–253.
46. Bates, E. J., Heaton, G. M., Taylor, C., Kernohan, J. C., and Cohen, P. (1975): Debranching enzyme from rabbit skeletal muscle; evidence for the location of two active centers on a single polypeptide chain. *FEBS Lett.,* 58:181–185.
47. Reed, G. B., Dixon, J. F. P., Neustein, H. B., Donnell, G. N., and Landing, B. H. (1968): Type IV glycogenosis. *Lab. Invest.,* 19:546–557.
48. Schochet, S. S., McCormick, W. F., and Zellweger, H. (1970): Type IV glycogenosis (amylopectinosis) *Arch. Pathol.,* 90:354–363.
49. Mercier, C., and Whelan, W. J. (1970): The fine structure of glycogen from type IV glycogen-storage disease. *Eur. J. Biochem.,* 16:579–583.

50. Mercier, C. (1973): Further characterization of glycogen from type IV glycogen storage disease. *Eur. J. Biochem.*, 40:221–223.
51. Illingworth-Brown, B., and Brown, D. H. (1966): Lack of an α-1,4-glucan: α-1,4-glucan 6-glycosyltransferase in a case of type IV glycogenosis. *Proc. Natl. Acad. Sci. U.S.A.*, 56:725–729.
52. Legum, C. P., and Nitowsky, H. M. (1969): Studies on leukocyte brancher enzyme activity in a family with type IV glycogenosis. *J. Pediatr.*, 74:84–89.
53. Howell, R. R., Kaback, M. M., and Illingworth-Brown, B. (1971): Type IV glycogen storage disease:branching enzyme deficiency in skin fibroblasts and possible heterozygote detection. *J. Pediatr.*, 78:638–642.
54. Schochet, S. S., McCormick, W. F., and Kovarsky, J. (1971): Light and electron microscopy of skeletal muscle in type IV glycogenosis. *Acta Neuropathol. (Berl.)*, 19:137–144.
55. Huijing, F., Lee, E. Y. C., Carter, J. H., and Whelan, W. J. (1970): Branching action of amylo-1,6-glucosidase/oligo-1,4:1,4-glucan-transferase. *FEBS Lett.*, 7:251–254.
56. Mancall, E. L., Aponte, G. E., and Berry, R. G. (1965): Pompe's disease (diffuse glycogenosis) with neuronal storage. *J. Neuropathol. Exp. Neurol.*, 24:85–96.
57. Gambetti, P. L., DiMauro, S., and Baker, L. (1971): Nervous system in Pompe's disease. *J. Neuropathol. Exp. Neurol.*, 30:412–430.
58. Martin, J. J., DeBarsy, Th., Van Hoof, F., and Palladini, G. (1973): Pompe's disease: an inborn lysosomal disorder with storage of glycogen. *Acta Neuropathol. (Berl.)*, 23:229–244.
59. Araoz, C., Sun, C. N., Shenefelt, R., and White, H. J. (1974): Glycogenosis type II (Pompe's disease): ultrastructure of peripheral nerves. *Neurology (Minneap.)*, 24:739–742.
60. Curtecuisse, V., Royer, P., Habib, R., Monnier, C., and Demas, J. (1965): Glycogenose musculaire par deficit d'alpha-1,4-glucosidase simulant une dystrophie musculaire progressive. *Arch. Fr. Pediatr.*, 22:1153–1164.
61. Zellweger, H., Illingworth-Brown, B., McCormick, W. F., and Tu, J. B. (1965): A mild form of muscular glycogenosis in two brothers with alpha-1,4-glucosidase deficiency. *Ann. Paediatr.*, 205:413–437.
62. Smith, H. L., Amick, L. D., and Sidbury, J. B. (1966): Type II glycogenosis. Report of a case with four-year survival and absence of acid maltase associated with an abnormal glycogen. *Am. J. Dis. Child.*, 111:475–481.
63. Badoual, J., Lestradet, H., Vilde, J. L., and Ploussard, J. P. (1967): Une forme atypique de glycogenose par deficit en maltase acide. *Sem. Hop. Paris*, 43:1427–1434.
64. Smith, J., Zellweger, H., and Afifi, A. K. (1967): Muscular form of glycogenosis type II (Pompe). *Neurology (Minneap.)*, 17:537–549.
65. Roth, J. C., and Williams, H. E. (1967): The muscular variant of Pompe's disease *J. Pediatr.*, 71:567–573.
66. Swaiman, K. F., Kennedy, W. R., and Sauls, H. S. (1968): Late infantile acid maltase deficiency. *Arch. Neurol.*, 18:642–648.
67. Hudgson, P., Gardner-Medwin, D., Worsfold, M., Pennington, R. J. T., and Walton, J. N. (1968): Adult myopathy from glycogen storage disease due to acid maltase deficiency. *Brain*, 91:435–461.
68. Engel, A. G., Gomez, M. R., Seybold, M. E., and Lambert, E. H. (1973). The spectrum and diagnosis of acid maltase deficiency. *Neurology (Minneap.)*, 23:95–106.
69. Engel, A. G. (1970): Acid maltase deficiency in adults: Studies in four cases of a syndrome which may mimic muscular dystrophy or other myopathies. *Brain*, 93:599–616.
70. Chou, S. M., Gutman, L., Martin, J. D., and Kettler, H. L. (1974): Adult-type acid maltase deficiency: pathologic features. *Neurology (Minneap.)*, 24:394.
71. Mehler, M., and DiMauro, S. (1976): Residual acid maltase activity in late-onset acid maltase deficiency. *Neurology (Minneap.)* (*in press*).
72. Mehler, M., and DiMauro, S. (1976): Late-onset acid maltase deficiency: detection of patients and heterozygotes by urinary enzyme assay. *Arch. Neurol.*, 33:692–695.
73. Hers, H. G. (1963): α-Glucosidase deficiency in generalized glycogen-storage disease (Pompe's disease). *Biochem. J.*, 86:11–16.
74. Hers, H. G. (1965): Inborn lysosomal diseases. *Gastroenterology*, 48:625–633.
75. Hers, H. G. (1973): The concept of inborn lysosomal disease. In: *Lysosomes and*

Storage Diseases, edited by H. G. Hers and F. Van Hoof, pp. 147–171. Academic Press, New York.

76. Illingworth-Brown, B., Brown, D. H., and Jeffrey, P. L. (1970): Simultaneous absence of α-1,4-glucosidase and α-1,6-glucosidase activities (ph 4) in tissues of children with type II glycogen storage disease. *Biochemistry,* 9:1423–1428.

77. Angelini, C., and Engel, A. G. (1973): Subcellular distribution of acid and neutral α-glucosidase in normal, acid maltase deficient, and myophosphorylase deficient human skeletal muscle. *Arch. Biochem. Biophys.,* 156:350–355.

78. Angelini, C., and Engel, A. G. (1972): Comparative study of acid maltase deficiency. *Arch. Neurol.,* 26:344–349.

79. Dreyfus, J. C., and Alexandre, Y. (1972): Electrophoretic characterization of acidic and neutral amylo 1-4 glucosidase (acid maltase) in human tissues and evidence for two electrophoretic variants in acid maltase deficiency. *Biochem. Biophys. Res. Commun.,* 48:914–920.

80. Dreyfus, J. C., Proux, D., and Alexandre, Y. (1974): Molecular studies on glycogen storage diseases. *Enzyme,* 18:60–72.

81. Illingworth-Brown, B., and Zellweger, H. (1966): α-1,4-Glucosidase activity in leukocytes from the family of two brothers who lack this enzyme in muscles. *Biochem. J.,* 101:16c–18c.

82. Koster, J. F., Slee, R. G., and Hulsmann, W. C. (1974): The use of leukocytes as an aid in the diagnosis of glycogen storage disease type II (Pompe's disease). *Clin. Chim. Acta,* 51:319–325.

83. Hug, G., Schubert, W. K., and Soukup, S. (1973): Treatment related observations in solid tissues, fibroblast cultures and amniotic fluid cells of type II glycogenosis, Hurler disease and metachromatic leukodystrophy. Enzyme therapy in genetic diseases. *Birth Defects,* 9:160–183.

84. Baudhuin, P., Hers, H. G., and Loeb, H. (1946): An electron microscopic and biochemical study of type II glycogenosis. *Lab. Invest.,* 13:1139–1152.

85. DeBarsy, Th., Jacquemin, P., Van Hoof, F., and Hers, H. G. (1973): Enzyme replacement in Pompe's disease: An attempt with purified human acid α-glucosidase. Enzyme therapy in genetic diseases. *Birth Defects,* 9:184–190.

86. Newsholme, E. A., and Start, C. (1973): *Regulation in Metabolism.* John Wiley & Sons, London.

87. Kopek, B., and Fritz, I. B. (1973): Comparison of properties of carnitine palmityltransferase 1 with those of carnitine palmityltransferase II. *J. Biol. Chem.,* 248:4069–4074.

88. DiMauro, S., and Melis-DiMauro, P. M. (1973): Muscle carnitine palmityltransferase deficiency and myoglobinuria. *Science,* 182:929–931.

89. Bank, W. J., DiMauro, S., Bonilla, E., Capuzzi, D. M., and Rowland, L. P. (1975): A disorder of muscle lipid metabolism and myoglobinuria. *N. Engl. J. Med.,* 292:443–449.

90. Engel, W. K., Vick, N. A., Glueck, C. J., and Levy, R. I. (1970): A skeletal muscle disorder associated with intermittent symptoms and a possible defect in lipid metabolism. *N. Engl. J. Med.,* 282:697–704.

91. Engel, A. G., and Siekert, R. G. (1972): Lipid storage myopathy responsive to prednisone. *Arch. Neurol.,* 27:174–181.

92. Engel, A. G., and Angelini, C. (1973): Carnitine deficiency of human skeletal muscle with associated lipid storage myopathy: A new syndrome. *Science,* 179:899–902.

93. Engel, A. G., Angelini, C., and Nelson, R. A. (1974): Identification of carnitine deficiency as a cause of human lipid storage myopathy. In: *Exploratory Concepts in Muscular Dystrophy, 11,* edited by A. T. Milhorat, pp. 601–618. Excerpta Medica, Amsterdam.

94. Markesbery, W. R., McQuillen, M. P., Procopis, P. G., Harrison, A. R., and Engel, A. G. (1974): Muscle carnitine deficiency. *Arch. Neurol.,* 31:320–324.

95. Karpati, G., Carpenter, S., Engel, A. G., Watters, G., Allen, J., Rothman, S., Klassen, G., and Mamer, O. A. (1975): The syndrome of systemic carnitine deficiency. *Neurology (Minneap.),* 25:16–24.

96. VanDyke, D. H., Griggs, R. C., Markesbery, W., and DiMauro, S. (1975): Hereditary carnitine deficiency of muscle. *Neurology (Minneap.),* 25:154–159.

97. Smyth, D. P. L., Lake, B. D., MacDermot, J., and Wilson, J. (1975): Inborn error of carnitine metabolism ("carnitine deficiency") in man. *Lancet,* 1:1198–1199.

98. Angelini, C., Pierobon, S., Lucke, S., and Cantarutti, F. (1975): Carnitine deficiency: Report of a treated case. *Neurology (Minneap.)*, 25:374.

99. Wittels, B., and Bressler, R. (1964): Biochemical lesion of diptheria toxin in the heart. *J. Clin. Invest.*, 43:630–637.

100. Corredor, C., Mansbach, C., and Bressler, R. (1967): Carnitine depletion in the choline-deficient state. *Biochem. Biophys. Acta*, 144:366–374.

101. Tanphaichitr, V., and Broquist, H. P. (1973): Lysine deficiency in the rat: Concomitant impairment in carnitine biosynthesis. *J. Nutr.*, 103:80–87.

102. Blass, J. P., Kark, P., and Engel, W. K. (1971): Clinical studies of a patient with pyruvate decarboxylase deficiency. *Arch. Neurol.*, 25:449–460.

103. Jerusalem, F., Spiess, H., and Baumgartner, G. (1975): Lipid storage myopathy with normal carnitine levels. *J. Neurol. Sci.*, 24:273–282.

104. Chanarin, I., Patel, A., Slavin, G., Wills, E. J., Andrews, T. M., and Stewart, G. (1975): Neutral-lipid storage disease: A new disorder of lipid metabolism. *Br. Med. J.*, 5957:553–555.

105. Miranda, A. F., DiMauro, S., Eastwood, A. B., Hays, A. P., and Johnson, W. G. (1976): The expression of a triglyceride storage disease in tissue culture. *In Vitro*, 12:326.

106. Martonosi, A., and Feretos, R. (1964): Sarcoplasmic reticulum. I: The uptake of Ca^{++} by sarcoplasmic reticulum fragments. *J. Biol. Chem.*, 239:648–658.

107. Margreth, A., Salviati, G., DiMauro, S., and Turati, G. (1972): Early biochemical consequences of denervation in fast and slow skeletal muscles and their relationship to neural control over muscle differentiation. *Biochem. J.*, 126:1099–1110.

108. Norum, K. (1964): Palmityl-CoA: carnitine palmityltransferase. Purification from calf-liver mitochondria and some properties of the enzyme. *Biochem. Biophys. Acta*, 89:95–108.

109. Mellman, W. J., and Tedesco, T. A. (1965): An improved assay of erythrocytes and leukocytes galactose-1-phosphate uridyl transferase: stabilization of the enzyme by a thiol protective reagent. *J. Lab. Clin. Med.*, 66:980–986.

110. Richards, G. M. (1974): Modification of the diphenylamine reaction giving increased sensitivity and simplicity in the estimation of DNA. *Anal. Biochem.*, 57:369–376.

Advances in Neurology, Vol. 17, edited by
R. C. Griggs and R. T. Moxley, III. Raven Press,
New York © 1977.

The Myotonic Disorders and the Periodic Paralyses

Robert C. Griggs

*Departments of Neurology, Medicine, and Pediatrics, University of Rochester
School of Medicine and Dentistry, 601 Elmwood Avenue,
Rochester, New York 14642*

This chapter reviews briefly the myotonic disorders and the periodic paralyses and focuses on the treatment of each. The myotonic disorders and periodic paralysis are considered together because several of these diseases have a number of common features: myotonia occurs in patients with both types of disorders; the hereditary pattern is autosomal dominant in most instances; a membrane abnormality seems likely to be present in each; and both respond to the same therapeutic agent—acetazolamide.

THE MYOTONIC DISORDERS

Types of Myotonia

Clinical myotonia is *the delayed relaxation of muscle after voluntary contraction or mechanical stimulation which is accompanied by repetitive muscle electrical activity* (action potentials on electromyography). This physical finding can be separated into two categories, action myotonia and percussion myotonia. Each type requires separate procedures to elicit its presence. Because action myotonia and percussion myotonia are not equally expressed in myotonic patients, a specific search for each type is necessary on routine physical examination. Action myotonia is the delay in relaxation after voluntary movement. This myotonia may be a source of embarrassment such as in the eyelids (Fig. 1A and B) or may limit muscle function such as in the hands where grip cannot be released. Generalized action myotonia is often disabling as shown in Fig. 1C and D where virtually complete immobility because of generalized stiffness follows muscle contraction. Although action myotonia typically improves with repeated activity, occasional patients may have myotonia that paradoxically worsens with repeated activity. Such a sequence is shown in Fig. 3. This type of myotonia has been termed "paradoxical myotonia" (42). Percussion myotonia, on the other hand, is useful diagnostically when elicited by the examiner but does not cause symptoms. Percussion myotonia may be elicited in the thenar eminence (Figs. 2A and B), tongue (Fig. 2C),

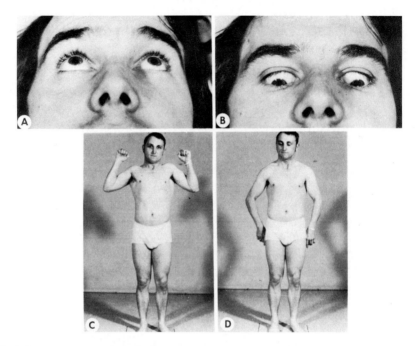

FIG. 1. Action myotonia. **A, B:** Elicitation of myotonic lid lag. After a brief period of upward gaze **(A)** the patient looks downward **(B)** and a large rim of sclera is exposed. The lid then gradually descends to a normal position. **C, D:** Patient with myotonia congenita virtually immobilized **(D)** after muscle contraction **(C).**

or wrist extensors. Patients with generalized myotonia may have myotonia elicited by percussion in virtually any muscle.

Clinical myotonia must be distinguished from electrically silent delayed relaxation, such as that seen in hypothyroidism (3), "relaxing factor deficiency" (9), and occasionally in other unusual syndromes (3,33). On the other hand, repetitive electrical discharges resembling myotonia may be seen by electromyography in patients who do not have clinical myotonia. The term "pseudomyotonia" has been applied to this phenomenon, but since this term has occasionally been used to describe electrically silent muscle contraction, it is probably wise to avoid this term and refer simply to "electrical myotonia."

Percussion myotonia must also be distinguished from the percussion responses of normal individuals. After percussion of a muscle belly, there is a brief electrical discharge accompanied by a generalized muscle contraction. This contraction is brief in normals and is accentuated in patients with denervating illness (10,46). In addition to the electrically active contraction, an electrically silent local "mound" of myoedema is frequently observed (10). Myoedema is particularly apparent in thin individuals.

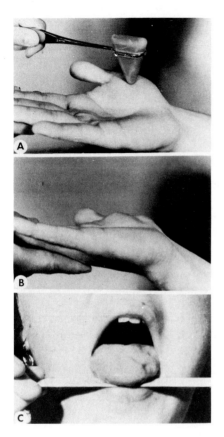

FIG. 2. Percussion myotonia. Percussion of the thenar eminence **(A)** with the patient actively extending and abducting the thumb results in a persistent dimple **(B). C:** A "napkin ring" sign after horizontal percussion of the tongue.

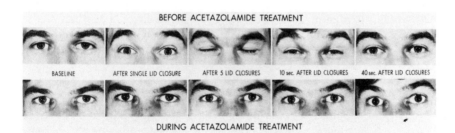

FIG. 3. Paradoxical action myotonia of the orbicularis oculi muscle in a patient with paramyotonia congenita. **Baseline:** Before lid closure. **After single lid closure:** Patient is attempting to open his eyes maximally. The patient then closed his eyes forcibly 4 additional times and is shown attempting to open his eyes immediately, 10 sec, and 40 sec after 5 lid closures. Acetazolamide abolished myotonia. [Reproduced by permission of *Ann. Intern. Med.* (52).]

Diseases Associated with Myotonia

Table 1 lists the major conditions associated with myotonia. Although myotonic dystrophy is the most common disease associated with clinically detectable myotonia, myotonia congenita is the disorder that most frequently requires treatment of symptomatic myotonia. Although the periodic paralyses are associated with myotonia, only the hyperkalemic (potassium-sensitive) form of the disease has clinical and electrical myotonia documented with any frequency (14,51). Symptomatic clinical or electrical myotonia is rare in all forms of periodic paralysis, but a myotonic lid lag can occur in both hypo- and hyperkalemic periodic paralyses (51).

TABLE 1. *Diseases associated with clinical myotonia*

Myotonic dystrophy
Myotonia congenita
Paramyotonia congenita
Myotonia, myokymia, hyperhidrosis, distal wasting syndrome
Chondrodystrophic myotonia
Hyperkalemic (myotonic) periodic paralysis
Rarely occurs with:
   Drug toxicity—clofibrate
            diazocholesterol
            2,4-dichlorphenoxyacetate (2,4-D)
   Carcinoma of the lung

MYOTONIC DYSTROPHY

Myotonic dystrophy is a multisystemic illness and is the commonest adult muscular dystrophy. The myotonia of these patients is helpful in diagnosis but is frequently asymptomatic, and the clinical picture is usually dominated by either skeletal muscle weakness or one of the other manifestations of the illness including cardiac conduction abnormalities, gonadal failure, cataracts, hypersomnia, or mental deterioration. The myotonia of these patients responds to treatment, but of the series of patients which we have treated recently, only 2 of 13 have elected to continue therapy (21).

MYOTONIA CONGENITA

Myotonia congenita occurs with a frequency of approximately $\frac{1}{50,000}$ (4) and appears to include at least two and possibly more disorders. There are two distinct hereditary patterns—an autosomal dominant and an autosomal recessive form (4,23). Most patients with myotonia congenita have painless action myotonia, but there appears to be a variant form with painful muscle stiffness also inherited as an autosomal dominant (5).

The action myotonia of these patients is often disabling, frequently more severe in males, and gradually improves with age. Although weakness may appear to be present on initial examination, strength may improve with "warm-up." Patients do not usually develop the weakness and multisystemic involvement of myotonic dystrophy (11).

PARAMYOTONIA CONGENITA

As described by Eulenburg (16), paramyotonia congenita is characterized by (a) autosomal dominant inheritance, (b) paradoxical myotonia that is markedly exacerbated by cold, (c) flaccid paralysis precipitated by prolonged exposure to cold, and (d) flaccid paralysis occurring spontaneously and unassociated with cold. Paradoxical myotonia is often a significant symptom, but the episodic weakness usually dominates the clinical picture and the treatment of paramyotonia is considered in the section on the periodic paralyses.

MYOTONIA, MYOKYMIA, HYPERHIDROSIS, AND DISTAL WASTING

This rare condition includes myotonia as part of a symptom complex characterized by distal muscle wasting and weakness, widespread fasciculations usually most prominent distally, excessive sweating, hypermetabolism, and occasionally other abnormalities (18,20). Although myotonia is significant in these patients, it is usually less symptomatic than the more evident symptoms of denervating illness.

OTHER CONDITIONS ASSOCIATED WITH MYOTONIA

Myotonia has been associated with malignancy and responded to its removal (27). A number of drugs have been associated with electrical and occasionally clinical myotonia and improved when the agent was withdrawn (15). The chondrodystrophic myotonia syndrome has diagnostically helpful myotonia, but the clinical picture is usually dominated by the underlying joint disability (1).

CONDITIONS RESEMBLING MYOTONIA

The majority of patients with complaints such as muscle "stiffness" suggesting myotonia do not, in fact, have myotonia. Occasionally the observation of a normal muscle percussion response or myoedema may be misinterpreted as myotonia. Table 2 lists some causes of muscle stiffness and cramps. Although patients with episodic cramps may have one of the syndromes associated with a defect of substrate utilization (35) or anterior horn cell disease, the majority of patients do not have a definable diagnosis.

TABLE 2. *Differential diagnosis of painful muscle stiffness*

Vascular insufficiency
Spasticity — disease of corticospinal tracts
Stiff man syndrome
Motor neuron disease
Peripheral neuropathy
Toxins — alcohol, clofibrate
Defective substrate utilization (glycogen, lipid)
Electrolyte disorders (hyponatremia, hypokalemia, hypocalcemia)
Myotonic disorders

Biopsy and electromyogram may give evidence of subtle denervation (M. Brooke, *unpublished observations*). Similarly, we studied a series of 30 patients who complained of "aching" or "cramping" and in whom the conditions listed in Table 2 were excluded. The majority had evidence of denervation by muscle biopsy — including small angular fibers, type grouping, and fibrotic nerve twigs. More severe changes of denervation such as marked grouped atrophy were usually not seen.

Agents Useful in Treating Myotonia

Table 3 lists agents that have been used successfully in the treatment of myotonia. Quinine and procainamide usually represent the most satisfactory intermittent treatment of myotonia, although their usefulness is often limited by side effects related to regular drug use (11). Thus, a patient can take such agents shortly before engaging in physical activity. In patients requiring chronic antimyotonic treatment, phenytoin is often the agent of choice in view of its relatively low incidence of side effects (45,58). In patients with cardiac conduction abnormalities, such as occur in myotonic dystrophy, phenytoin is at least theoretically preferable, since both quinine and procainamide slow conduction through the atrioventricular (AV) node (53). Phenytoin, on the other hand, speeds conduction through the AV node (13). Even in the patient who already has a cardiac pacemaker, procainamide

TABLE 3. *Agents used in treatment of myotonia*

Commonly useful
   Quinine
   Procainamide
   Phenytoin
Possibly useful
   Acetazolamide (see text)
   Corticosteroids, ACTH
   Thiazide diuretics
   Diazepam
   Lioresal

use may be hazardous since it can decrease response to the generated impulse (19). Fortunately, myotonia congenita, for which therapy is most frequently necessary, is not associated with an increased incidence of cardiac conduction abnormalities (11).

In some patients therapy with quinine, procainamide, or phenytoin is ineffective or limited by drug toxicity. In this situation, one of the other agents listed in Table 3 may be necessary. Acetazolamide has been found to be effective in occasional reported patients (31), and we have found this agent to be of benefit in several patients with myotonia.

One patient is illustrative. A 29-year-old woman with autosomal dominant myotonia congenita associated with severe, painful muscle stiffness had severe thrombocytopenia with quinine, a lupus syndrome precipitated by chronic procainamide, and a severe skin rash with phenytoin. Acetazolamide therapy in a dose of 125 mg b.i.d. has been associated with complete loss of symptoms of myotonia. On examination, myotonia has persisted but is much diminished. A single-blind therapeutic trial has confirmed the beneficial effects of acetazolamide.

Table 4 summarizes our experience with acetazolamide in myotonia. A single-blind, placebo-controlled trial of therapy has been conducted in each instance except in the patient with paramyotonia congenita. An example of the response of myotonia to acetazolamide is shown for the patient with paramyotonia congenita (Fig. 3). This patient has marked paradoxical myotonia. Within hours after acetazolamide was started, myotonia was virtually abolished. As shown in Fig. 3, lid myotonia was markedly decreased. Although this patient developed weakness and has not continued on therapy, strength has not been affected in any of the other patients treated. Long-term therapy has been continued in only three patients because of the occurrence of paresthesias in two patients with myotonia congenita and weakness in the patient with paramyotonia congenita. In three treated patients, however, acetazolamide provides the only satisfactory alternative form of therapy.

Other agents used in the treatment of myotonia include corticosteroids

TABLE 4. *Treatment of myotonia with acetazolamide* (single-blind)

Myotonia	Effect on myotonia	Side effects
Myotonia congenita		
13-yr-old male (250 mg/day)	Diminished	Paresthesias
40-yr-old male (500 mg/day)	Diminished	Paresthesias
29-yr-old female (125 mg/day)	Abolished	Paresthesias
33-yr-old female (125 mg/day)	Diminished	Paresthesias
Paramyotonia congenita		
25-yr-old male (750 mg/day)	Abolished	Weakness
Myotonic syndrome		
19-yr-old female (500 mg/day)	Diminished	None

(11), adenocorticotropic hormone (11), and lioresal (28). The long-term hazards of corticosteroids and the uncertain nature of long-term side effects of lioresal limit their usefulness. Occasional patients have also responded to diazepam (37) or thiazides (56).

Mechanism of Action

The basis for the therapeutic effect of phenytoin and other therapeutic agents in myotonia is not fully understood. It has been suggested that phenytoin produces its effect by stabilizing muscle membranes (57), and it has been shown that it decreases net sodium influx during membrane excitation (49). The observation that phenytoin alters membrane fluidity in patients with myotonic dystrophy, returning abnormal erythrocyte membrane fluidity to normal, suggests a direct membrane effect for the agent (54). Similarly, procainamide and quinine are believed to act by their effect on stabilizing muscle membranes (2).

Since muscle has no carbonic anhydrase activity (41), the effect of acetazolamide seems likely to be due to either to some other action of the agent or to a generalized metabolic alteration. Acetazolamide causes a modest kaliuresis (22) and produced a slight decline in serum potassium in each patient responding to therapy. Since myotonia has been noted to be increased by potassium administration (38), it is possible that the diminution of myotonia reflects the slight change in serum potassium level.

Agents to be Avoided in Patients with Myotonia

Particularly in myotonia congenita, succinyl choline and anticholinesterase agents should be avoided since they aggravate myotonia (11,47). If muscle relaxation is necessary during anesthesia, d-tubocurarine is preferable. Myotonia is not prevented by curare but is not worsened by it (11).

Hyperthermic responses to general anesthesia have become a matter of increasing concern in patients with myotonic disorders (8). It is unclear whether or not patients with myotonia congenita or myotonic dystrophy are likely to develop malignant hyperpyrexia. As pointed out by Field and Shenton (17), only one reported patient appears to have had malignant hyperpyrexia complicating myotonia congenita. Thus, although malignant hyperpyrexia may also be inherited as an autosomal dominant disorder, the majority of patients with this syndrome do not have an underlying myotonic disorder (8,29). Nonetheless, it seems prudent not to use succinyl choline and to avoid general anesthesia when possible in patients with myotonia.

Because potassium administration worsens myotonia (38), intravenous and oral potassium supplementation should be given with caution and with careful observation. "Potassium-sparing" diuretic agents such as spironolactone and triamterene might be expected to be deleterious.

Management of Myotonic Dystrophy

Although occasional patients benefit remarkably from treatment of myotonia, most are not helped significantly. Moreover, the weakness of these patients is not amenable to therapy. On the other hand, some complications of the disease may be treatable: cardiac disease can be managed with pacemaker insertion or antiarrhythmic agents; cataract removal can restore vision; and gonadal failure because of testicular degeneration can be treated with androgen replacement. A recent study of the hypersomnia and mental deterioration of myotonic dystrophy suggests that they respond, at least in short-term treatment, to methylphenidate (48).

THE PERIODIC PARALYSES

Classification

Table 5 lists a provisional classification for the periodic paralyses. Another classification may prove more valid when the etiology of periodic paralysis is better defined. All forms of periodic paralysis have some similar features and are characterized by episodic attacks of limb weakness. Attacks almost invariably begin by the third decade and are more severe in men. Attacks typically occur after the rest that follows exercise. Also common in all forms is the occurrence of "fixed" proximal weakness during attack-free intervals after many years of the illness (6,22,62).

The term "hyperkalemic" periodic paralysis is often a misnomer since although the potassium rises, it may remain within the normal range during attacks of weakness (15). Whereas in the attacks of hypokalemic periodic paralysis the serum potassium is virtually always abnormally low, in the "hyperkalemic" form of the disease, the response of the patient to potassium loading rather than the absolute potassium level of serum best characterizes the illness. For this reason, "normokalemic" periodic paralysis has been included as a subgroup of hyperkalemic (potassium-sensitive) periodic paralysis since many of these patients are, in fact, potassium sensitive (50). Similarly, although hyperkalemic periodic paralysis does not usually have clinical or electrical myotonia, some patients with myotonic symptoms

TABLE 5. *Classification of periodic paralysis*

Hypokalemic periodic paralysis
    Familial
    Sporadic
    Thyrotoxic
"Hyperkalemic" (potassium-sensitive) periodic paralysis
    May include: normokalemic, myotonic periodic paralysis
Paramyotonia congenita

---

develop weakness with potassium challenge and may fall into the same category of disease. Paramyotonia congenita is separated from hyperkalemic periodic paralysis because at least certain of these patients have increased myotonia but *improved* strength with potassium loading and, in fact, are relatively *hypokalemic* during attacks of weakness (39,52).

Evaluation of the Patient with Episodic Weakness

The periodic paralyses are uncommon disorders. Patients presenting for the first time with an episode of weakness accompanied by hypo- or hyperkalemia usually do not have primary periodic paralysis. Even if a patient has a history of recurrent episodes of paralysis, the diagnosis is relatively unlikely. Table 6 lists some conditions that must be considered in the differential diagnosis of recurrent episodic weakness. Particularly common are the electrolyte disturbances associated with diuretic use, alcoholism, and increased or decreased adrenocortical hormone levels.

If a patient has historical and laboratory evidence that excludes secondary causes of periodic paralysis, the evaluation should proceed as noted in Table 7. Of utmost importance is documentation of potassium, EKG, and clinical signs during a presenting attack. Sequential analysis of serum for electrolytes is indicated. All too often, however, attacks are not well characterized or do not occur under observation. In such a situation provocative testing may be indicated (55). Since administration of glucose and insulin or potassium can be associated with potentially life-threatening arrhythmias,

TABLE 6. *Disorders causing episodic paralysis*

Secondary
  Hypokalemic
    Primary hyperaldosteronism (Conn's syndrome)
    Renal tubular acidosis
    Juxtaglomerular apparatus hyperplasia (Bartter's
      syndrome)
    Villous adenoma
    Alcoholism
    Diuretics, licorice, PAS, amphotericin B,
      corticosteroids
  Hyperkalemic
    Addison's disease
    Chronic renal failure
    Isolated aldosterone deficiency
    Chronic heparin therapy
    Rhabdomyolysis (e.g., McArdle's syndrome)
  Normokalemic
    Guanidine
    Sleep paralysis
    Myasthenia gravis, multiple sclerosis, Eaton-Lambert
      syndrome
    Transient ischemic attacks

TABLE 7. *Evaluation of the patient with suspected periodic paralysis*

Exclusion of other disorders (Table 6); thyrotoxicosis
Careful documentation of strength, EKG, and
    electrolytes during attack
Electromyography
(Muscle biopsy) — may be abnormal in attack-free interval
Provocative testing (carefully monitored)
    Hypokalemic — up to 200 g glucose; 20 units regular
    insulin intravenously
    Hyperkalemic — up to 12 g KCl orally
    Paramyotonia — cold provocation

---

careful monitoring is essential during these tests. In some patients, such as those with cardiac or renal disease, they are totally unwarranted.

Since the serum potassium level often drops below normal with glucose and insulin loading or rises above normal with potassium loading even in normal individuals, it is important to monitor strength closely during provocative testing. Functional testing is essential. Unless weakness is marked enough to interfere with the ability to raise the arms above the head, sit up from supine, rise from a squat, walk on heel or toe, or other objective parameters, it may not be possible to state with certainty that an attack was precipitated.

Treatment of Hypokalemic Periodic Paralysis

ACUTE

Our approach to patients with hypokalemic periodic paralysis is summarized in Table 8. During the acute attack, oral potassium salts (20–100 mEq) are useful. Intravenous potassium is particularly difficult to administer since concentrated potassium therapy is hazardous; even oral therapy can have complications (34). More dilute potassium solutions, on the other hand, often *decrease* serum potassium even when administered at a concentration as high as 40 mEq/liter in 5% glucose or physiologic saline (30). If nausea, vomiting, or dysphagia prevents the use of oral potassium, solutions containing potassium chloride 60–80 mEq/liter should be administered slowly. A possible alternative therapy, which at least theoretically would be expected to be effective, is the use of mannitol as a diluent. Since mannitol administration is associated with a rise in serum potassium (44) and when used with potassium in diluent solutions has resulted in a prompt rise in serum potassium (R. C. Griggs and J. Resnick, *unpublished observations*), this agent may hold promise for intravenous treatment of hypokalemic states.

TABLE 8. *Treatment of periodic paralysis*

Hypokalemic
  Acute
    Oral potassium salts safest
    Intravenous diluents (glucose, saline)
      potentially hazardous, use at least 60 mEq/liter of potassium
  Chronic
    Acetazolamide 125–1,000 mg/day
    Spironolactone 25–100 mg/day
    Triamterene
    Diet—avoid high carbohydrate
Hyperkalemic
  Acute
    Oral glucose, carbohydrate
    Intravenous glucose, insulin, calcium, sodium bicarbonate
  Chronic
    Chlorothiazide 500–1,000 mg/day
    Acetazolamide 125–1,000 mg/day
    Diet—high carbohydrate; sodium restriction
    (Salbutamol)

CHRONIC

Acetazolamide appears to be the agent of choice in hypokalemic periodic paralysis. The prophylactic administration of potassium does not prevent recurrent attacks of weakness (22). Although attack frequency was observed to decrease with spironolactone administration or dietary restriction of carbohydrates or sodium, the most consistent results have been obtained with acetazolamide used as a prophylactic agent for attacks (22). Although this agent was first used successfully in hyperkalemic periodic paralysis (43), its prophylactic use in hypokalemic periodic paralysis has been attended by dramatic improvement (22). Subsequently, 21 of 23 cases (12,22, 59,60) have been treated successfully. One additional possible benefit of chronic therapy with acetazolamide is an apparent reversal of the chronic interattack weakness of hypokalemic periodic paralysis (22).

The response to acetazolamide has been prompt. In responsive patients, attacks have ceased within 24 hr in each case and returned, in patients with frequent episodes, within 24 to 96 hr. Chronic use of acetazolamide has been attended by several problems. Although patients do not become refractory to therapy as has been reported for management of seizure disorders, many patients complain of paresthesias. Interestingly, patients with hypokalemic periodic paralysis seem to have much less of a problem with paresthesias than those with myotonia or hyperkalemic periodic paralysis treated with the drug.

The major limiting factor appears to be nephrotoxicity. Renal calculi can follow treatment with acetazolamide (26). A sulfonamide neuropathy and reversible renal failure have also been reported (26). One patient who was treated with acetazolamide for a mistaken diagnosis of periodic paralysis developed renal calculi and reversible renal failure on acetazolamide (32). A patient with myotonia congenita whom we treated with acetazolamide was found to have a renal calculus during acetazolamide therapy. For this reason, patients should have an abdominal film before long-term therapy; sequential abdominal X-rays should be obtained; fluid intake should be kept high; and sulfonamides should not be administered concurrently. Marrow suppression, skin rash, and hepatotoxicity have occurred in other settings but not in patients treated for periodic paralysis. The possibility that acetazolamide may worsen phenytoin-induced osteomalacia has also been raised (40).

Treatment of Hyperkalemic Periodic Paralysis

ACUTE

As with hypokalemic periodic paralysis, oral treatment is preferable to intravenous therapy except in unusual circumstances (Table 8). High-carbohydrate foods or fluids are usually promptly effective. Rarely in severe attacks when a patient is vomiting or cannot swallow, intravenous glucose, insulin, calcium, or bicarbonate may be warranted. The electrocardiogram must be monitored throughout such therapy.

CHRONIC

Although the beneficial effect of acetazolamide in periodic paralysis was first noted in hyperkalemic periodic paralysis (43), thiazide therapy may be preferable since it is at least as effective and may be associated with fewer side effects. Combining our own experience with those reported (36,43) reveals that a more marked reduction in attack frequency has been observed with thiazides than with acetazolamide. Dietary management with high carbohydrate or low sodium intake has also been reported to be effective, the latter in a particularly difficult patient (7). A recent report suggests that the beta-adrenergic blocking agent salbutamol may be effective in preventing severe attacks (61). It is not yet clear whether or not chronic treatment with any regimen will prevent or reverse the potentially disabling weakness that these patients may develop.

Treatment of Paramyotonia Congenita

Since paramyotonia congenita has been related in terms of classification to both hyperkalemic (14) and hypokalemic (39,52) periodic paralysis, acetazolamide therapy has been tried in a patient with the classic features of this disorder as described by Eulenberg (16). Although acetazolamide therapy virtually abolished myotonia, severe weakness was precipitated on each occasion when the agent was administered. The improvement of the myotonia is shown in Fig. 3. It would appear, therefore, that this deleterious effect of acetazolamide distinguishes paramyotonia congenita from both hypo- and hyperkalemic periodic paralysis, in which conditions acetazolamide prevents weakness.

Mechanism of Effectiveness of Acetazolamide in Periodic Paralysis

Paradoxically, acetazolamide is the most effective therapy for hypokalemic periodic paralysis while providing a substantial benefit in many patients with hyperkalemic periodic paralysis. In each patient with hypokalemic periodic paralysis who has been treated with acetazolamide (22,60), a slight metabolic acidosis has developed at the effective dose used. When the therapeutic effect was first noted, it was postulated that this metabolic acidosis might prevent pathological ingress of potassium into muscle in this condition (22). Recent studies have documented that acetazolamide does prevent the lowering of serum potassium seen during glucose and insulin loading in patients with hypokalemic periodic paralysis (60). Studies attempting to produce a similar therapeutic effect by inducing metabolic acidosis with the administration of ammonium chloride have been inconclusive (22,59). The slight lowering of serum potassium that has occurred in most patients we have treated with acetazolamide may be related to the beneficial effects in hyperkalemic periodic paralysis. On the other hand, the observation that acetazolamide administration corrects a defect in potassium flux in red blood cells from patients with hyperkalemic periodic paralysis (24,25) has suggested an effect on the cell membrane. Whatever the mechanism of action, it is apparent that acetazolamide is the agent of choice for prophylactic therapy for hypokalemic periodic paralysis, may be effective in hyperkalemic periodic paralysis, and may be deleterious in paramyotonia congenita.

SUMMARY

The myotonic disorders and periodic paralyses are among the most treatable of the muscular diseases. Disabling myotonia is most frequent in myotonia congenita and usually responds to intermittent treatment with quinine or procainamide or to chronic treatment with phenytoin. If these agents are ineffective or are contraindicated because of side effects, acetazolamide, corticosteroids, or other agents may provide an alternative therapy. Although myotonic dystrophy is the commonest myotonic disorder, patients seldom derive much symptomatic benefit from treatment and are usually more disabled by weakness or one of the other manifestations of the disease.

The primary periodic paralyses are relatively uncommon and a large number of secondary causes need to be excluded in the evaluation of patients with episodic weakness. Both hypokalemic and hyperkalemic (potassium-sensitive) periodic paralysis respond to acetazolamide, and this drug appears to be the agent of choice in the hypokalemic form. The hyperkalemic form may derive more benefit from thiazides. Paramyotonia congenita differs from both hyperkalemic and hypokalemic periodic paralysis since acetazolamide treatment precipitates weakness. The chronic interattack weakness of hypokalemic periodic paralysis may be prevented by acetazolamide therapy. It is not clear if therapy for hyperkalemic periodic paralysis prevents weakness, and no treatment is available for the muscle weakness developing in the course of paramyotonia congenita.

ACKNOWLEDGMENT

Drs. Richard T. Moxley and Jack Riggs assisted in these studies. Supported in part by grants from the Muscular Dystrophy Association and NIH grant RR00044.

REFERENCES

1. Aberfeld, D. C., Namba, T., Vye, M. V., et al. (1970): Chondrodystrophic myotonia: Report of two cases. *Arch. Neurol.*, 22:455–462.
2. Barchi, R. L. (1975): Myotonia. An evaluation of the chloride hypothesis. *Arch. Neurol.*, 32:175–180.
3. Bastron, J. A. (1960): Myotonia and other abnormalities of muscular contraction arising from disorders of the motor unit. In: *Neuromuscular Disorders, Vol. 35*, edited by R. D. Adams, L. M. Eaton, and G. M. Shy. Williams & Wilkins Co., Baltimore.
4. Becker, P. E. (1971): Genetic approaches to the nosology of muscle disease: myotonias and similar diseases. *Birth Defects*, 7:52–62.
5. Becker, P. E. (1977): Syndromes associated with myotonia: clinical-genetic. In: *Pathogenesis of the Human Muscular Dystrophies*. Excerpta Medica, Amsterdam (*in press*).
6. Bradley, W. G. (1969): Adynamia episodica hereditaria. Clinical, pathological, and electrophysiological studies in an affected family. *Brain*, 92:345–378.
7. Brillman, J., and Pincus, J. H. (1973): Myotonic periodic paralysis improved by negative sodium balance. *Arch. Neurol.*, 29:67–69.
8. Britt, B. A. (1974): Malignant hyperthermia: a pharmacogenetic disease of skeletal and cardiac muscle. *N. Engl. J. Med.*, 290:1140–1142.
9. Brody, I. A. (1969): Muscle contracture induced by exercise. A syndrome attributable to decreased relaxing factor. *N. Engl. J. Med.*, 281:187–192.
10. Brody, I. A., and Rozear, M. P. (1970): Contraction response to muscle percussion. Physiology and clinical significance. *Arch. Neurol.*, 23:259–265.
11. Caughey, J. E., and Myrianthopoulos, N. C. (1963): *Dystrophica Myotonica and Related Disorders*. Charles C Thomas, Springfield, Illinois.
12. Corbett, V. A., and Nuttall, F. Q. (1975): Familial hypokalemic periodic paralysis in blacks. *Ann. Intern. Med.*, 83:63–65.
13. Damato, A. N., Berkowitz, W. D., Patton, R. D., and Lau, S. H. (1970): The effect of diphenylhydantoin on atrioventricular and intraventricular conduction in man. *Am. Heart J.*, 79:51–56.
14. Drager, G. A., Hammill, J. F., and Shy, G. M. (1958): Paramyotonia congenita. *Neurology (Minneap.)*, 80:1–9.
15. Engel, W. K. (1971): Myotonia—A different point of view. *California Med.*, 114:32–37.

16. Eulenberg, A. (1886): Ueber eine familiare durch 6 generationen verfolgbare form congenitaler paramyotonia. *Neurologisches Centralblatt,* 5:265–272.
17. Field, E. J., and Shenton, B. K. (1975): Malignant hyperpyrexia. *Lancet,* 1:92.
18. Gamstorp, I., and Wohlfart, G. (1959): A syndrome characterized by myokymia, myotonia, muscular wasting and increased perspiration. *Acta Psychiatr. Scand.,* 34:181–194.
19. Gay, R. J., and Brown, D. F. (1974): Pacemaker failure due to procainamide toxicity. *Am. J. Cardiol.,* 34:728–732.
20. Greenhouse, A. H., Bicknell, J. M., Pesch, R. N., and Seelinger, D. F. (1967): Myotonia, myokymia, hyperhidrosis, and wasting of muscle. *Neurology (Minneap.),* 17:263–268.
21. Griggs, R. C., Davis, R. J., Anderson, D. C., and Dove, J. T. (1975): Cardiac conduction in myotonic dystrophy. *Am. J. Med.,* 59:37–42.
22. Griggs, R. C., Engel, W. K., and Resnick, J. S. (1970): Acetazolamide treatment of hypokalemic periodic paralysis. *Ann. Intern. Med.,* 73:39–48.
23. Harper, P. S., and Johnston, D. M. (1971): Recessively inherited myotonia congenita. *J. Med. Genet.,* 9:213–215.
24. Hoskins, B., Maren, T. H., Vroom, F. Q., and Jarrell, M. A. (1974): Acetazolamide and potassium flux in red blood cells. Studies in patients with hyperkalemic periodic paralysis. *Arch. Neurol.,* 31:187–191.
25. Hoskins, B., Vroom, F. Q., and Jarrell, M. A. (1975): Hyperkalemic periodic paralysis. Effects of potassium, exercise, glucose, and acetazolamide on blood chemistry. *Arch. Neurol.,* 32:519–523.
26. Howlett, S. A. (1975): Renal failure associated with acetazolamide therapy for glaucoma. *South. Med. J.,* 68:504–506.
27. Humphrey, J. G., Hill, M. E., Gordon, A. S., and Kalow, W. (1974): Myotonia associated with small cell carcinoma of the lung. *Excerpta Medica,* 334:152.
28. Karli, P., and Bergstrom, L. (1974): Effect of baclofen on myotonia. *Lancet,* 1:1285.
29. King, J. O., Denborough, M. A., and Zapf, P. W. (1972): Inheritance of malignant hyperpyrexia. *Lancet,* 1:365–370.
30. Kunin, A. S., Surawicz, B., and Sims, E. A. H. (1962): Decrease in serum potassium concentrations and appearance of cardiac arrhythmias during infusion of potassium with glucose in potassium-depleted patients. *N. Engl. J. Med.,* 5:228–233.
31. Kusakabe, T., Shiotu, H., and Nishikawa, M. (1974): Metabolic studies on a case of paroxysmal myotonia with periodic paralysis. *Metabolism,* 23:215–223.
32. Lafrance, R., Griggs, R. C., Moxley, R. T., and McQuillen, J. (1977): *Hereditary paroxysmal ataxia responsive to acetazolamide. Neurology, (in press).*
33. Lambert, E. H., and Goldstein, N. P. (1957): Unusual form of "myotonia." *Physiologist,* 1:51.
34. Lawson, D. H. (1974): Adverse reactions to potassium chloride. *Q. J. Med.,* 43:433–440.
35. Layzer, R. B., and Rowland, L. P. (1971): Cramps. *N. Engl. J. Med.,* 285:31–40.
36. Layzer, R. B., Lovelace, R. E., and Rowland, L. P. (1967): Hyperkalemic periodic paralysis. *Arch. Neurol.,* 16:455–472.
37. Lewis, I. (1966): Trial of diazepam in myotonia. *Neurology (Minneap.),* 16:831–836.
38. Leyburn, P., and Walton, J. N. (1960): The effect of changes in serum potassium upon myotonia. *J. Neurol. Neurosurg. Psychiatry,* 23:119–126.
39. Lundberg, P. O., Stalberg, E., and Thiele, B. (1974): Paralysis periodica paramyotonica. A clinical and neurophysiological study. *J. Neurol. Sci.,* 21:309–321.
40. Mallette, L. E. (1975): Anticonvulsants, acetazolamide and osteomalacia. *N. Engl. J. Med.,* 93:668.
41. Maren, T. H. (1967): Carbonic anhydrase: chemistry, physiology, and inhibition. *Physiol. Rev.,* 47:595–781.
42. Marshall, J. (1952): Observations of myotonia paradoxa. *J. Neurol. Neurosurg. Psychiatry,* 15:206–210.
43. McArdle, B. (1962): Adynamia episodica hereditaria and its treatment. *Brain,* 85:121–148.
44. Moreno, M., Murphy, C., and Goldsmith, C. (1969): Increase in serum potassium resulting from the administration of hypertonic mannitol and other solutions. *J. Lab. Clin. Med.,* 73:291–298.
45. Munsat, T. L. (1967): Therapy of myotonia. *Neurology (Minneap.),* 17:359–367.
46. Patel, A., and Swami, R. K. (1969): Muscle percussion and neostigmine test in the clinical evaluation of neuromuscular disorders. *N. Engl. J. Med.,* 281:523.

47. Paterson, I. S. (1962): Generalized myotonia following suxamethonium. A case report. *Br. J. Anaesth.,* 34:340–341.
48. Penovich, P., Griggs, R. C., Moxley, R. T., and Charlton, M. (1977): Hypersomnia in myotonic dystrophy Neurology, (*in press*).
49. Pincus, J. H. (1972): Diphenylhydantoin and ion flux in lobster nerve. *Arch. Neurol.,* 26:4–10.
50. Poskanzer, D. C., and Kerr, D. N. S. (1961): A third type of periodic paralysis, with normokalemia and favourable response to sodium chloride. *Am. J. Med.,* 31:328–342.
51. Resnick, J. S., and Engel, W. K. (1967): Myotonic lid lag in hypokalaemic periodic paralysis. *J. Neurol. Neurosurg. Psychiatry,* 30:47–51.
52. Riggs, J. E., Griggs, R. C., and Moxley, R. T. (1977): Acetazolamide induced weakness in paramyotonia congenita. *Ann. Intern. Med.* (*in press*).
53. Rosen, K. M., Lisi, K. R., Berkowitz, W. D., Lau, S. H., and Damato, A. N. (1969): The effects of procaine amide on atrioventricular and intraventricular conduction in man. *Circulation (Suppl. III),* 39,40:173.
54. Roses, A. D., Butterfield, A., Appel, S. H., and Chestnut, D. B. (1975): Phenytoin and membrane fluidity in myotonic dystrophy. *Arch. Neurol.,* 32:535–538.
55. Rowland, L. P., and Layzer, R. B. (1975): Muscular dystrophies, atrophies, and related diseases. In: *Clinical Neurology, Vol. 3,* edited by A. B. Baker and L. H. Baker. Harper & Row Publishers, New York.
56. Samaha, F. J. (1964): Von Eulenburg's paramyotonia, a clinical study of restricted myotonia and episodic paralysis successfully controlled by chlorothiazide. *Trans. Am. Neurol. Assoc.,* 89:87.
57. Su, P. C., and Feldman, D. S. (1973): Motor nerve terminal and muscle membrane stabilization by diphenylhydantoin administration. *Arch. Neurol.,* 28:376–379.
58. Thompson, C. E. (1972): Diphenylhydantoin for myotonia congenita. *N. Engl. J. Med.,* 16:893.
59. Viskoper, R. J., Fidel, J., Horn, T., Tzivoni, D., and Chaco, J. (1973): On the beneficial action of acetazolamide in hypokalemic periodic paralysis: study of the carbohydrate metabolism. *Am. J. Med. Sci.,* 266:125–129.
60. Vroom, F. Q., Jarrell, M. A., and Maren, T. H. (1975): Acetazolamide treatment of hypokalemic periodic paralysis. *Arch. Neurol.,* 32:385–392.
61. Wang, P., and Clausen, T. (1976): Treatment of attacks in hyperkalaemic familial periodic paralysis by inhalation of salbutamol. *Lancet,* 1:221–223.
62. Woolsey, R. M., Nelson, J. S., and Rossini, A. A. (1969): Paramyotonia and progressive neurogenic atrophy. *Neurology (Minneap.),* 19:909–914.

Advances in Neurology, Vol. 17, edited by
R. C. Griggs and R. T. Moxley, III. Raven Press,
New York © 1977.

Metabolic Studies in Muscular Dystrophy: A Role for Insulin

Richard T. Moxley, III

Departments of Neurology and Pediatrics, University of Rochester School of Medicine and Dentistry, Rochester, New York 14642

INTRODUCTION

Insulin is a hormone with important anabolic effects on skeletal muscle (25). However, relatively few metabolic studies examining the release and action of this hormone in the muscular dystrophies (3,10,13,16,19,27) or neuropathies (8,11) are available. Muscle wasting is the hallmark of the muscular dystrophies and many of the neuropathies. No specific muscle enzyme deficiency or intracellular toxin has been found that explains the muscle loss characteristic for these diseases. It may be that the muscle wasting and certain of the other clinical features typically observed in muscular dystrophies may result from an abnormal regulation of cellular metabolism. Such a regulatory derangement might be secondary to a defect in some portion of the cell membrane or owing to a defective regulatory function of the cell nucleus in its complex interactions with the various cytoplasmic organelles. Such an abnormality would not necessarily be associated with enzyme deficiency. Cellular metabolic regulatory functions are usually the responsibility of circulating hormones, and this indicates the potential importance of hormone studies in muscular dystrophy. Table 1 lists some of the metabolic effects of insulin on skeletal muscle. It is easy to see that if these actions were significantly diminished, one of the sequellae would be the development of muscle wasting. A closer examination of insulin regulation and its metabolic action in the various muscular dystrophies and peripheral neuropathies appears to be indicated.

TABLE 1. *Insulin action on skeletal muscle*

Increases glucose uptake
Causes retention of certain amino acids
Stimulates protein synthesis
Enhances net K^+ uptake
Inhibits lipolysis

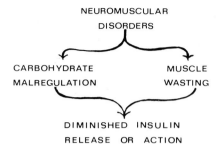

FIG. 1. Hypothetical scheme to demonstrate the interrelationship between insulin, carbohydrate regulation, muscle wasting, and neuromuscular diseases.

Insulin is of foremost importance in carbohydrate as well as protein metabolism, and it is important to recognize that many neuromuscular disorders demonstrate carbohydrate intolerance or malregulation of carbohydrate metabolism as well as muscle wasting (8,11,15). As Fig. 1 depicts, insulin is an important link between altered carbohydrate metabolism and decreased skeletal muscle mass.

An indication of the likelihood that insulin is of etiologic significance in the carbohydrate intolerance and muscle wasting seen in certain neuromuscular disorders can be gained by considering some studies performed in the primary endocrine disorders (Table 2).

With the exception of Addison's disease and primary hyperaldosteronism, each of the diseases in Table 2 has been associated with carbohydrate intolerance and muscle wasting. For example, in hyperthyroidism striking muscle wasting may develop (15). Although the detailed mechanism of action of thyroid hormone excess in producing the muscular symptoms in this disease is unclear, it is of interest that these patients have diminished pancreatic insulin release on glucose tolerance testing (7,24). Decreased insulin output may be an important factor not only in explaining the glucose intolerance in hyperthyroid patients, but also in accounting for their decreased muscle mass. In Cushing's syndrome often there is carbohydrate intolerance, and this occurs in the presence of greater-than-normal amounts of circulating insulin (28). These findings have suggested that decreased effectiveness of insulin's action in stimulating peripheral glucose uptake has necessitated the greater-than-normal pancreatic insulin release. Muscle

TABLE 2. *Endocrine disorders with skeletal muscle weakness*

Hyperthyroidism
Hypothyroidism
Hyperparathyroidism
Acromegaly
Cushing's syndrome
Addison's disease
Hyperaldosteronism (Conn's syndrome)

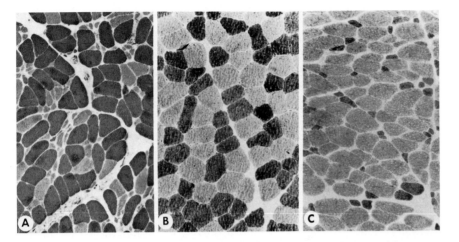

FIG. 2. A: Type II muscle fiber atrophy typical of Cushing's disease and steroid myopathy, showing both atrophy and a paucity of the type II fibers (*dark*), compared to the normal size and proportion seen in **B. C:** Characteristic type I fiber atrophy in myotonic dystrophy with a decrease of type I (*light*) fibers. (Myofibrillar ATPase, pH 9.4; original magnification 14X.)

wasting also occurs in Cushing's syndrome, which may be another sign of decreased peripheral insulin action. Type II fiber atrophy may be pronounced in Cushing's disease. Figure 2 demonstrates the paucity of darkly staining type II fibers in a muscle biopsy from a patient with steroid myopathy.

In summary, it can be seen that endocrine disorders, which often have an evaluation of carbohydrate tolerance and insulin release as a part of the clinical work-up, not infrequently show diminished insulin release or decreased peripheral insulin effectiveness. These alterations may cause the often observed carbohydrate intolerance and muscle wasting.

This chapter presents and discusses the results of metabolic studies of insulin action in a specific muscular dystrophy, myotonic dystrophy. Selected laboratory investigations are reported that pertain to carbohydrate and protein metabolism in this disease. A review of the factors important in the release as well as the peripheral action of insulin is included. The last section reports our recent findings from forearm studies, which have evaluated the response of forearm muscle to intra-arterial insulin infusion in several myotonic dystrophy patients and selected myotonic and wasted disease control patients. These same laboratory methods can be used to evaluate insulin action in other neuromuscular diseases, and the investigative approach this chapter describes should have general applicability to any neuromuscular disorder manifesting muscle wasting or carbohydrate intolerance.

FACTORS REGULATING INSULIN RELEASE

Table 3 summarizes the primary regulatory events controlling insulin release (2,9,25,29). After a meal is ingested, such as glucose during an oral glucose tolerance test, the sympathetic nerves to the gastrointestinal tract and to the pancreatic beta cell are activated. This neural activity prepares the beta cell for optimum insulin release. At the same time certain gastrointestinal hormones are released which also prime the pancreas for insulin output. After these two activating steps, glucose, and in the case of meals amino acids and small peptides, directly stimulates the beta cell to release insulin. After this stimulation insulin enters the bloodstream, circulates, and attaches to its peripheral receptor site on the target organ's cell surface to produce its physiologic effect. Alteration of or damage to the steps of this sequence can lead to either inadequate insulin release or diminished peripheral action. Such an alteration in release or peripheral action leads to abnormal regulation of carbohydrate metabolism and might, if the defect persists, cause muscle wasting.

TABLE 3. *Factors regulating normal insulin release*

1. A meal is ingested
2. This activates:
   A. Autonomic nerves to gastrointestinal tract and pancreas
   B. Release of gastrointestinal hormones that stimulate insulin secretion (gastric inhibitory polypeptide, gastrin, secretin)
3. Absorbed glucose and amino acids further stimulate beta cell insulin release
4. Insulin circulates and attaches to peripheral receptors producing its physiologic effect

CLINICAL TESTS

Various clinical investigative techniques have been used to evaluate insulin release and carbohydrate regulation (Table 4). Oral glucose tolerance testing measures plasma glucose and plasma insulin levels after a standard oral dose of glucose. Intravenous glucose tolerance bypasses the gastrointestinal factors, which prime the pancreas for insulin release on oral testing. Intravenous insulin tolerance testing (ITT) provides information about the effectiveness of exogenous insulin in stimulating glucose utilization. The ITT is also useful in estimating insulin's plasma half-life. The intravenous tolbutamide and arginine tolerance tests demonstrate the pancreatic beta cell's ability to release insulin in response to secretagogues other than glucose. In addition to these studies, some patient investigations use an oral amino acid test to evaluate the effect of noncarbohydrate nutrients on pancreatic insulin release.

TABLE 4. *Clinical test results after evaluation of carbohydrate regulation in myotonic dystrophy*

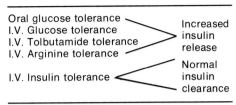

Oral glucose tolerance	Increased insulin release
I.V. Glucose tolerance	
I.V. Tolbutamide tolerance	
I.V. Arginine tolerance	
I.V. Insulin tolerance	Normal insulin clearance

STUDIES IN MYOTONIC DYSTROPHY

Myotonic dystrophy is the most common adult muscular dystrophy and is a multisystem disorder the major muscle symptoms of which are myotonia and skeletal muscle weakness and wasting (Figs. 2 and 3) (6,30). Myotonic dystrophy is an autosomal dominant disorder with variable degrees of clinical expression. Atrophy is a major feature of the condition and in most instances is typically most severe in type I muscle fibers (Fig. 2). The exact etiology of this disease, as is the case for the other muscular dystrophies, remains obscure. Recently, abnormalities in membrane protein phosphorylation have been described in red blood cells and skeletal muscle of patients with myotonic dystrophy (4,5,22,23). These findings have prompted the hypothesis that myotonic dystrophy is a diffuse membrane disease. This membrane hypothesis can be related to the abnormalities in carbohydrate tolerance and excessive insulin release often seen in myotonic dystrophy.

Table 4 records the laboratory tests that depict hypersecretion of insulin in myotonic dystrophy. In the majority of patients with myotonic dystrophy,

PRESENTING FEATURES
OF MYOTONIC DYSTROPHY

DISTAL WEAKNESS
MYOTONIA
RETARDATION
DYSPHAGIA
DYSPHONIA
CATARACTS
CARDIAC DISEASE
PULMONARY INSUFFICIENCY
FRONTAL BALDING
GONADAL ATROPHY
LETHARGY
DIABETES
INFECTION

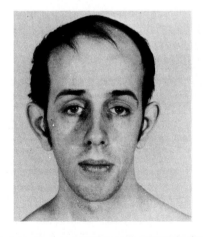

FIG. 3. Typical facial appearance and clinical signs in a patient with myotonic dystrophy.

there is hypersecretion of insulin in response to both oral and intravenous glucose loads as well as to other insulin secretagogues, such as tolbutamide and the amino acid arginine (3,10,12,13,16,19,27). These results demonstrate that the excessive insulin release is not a response limited to one specific secretagogue, and that the large insulin output seen does not demand the priming effects of gastrointestinal hormones.

Intravenous insulin tolerance studies in myotonic dystrophy indicate a normal plasma half-life for insulin. This argues against a slowed insulin removal rate as the explanation for the prolonged elevations of insulin observed in the four tests cited in Table 4. Why is insulin output excessive in many myotonic dystrophy patients? One possible answer is that there is a decreased peripheral response to the insulin released, and that for insulin to accomplish its usual effects, supranormal amounts are required.

If such diminished peripheral insulin sensitivity is present, how then does this phenomenon relate to abnormal carbohydrate regulation and muscle wasting? The major portion of the answer to this question can be seen by considering the specific effects of insulin on skeletal muscle (see Table 1). Insulin has several actions that follow its attachment to the muscle cell surface: it increases glucose uptake (31), causes retention of certain amino acids (20), stimulates protein synthesis (17,21), enhances net potassium uptake (31), and inhibits lipolysis (31). Not all of these actions occur with equal vigor at the same concentration of insulin. With mildly elevated levels of insulin, the effects on glucose uptake and amino acid retention are minimal, although the effects on potassium uptake and lipolysis are quite evident. Facilitation of glucose uptake and amino acid retention requires higher insulin concentrations, such as the peak levels achieved during an oral glucose tolerance test.

On oral glucose tolerance testing, the majority of patients with myotonic dystrophy have excessive release of insulin. Despite these supernormal insulin levels these same patients show either an abnormally elevated or normal plasma glucose level. There has been no indication that a structurally abnormal form of insulin is present in myotonic dystrophy, nor has there been evidence that excessive amounts of proinsulin (the less active precursor of insulin) are released (18). A logical inference is that the peripheral actions of insulin have been diminished in myotonic dystrophy. Such a finding supports the hypothesis that myotonic dystrophy is a diffuse membrane disease. The large insulin output in these patients may reflect the presence of an abnormality in the peripheral skeletal muscle membrane receptor for insulin.

Figure 4 presents data collected during a standard oral glucose tolerance test in a group of moderately affected myotonic dystrophy patients and compares these results to a group of age-, weight-, and sex-matched normal volunteers. All the patients are ambulatory and fully able to perform activities of daily living, and most have only mild muscular atrophy. The data

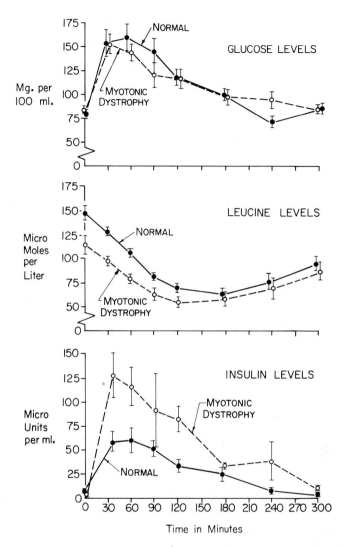

FIG. 4. Glucose, leucine, and insulin concentration changes after a standard oral glucose tolerance test in 5 normal subjects and 10 myotonic dystrophy patients. Each point represents the mean ± SEM.

presented are glucose, insulin, and leucine values obtained from serial blood samples collected during the standard oral glucose tolerance test.

The rise and fall in plasma glucose levels for the patients and the controls are very similar with only the 240-min point being statistically higher in the myotonic dystrophy group. On the other hand, the simultaneous insulin values are significantly higher for the myotonic dystrophy group. This pattern suggests that two or three times the normal amount of insulin is required in these patients to give a normal glucose tolerance curve. One interpretation of these findings is that insulin's peripheral action of facilitating glucose uptake is diminished in these myotonic dystrophy patients.

Figure 4 also presents leucine levels obtained with the glucose and insulin values during these same oral glucose tolerance tests. Leucine has been plotted as a representative of the amino acids whose retention by muscle is significantly stimulated by insulin. This group of insulin-sensitive amino acids is composed of threonine, glycine, isoleucine, leucine, tyrosine, and phenylalanine. These amino acids are retained at high physiologic concentrations of insulin (20), such as those reached during the peak release of a standard oral glucose tolerance test (1,26).

The changes in concentration of leucine provide an indirect assessment of another action of insulin on peripheral tissue, the retention of amino acids. As can be seen in Fig. 4, the decline in leucine concentration during the oral glucose tolerance test is virtually identical in shape for both the myotonic dystrophy patients and the control group. No significant difference in rate or degree of fall of leucine levels is observed on comparing the myotonic dystrophy and control groups. Nevertheless, the insulin output for the patients is two to three times greater than for the controls. It again appears that supernormal levels of insulin are needed to facilitate peripheral glucose uptake and amino acid retention, giving further support to the hypothesis that peripheral insulin insensitivity may be an important factor in myotonic dystrophy.

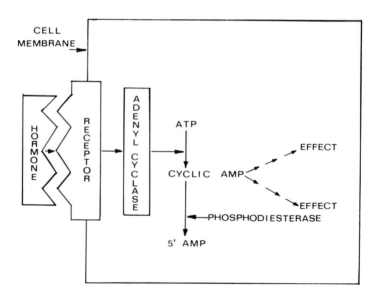

FIG. 5. Hypothetical model for regulation of cellular metabolism by surface-active hormones. Specific hormones may either stimulate or inhibit the intracellular accumulation of cyclic AMP by attaching to their designated cell surface receptor.

Figure 5 depicts a conceptual representation of the hypothesized mechanism of action for insulin. Insulin is believed to exert its effect by attaching to its receptor on the muscle cell surface. After this it is felt to suppress adenyl cyclase activity and to enhance the activity of the phosphodiesterase (14). The net effect of these two actions is to decrease intracellular cyclic AMP. If there is a defect in the muscle cell membrane affecting the insulin attachment site, this could hamper its physiologic effectiveness.

FOREARM INSULIN INFUSION STUDIES

A more direct method is available to evaluate the hypersection of insulin observed in myotonic dystrophy. It allows a direct examination of the sensitivity of peripheral skeletal muscle to intra-arterially infused insulin. This method, known as the human forearm technique, has been used to study the same myotonic dystrophy and control patients whose data are presented in the oral glucose tolerance study in Fig. 4.

During a typical forearm study an intrabrachial arterial line is established, allowing the investigator to measure simultaneously the forearm blood flow by dye dilution principles and to infuse insulin at a rate that produces physiologic elevations (20,31). Blood samples are collected simultaneously from the brachial artery and the deep venous system of the forearm to allow the determination of an arteriovenous concentration difference of the various metabolites that insulin affects. The AV difference for metabolites such as glucose, amino acids, potassium, free fatty acids, and oxygen can be measured and multiplied by the simultaneously measured blood flow. The product of flow times the AV difference is the net amount of a given substance moving into or out of muscle. Such determinations have been made in the persons noted above, and selected results of three representative forearm studies appear in Table 5.

TABLE 5. *Effects on glucose uptake of intrabrachial arterial insulin infusion (100 μunits/ kg/min) in 3 people*

	Glucose uptake by muscle (μmoles/min/100 ml forearm)		Venous insulin level (μunits/ml) — peak level after infusion completed
	Before insulin infusion	Peak uptake after insulin	
Normal volunteer (CH, male, age 24 yr)	0.66	3.95	170
Myotonic dystrophy (NB, male, age 33 yr)	0.44	0.94	165
Chronic anterior horn cell disease (GW, male, age 33 yr)	0.31	7.16	128

Insulin has been infused intra-arterially at a rate of 100 μunits/kg/min for 20 min and discontinued. At the end of the insulin infusion the deep venous levels are comparable for the normal control subject and the myotonic dystrophy patient (Table 5). Deep venous insulin concentration is slightly lower for the disease control patient who has a chronic anterior horn cell disorder. Each of these insulin levels is within the physiologic range. As can be seen by comparing zero time control glucose uptake to the peak uptake after insulin infusion, there is a sixfold increase in the normal subject while only a twofold increase has occurred in the myotonic dystrophy patient. The disease control patient shows a 23-fold rise in his glucose uptake. This disease control patient has wasting of forearm muscle similar to that seen in the myotonic dystrophy subject. It is clear that atrophy alone does not account for the decreased glucose uptake in the myotonic dystrophy patient.

The data in Table 5 provide direct evidence that this myotonic dystrophy patient has decreased peripheral responsiveness to insulin. If hyporesponsiveness is a constant finding in subsequent patient studies, what does it tell us about the excessive release of insulin seen in our myotonic dystrophy patients? This suggests that the high levels are owing to diminished peripheral response, and that this might account for the glucose intolerance and muscle wasting often seen in this disease. It is also consistent with an abnormal membrane theory of the disease etiology.

Is this hyporesponsiveness to insulin confined to myotonic dystrophy? To determine the specificity of the resistance to insulin-mediated glucose uptake in myotonic dystrophy, we have planned additional forearm studies. These investigations will evaluate not only other myotonic dystrophy subjects, but also patients with paramyotonia congenita, myotonia congenita, and various nonmyotonic neuromuscular diseases having mild involvement of forearm muscle. Preliminary oral glucose tolerance evaluations and other clinical tests described earlier have already been performed in these disease control patients, and no excessive release of insulin has occurred.

DISCUSSION

If peripheral skeletal muscle insulin insensitivity can be shown as a frequent occurrence in symptomatic myotonic dystrophy patients, treatment directed toward bypassing insulin insensitivity should be given a trial in these patients. One approach might be to administer exogenous insulin, timing the dosage to coincide with the peak levels of insulin after each meal. This would allow the maximum uptake of amino acids, glucose, and other nutrients whose transport into the cell is facilitated by insulin. Another approach to bypassing peripheral muscle insulin insensitivity would be the administration of a medication that mimicks some of the actions insulin has on skeletal muscle. Such an agent is not readily available; but, for example, perhaps in the near future the hormone somatomedin C will become available and can be used in this capacity. Alternatively, such myotonic dystrophy patients could be studied to see if they have greater-than-normal levels of catecholamines or corticosteroids, which are known to antagonize the effectiveness of endogenous insulin. If such abnormal elevations of antagonists are detected, therapy could be directed toward them.

This last approach, which depends on measurement of circulating hormonal antagonists to insulin, has some applicability to acute medical illness as well as to the muscular dystrophies. Certain common medical conditions with high circulating catecholamine levels—such as burns, hypoxia, and acute myocardial infarction—may all demonstrate significantly diminished pancreatic insulin release (14). If such decreased release is maintained, carbohydrate intolerance and muscle wasting can develop. As a somewhat different example, Cushing's disease has excessive levels of corticosteroids, which appear to decrease the effectiveness of normal amounts of circulating insulin. These patients have glucose intolerance and type II muscle fiber atrophy. Perhaps various types of defects that affect insulin release and action will explain the carbohydrate malregulation and muscle wasting often noted in many neuromuscular diseases.

SUMMARY

Insulin is important in maintaining carbohydrate tolerance and normal muscle mass. Carbohydrate intolerance and muscle wasting are frequent in the neuromuscular disorders associated with endocrinopathy and in myotonic dystrophy. Studies of the systemic factors that regulate insulin release in myotonic dystrophy have shown that excessive insulin release occurs on oral glucose tolerance testing with diminished peripheral effectiveness. Study of the peripheral action of insulin by forearm investigations of myotonic dystrophy patients and disease controls has suggested that the peripheral skeletal muscle insulin receptor may be relatively insensitive in myotonic dystrophy.

It is possible that an evaluation of insulin regulation and action in myotonic dystrophy or many neuromuscular disorders may have eventual therapeutic implications. If neuromuscular disorders other than myotonic dystrophy have evidence of peripheral insulin ineffectiveness, reasonable causes could be an excessive level of an antagonistic hormone, a faulty insulin receptor, or inadequate pancreatic insulin release.

ACKNOWLEDGEMENTS

The author wishes to acknowledge the excellent technical support of Vincent VanGelder, Barbara Herr, and Marjorie Shoemaker. This work was supported in part by grants from the Muscular Dystrophy Association, NIH RR00044, and the Leonard A. Waasdorp Memorial Fund.

REFERENCES

1. Adibi, S., Morse, E. L., and Amin, P. M. (1975): Role of insulin and glucose in the induction of hypoaminoacidemia in man: Studies in normal, juvenile diabetic, and insuloma patients. *J. Lab. Clin. Med.,* 86:395–409.
2. Andersen, D. K., Tobin, J. D., and Andres, R. (1976): Gastric inhibitory polypeptide release after oral glucose and quantification of its role in insulin secretion in states of glucose intolerance. *Clin. Res.,* 24:355.
3. Barbosa, J., Nuttall, F. Q., Kennedy, W., and Goetz, F. (1974): Plasma insulin in patients with myotonic dystrophy and their relatives. *Medicine (Baltimore),* 53:307.
4. Butterfield, D. A., Chesnut, D. B., Roses, A. D., and Appel, S. H. (1974): Electron spin resonance studies of erythrocytes from patients with myotonic muscular dystrophy. *Proc. Natl. Acad. Sci. (U.S.A.),* 71:909.
5. Butterfield, D. A., Roses, A. D., Cooper, M., Appel, S. H., and Chestnut, D. B. (1974): A comparative electron spin resonance study of the erythrocyte membrane in myotonic muscular dystrophy. *Biochemistry,* 43:5078.
6. Caughey, J. E., and Myrianthopoulos, N. C. (Eds.) (1963): *Dystrophica Myotonica and Related Disorders.* Charles C. Thomas, Publisher, Springfield, Ill.
7. Cavagnini, F. (1974): Impairment of growth hormone and insulin secretion in hyperthyroidism. *Eur. J. Clin. Invest.,* 4:71–77.
8. Collis, W. J., and Engel, W. K. (1968): Glucose metabolism in five neuromuscular disorders. *Neurology (Minneap.),* 18:915–925.
9. Fajans, S. S., and Floyd, J. C., Jr. (1972): Simulation of islet cell secretion by nutrients and by gastrointestinal hormones related during ingestion. In: *Handbook of Physiology: Endocrinology, Sec. 7, Vol. I,* edited by R. O. Greep and E. B. Astwood, pp. 473–494. American Physiological Society, Washington, D.C.
10. Gordon, P., Griggs, R. C., Nissley, S. P., Roth, J., and Engel, W. K. (1969): Studies of plasma insulin in myotonic dystrophy. *J. Clin. Endocrinol.,* 29:684.
11. Gotoh, F., Kitamura, A., Koto, A., Kataoka, K., and Atsuji, H. (1972): Abnormal insulin secretion in amyotrophic lateral sclerosis. *J. Neurol. Sci.,* 16:201–207.
12. Huff, T. A., and Lebovitz, H. E. (1968): Dynamics of insulin secretion in myotonic dystrophy. *J. Clin. Endocrinol.* 28:992.
13. Huff, T. A., Horton, E. S., and Lebovitz, H. E. (1967): Abnormal insulin secretion in myotonic dystrophy. *N. Engl. J. Med.,* 277:837.
14. Kones, R. J. (1974): Insulin, adenylcyclate, ions, and the heart. *Trans. N. Y. Acad. Sci.,* 36:738–774.
15. McArdle, B. (1974): Metabolic and endocrine myopathies. In: *Disorders of Voluntary Muscle,* edited by J. N. Walton. Churchill Livingstone, Edinburgh.
16. Mendelsohn, L. V., Friedman, L. M., Corredor, D. C., Sieracki, J. C., Sabeh, G., Vester, J. W., and Danowski, T. S. (1969): Insulin responses in myotonia dystrophica. *Metabolism,* 18:764.
17. Morgan, H. E., Jefferson, L. S., and Wolpot, E. B. (1971): Regulation of protein synthesis in muscle. II. Effects of amino acid levels and insulin or ribosomal aggregation. *J. Biol. Chem.,* 246:2163–2170.
18. Poffenbarger, P. L., Pozefsky, T., and Soeldner, J. S. (1976): The direct relationship of proinsulin-insulin hypersecretion to basal serum levels of cholesterol and triglyceride in myotonic dystrophy. *J. Lab. Clin. Med.,* 87:384–396.
19. Polgar, J. G., Bradley, W. G., Upton, A. R. M., Anderson, J., Howat, J. M. L., Petito, F., Roberts, D. F., and Scopa, J. (1972): The early detection of dystrophica myotonica. *Brain,* 95:761–766.
20. Pozefsky, T., Felig, P., Tobin, J. D., Soeldner, J. S., and Cahill, G. F. (1969): Amino acid balance across tissues of the forearm in postabsorptive man. Effects of insulin at two dose levels. *J. Clin. Invest.,* 48:2273–2282.
21. Rannels, D. E., Jefferson, L. S., and Hjalmarson, A. C. (1970): Maintainance of protein synthesis in hearts of diabetic animals. *Biochem. Biophys. Res. Commun.,* 40:1110–1116.

22. Roses, A. D., and Appel, S. H. (1973): Protein kinase activity in erythrocyte ghosts of patients with myotonic muscular dystrophy. *Proc. Natl. Acad. Sci. U.S.A.,* 70:1855.
23. Roses, A. D., and Appel, S. H. (1974): Muscle membrane protein kinase in myotonic muscular dystrophy. *Nature,* 250:245.
24. Seino, Y., Goto, Y., Taminato, T., Ikeda, M., and Imura, H. (1974): Plasma insulin and glucagon responses to arginine in patients with thyroid dysfunction. *J. Clin. Endocrinol. Metab.,* 38:1136–1140.
25. Shafrir, E. (Ed.) (1971): *Impact of Insulin on Metabolic Pathways.* Academic Press, New York.
26. Swendseid, M. E., Tuttle, S. G., Drenick, E. J., Joven, C. B., and Massey, F. J. (1967): Plasma amino acid response to glucose administration in various nutritive states. *Am. J. Clin. Nutr.,* 20:243–249.
27. Walsh, J. C., Turtle, J. R., Miller, S., and McLeod, J. G. (1970): Abnormalities of insulin secretion in dystrophica myotonica. *Brain,* 93:731.
28. Wise, J. K., Hendler, R., and Felig, P. (1973): Influence of glucocorticoids on glucagon secretion and plasma amino acid concentrations in man. *J. Clin. Invest.,* 52:2774–2782.
29. Woods, S. C., and Porte, D. (1974): Neural control of the endocrine pancreas. *Physiol. Rev.,* 54:596–619.
30. Zellweger, H., and Ionasecu, V. (1973): Myotonic dystrophy and its differential diagnosis. *Acta. Neurol. Scand. Suppl. 55,* 49:1.
31. Zierler, K. L., and Rabinowitz, D. (1963): Roles of insulin and growth hormone, based on studies of forearm metabolism in man. *Medicine (Baltimore),* 42:385.

Advances in Neurology, Vol. 17, edited by
R. C. Griggs and R. T. Moxley, III. Raven Press,
New York © 1977.

Pathology of Muscular Dystrophy and Related Disorders

William R. Markesbery

Departments of Neurology and Pathology, University of Kentucky College of Medicine, Lexington, Kentucky 40506

INTRODUCTION

Although Duchenne (11) is generally given credit for describing the first case of muscular dystrophy in 1861, it was Meryon (40) in 1852 who initially characterized muscular dystrophy in four boys from the same family and suggested that it was a primary muscle disorder. Griesinger (25), in 1865, performed the first surgical muscle biopsy. Subsequently, Duchenne (12) designed and used the first biopsy needle to obtain muscle from a patient with muscular dystrophy in which he described increased connective tissue and fat. In the later nineteenth century the major forms of muscular dystrophy were described, and in 1891 Erb (21) outlined the major histologic findings in the different dystrophic disorders and pointed out their general similarity.

In general, advances in the pathology of muscle disease moved at a slow pace until the 1950s when enzyme histochemistry and subsequently electron microscopy were applied to these disorders. In recent years the ultrastructural study of muscle disease has accelerated at a remarkable rate. Electron microscopic studies have led to an understanding of the subcellular details of muscle fibers and how they react in different disease processes. Basically what has been learned is that muscle reacts in a limited number of ways, a few of which are relatively specific and the majority of which are nonspecific. Indeed, as our knowledge of muscle ultrastructure increases we are finding that some of the specific alterations are not as specific as initially thought.

The purpose of this chapter is to outline some of the light and electron microscopic alterations found in the muscular dystrophies and several related disorders, the congenital myopathies and lipid myopathies. The classification of the dystrophies to be followed is that outlined by Gardner-Medwin and Walton (23) and includes: Duchenne dystrophy, facioscapulohumeral dystrophy, limb-girdle dystrophy, distal myopathy, ocular myopathy, and oculopharyngeal dystrophy.

DUCHENNE MUSCULAR DYSTROPHY

Duchenne or pseudohypertrophic dystrophy is the most common dystrophy and is inherited in a sex-linked recessive pattern, although sporadic cases are common. Onset of pelvic girdle weakness usually occurs in the first few years and progresses steadily, leading to inability to walk. Death occurs by the second or early third decade. A form of sex-linked dystrophy with clinical manifestations similar to those of Duchenne's but with a much milder course has been called the Becker type.

Muscle biopsy findings in all forms of dystrophy vary with the stage of the disease in which the biopsy is obtained. The classic histopathological alterations in Duchenne dystrophy are: (a) pronounced random variation in fiber size (Fig. 1); (b) slight internalization of sarcolemmal nuclei; (c) degeneration, necrosis, and phagocytosis of fibers; (d) regeneration of fibers; and (e) proliferation of endomysial and perimysial connective tissue. These abnormalities do not differ significantly from those seen in many other forms of myopathy. It has been pointed out that the grouped pattern of degenerating (Fig. 2) and regenerating fibers early in the disease and subsequent increase in endomysial and perimysial connective tissue are characteristic findings of Duchenne dystrophy (19). Considerable emphasis has been

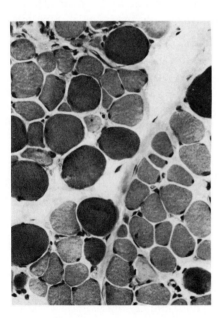

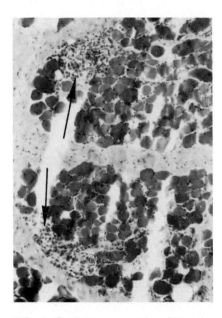

FIG. 1. Duchenne muscular dystrophy. Light micrograph showing striking variation in fiber size and several hyaline fibers. Modified Gomori trichrome stain (trichrome); ×160.

FIG. 2. Duchenne muscular dystrophy. Light micrograph showing two groups of degenerating fibers. H&E;×63.

placed on the large, dark, rounded hyaline or opaque fibers (Fig. 1) in Duchenne dystrophy. At the light microscopic level, these fibers have increased enzymatic activity (9). At the ultrastructural level, they have been found to be degenerated fibers containing homogenized contractile material (6). Regeneration of fibers is common in the early stages of this disorder, but the process becomes less efficient in later stages (59). Fiber typing in Duchenne muscular dystrophy is often less than ideal and some fibers cannot be categorized. However, it is generally held that there is no selective fiber type involvement and that often there is a predominance of type 1 fibers. In late stages of the disease, necrosis is less active and hypertrophied fibers are common. Eventually, there is striking replacement of muscle by abundant connective tissue and fat, remnants of small muscle fibers, and pyknotic nuclear clumps; during this stage Duchenne dystrophy is indistinguishable from other chronic myopathic disorders.

A number of studies of the ultrastructural features of the dystrophies are available (6,22,35,38,41,42,44,48). In these reports a wide variety of alterations have been described, including alterations and loss of Z- and I-bands, disorganization and loss of myofibrils, sarcoplasmic masses, increased glycogen granules and lipid droplets, mitochondrial inclusions, dilatation of the sarcoplasmic reticulum, formation of autophagic vacuoles and various other forms of lysosomes, alterations in basement and plasma membranes, formation of tubular aggregates, and migration and variation in location of nuclei. Few studies of the ultrastructural alterations in the various stages of Duchenne dystrophy are available. Milhorat et al. (41) divided fiber alteration into early, intermediate, and late stages based on the condition of groups of fibers. Cullen and Fulthorpe (6) divided the process of fiber breakdown into five sequential stages. Dividing the change into stages is helpful in understanding the fine structure, but it must be remembered that this disease is a continuing process and does not occur in a series of discrete stages.

In the early stages of fiber alteration in Duchenne dystrophy, there is discontinuity and streaming of the Z-line. There is dilatation of the sarcoplasmic reticulum (Fig. 3), a loss of continuity of myofibrils with widening of the intermyofibrillar space, and an increase in intermyofibrillar glycogen (Fig. 4). Undulation of the sarcolemma is often present. Nuclei occasionally are found in the center of fibers.

In intermediate stages there is more severe fragmentation and disorganization of the myofibrils (Fig. 5). Spaces in which there has been a complete loss of myofibrils are present. Swollen, degenerated mitochondria, dilatation of the T-system, variable-sized vesicles, and increasing amounts of glycogen are present between myofibrils or in areas free of contractile elements. Lipid droplets and lysosomes are also increased in these sites. The sarcolemma is often not in contact with the myofibrils. Clumps of disorganized organelles and granular material are often adjacent to the nucleus just

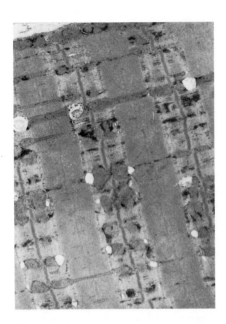 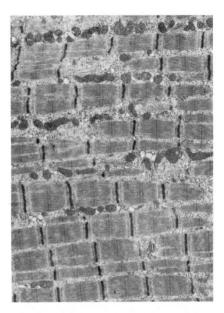

FIG. 3. Duchenne muscular dystrophy. Electron micrograph showing dilatation of sarcoplasmic reticulum. ×8,875.

FIG. 4. Duchenne muscular dystrophy. Electron micrograph showing loss of continuity of myofibers, widening of the intermyofibrillar space, and increased glycogen granules. ×6,300.

beneath the sarcolemma. Abundant connective tissue is between fibers.

In later stages of degeneration, fibers have numerous contraction clumps (Fig. 6). These are dark, dense, homogeneous masses of coalescent contractile material. They are occasionally adjacent to homogeneous, lightly osmophilic granular material (Fig. 6) containing lipid droplets, degenerating mitochondrial membranes, and organelle fragments of undetermined origin. Subsequently, the fiber becomes one shrunken mass of structureless cytoplasmic material that is invaded by macrophages.

Electron microscopists have long been concerned with defining the earliest detectable morphological alterations in dystrophic muscle. Early workers suggested that the initial change may be alteration in the sarcoplasmic reticulum (55). Others have hypothesized that the primary defect may be a vascular abnormality (19). Recently, Mokri and Engel (42) have described focal defects in the plasma membrane from patients with Duchenne dystrophy and have suggested that these defects may be the earliest lesions. It is of interest that by quantitative morphometric analysis the volume fraction of mitochondria is less and the relative volume of sarcoplasm is greater than normal in the earliest stages of Duchenne dystrophy (6).

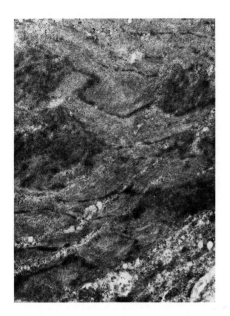

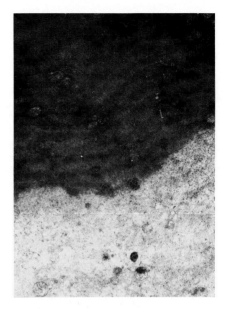

FIG. 5. Duchenne muscular dystrophy. Electron micrograph showing severe disorganization of myofibrils and smearing of the Z-band. ×12,400.

FIG. 6. Duchenne muscular dystrophy. Electron micrograph of late stages of fiber degeneration showing contraction clump at top and area of pale granular degeneration at bottom. ×7,200.

FACIOSCAPULOHUMERAL MUSCULAR DYSTROPHY

Facioscapulohumeral (FSH) muscular dystrophy is inherited in an autosomal dominant pattern, begins with weakness in facial and shoulder girdle muscles — usually by the end of the second decade — and often has a slow, benign course. It has been pointed out that facial and proximal shoulder girdle involvement is not limited to FSH dystrophy. van Wijngaarden and Bethlem (57) found cases of myotubular myopathy, nemaline myopathy, central core disease, and a mitochondrial myopathy in the FSH syndrome of early onset and several cases of myasthenia gravis in the FSH syndrome of late onset.

Although the light microscopic alterations in FSH dystrophy lack specificity, most authors agree that extreme variation in fiber size with scattered atrophic angular fibers, many hypertrophied fibers (Fig. 7), and few degenerating fibers are common findings (10,59). Munsat et al. (43) have drawn attention to the frequent mononuclear inflammatory response seen in biopsies from patients with this disorder. Ultrastructural studies on small numbers of cases have revealed no specific findings (22,35,38).

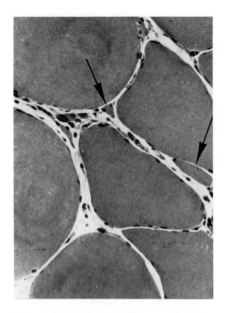 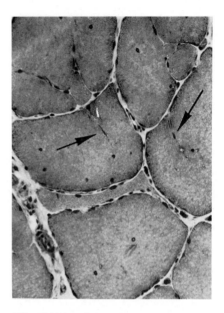

FIG. 7. Facioscapulohumeral muscular dystrophy. Light micrograph showing several hypertrophied fibers and small atrophic angular fibers (*arrows*). Trichrome; ×200.

FIG. 8. Limb-girdle muscular dystrophy. Light micrograph showing numerous split fibers (*arrows*), internal nuclei, and a single degenerating fiber. Trichrome; ×160.

LIMB-GIRDLE MUSCULAR DYSTROPHY

Limb-girdle muscular dystrophy, an autosomal recessive disorder with a variable age of onset and course, is less clearly defined than other forms of dystrophy. It has been suggested that some patients with this diagnosis may have slowly progressive spinal muscular atrophy of the Kugelberg-Welander form (59).

Many authors lump the histopathological alterations of limb-girdle dystrophy with those of the other dystrophies as a single group and point out their similarities. However, Dubowitz and Brooke (10) in a detailed analysis of biopsies from 18 patients with limb-girdle dystrophy showed numerous enlarged fibers, frequent ring fibers, pronounced fiber splitting, and internalization of sarcolemmal nuclei. They indicated that fiber splitting is more frequent in this form of dystrophy than in any other. Others have emphasized the frequency of ring fibers (59). Figure 8 demonstrates internalization of sarcolemmal nuclei and fiber splitting in a biopsy from a patient with limb-girdle dystrophy. Electron microscopic studies of the disorder have demonstrated no unique features (35,38,48).

DISTAL MUSCULAR DYSTROPHY (DISTAL MYOPATHY)

Although Gowers initially reported distal myopathy in 1902, it remained for Welander (60) in 1951 to define this entity clearly. She described 249 cases of distal myopathy in Sweden with the following characteristics: (a) dominant inheritance, (b) onset between 20 and 77 years, with an average of 47 years, (c) three to two male to female ratio, (d) onset of weakness and atrophy in small muscles of distal extremities, (e) slow progression, and (f) myopathic electromyograms and muscle biopsies.

This disorder is rarely reported in the United States. Recently, we have studied a family in which seven members developed a late-onset form of distal myopathy (36) with characteristics similar to those described by Welander. Autopsy was performed on two of these cases and revealed normal brains, spinal cords, and spinal and peripheral nerves. Cardiomyopathy was found in one case. Autopsy muscle and muscle biopsies during life revealed numerous myopathic changes. Subsequently, we have studied another member of this family and two sporadic cases of distal myopathy in younger people.

In general, the histologic changes in distal myopathy are similar to those described in other forms of dystrophy, including variation in muscle fiber size and the presence of central nuclei, necrotic fibers, and fibro-fatty replacement of muscle. Histochemistry studies demonstrated no unusual features. In our cases we found a large number of PAS- and Oil Red O–negative vacuoles in muscle fibers (Fig. 9). In our familial cases, in ad-

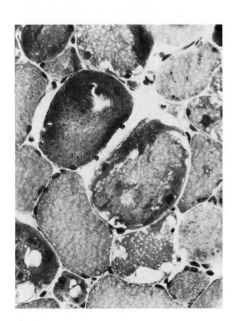

FIG. 9. Distal muscular dystrophy. Light micrograph showing numerous vacuolated fibers and areas of dark granular degeneration. Trichrome; ×200.

dition to extensive vacuolization, we encountered an unusual granular alteration in fibers (Fig. 9).

By electron microscopy, a wide spectrum of alterations were found including severe myofilament disorganization, striking Z-disk alterations, dilatation of the sarcoplasmic reticulum, proliferation of T-tubules, and necrosis and phagocytosis of fibers. Typical contraction clumps were observed in degenerated fibers in nonfamilial cases. The vacuoles in both

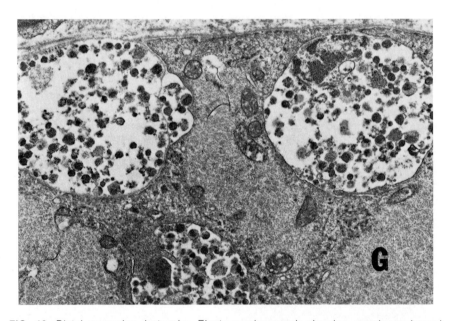

FIG. 10. Distal muscular dystrophy. Electron micrograph showing membrane-bound autophagic vacuoles containing small osmophilic granules, membranous structures, and debris. Also note areas of granular degeneration (G). ×13,500.

familial and sporadic cases were found to be autophagic vacuoles (Fig. 10), a nonspecific alteration which can occur in any myopathy. However, their excessive number in our cases was unusual. Myeloid figures were also prominent. The granular change noted in familial cases consisted of focal granular sarcoplasmic material generally devoid of other organelles (Fig. 10), usually near the surface of fibers. This material was composed of a homogeneous collection of dark and light granules 150 to 400 Å in diameter. Thus our findings indicate that the electron microscopic alterations in distal muscular dystrophy also lack specificity. However, the combination of extensive vacuolization and granular change found in our familial case is relatively unique.

OCULAR MUSCULAR DYSTROPHY (OCULAR MYOPATHY)

Disorders described under the names of ocular muscular dystrophy, progressive dystrophy of the extraocular muscles, ocular myopathy, ocular myopathy of von Graefe-Fuchs, progressive external ophthalmoplegia (PEO), and a number of other names comprise a complicated, poorly understood, wide spectrum of disorders. In this group of neuromuscular disorders the extraocular muscles are affected initially, and in many cases muscles of face, neck, and limbs are subsequently involved. Our knowledge of these

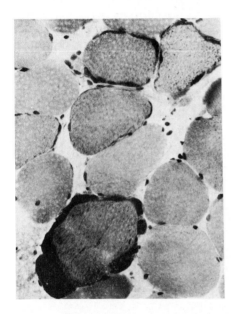

FIG. 11. Progressive external ophthalmoplegia. Light micrograph showing three ragged red fibers. Trichrome; ×200.

disorders is limited by a lack of understanding of the changes in eye muscles. Kiloh and Nevin (31) characterized the changes in eye muscles as myopathic, whereas others have thought the primary pathological alterations were in the cranial nerves or brainstem nuclei. Drachman's (8) review of PEO showed that it could be associated with a variety of neurologic degenerative disorders and emphasized the problem of classifying these disorders (8). In 1958 Kearns and Sayre (30) described a patient with progressive external ophthalmoplegia, heart block, and retinitis pigmentosa. Subsequently, a number of cases of this syndrome have been described, often with the added features of cerebellar ataxia, deafness, mental retardation, and small stature. Olson et al. (46) described a distinct morphological abnormality, ragged red fibers, in skeletal muscle from a group of patients with this syndrome, which they termed oculocraniosomatic neuromuscular disorder.

Recently we have described ragged red fibers in limb muscles in several members of a family with PEO (26). Our cases demonstrated only external ophthalmoplegia and face and shoulder girdle weakness without retinal changes, mental retardation, or cerebellar dysfunction. This syndrome occurred in four successive generations in females only in this family.

Ragged red fibers are characterized by subsarcolemmal and intramyofibrillar accumulations of granular material of irregular contour that stains red with the modified Gomori trichrome method (Fig. 11), deep blue with the NADH-TR reaction, and deep purple with succinic dehydrogenase. The fibers often contain a mild increase in lipid. In PEO the majority of ragged red fibers have been type 1 fibers, although they also have been reported in type 2 fibers. Others have noted small angular fibers suggestive of denervation in PEO, but they were not present in our familial cases.

By electron microscopy, ragged red fibers consist of large aggregates of mitochondria beneath the sarcolemmal membrane (Fig. 12), adjacent to nuclei, or between myofibrils. Mitochondria are large, irregularly shaped,

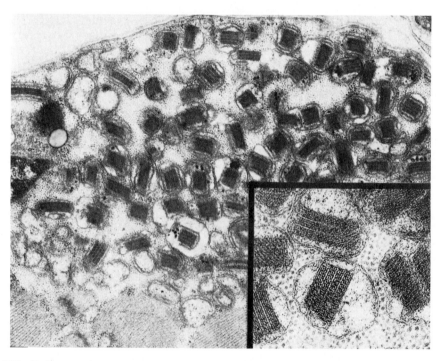

FIG. 12. Progressive external ophthalmoplegia. Electron micrograph of ragged red fiber showing subsarcolemmal collection of mitochondria containing paracrystalline inclusions. Glycogen present between mitochondria. ×10,800. **Inset:** Higher magnification (×60,500) of paracrystalline inclusions.

and often contain paracrystalline inclusions (Fig. 12 and inset, Fig. 12). Others contain concentric crystae, glycogen granules, or fine granular material. Lipid vacuoles and increased amounts of glycogen are also scattered between aggregates of mitochondria.

Ragged red fibers containing similar mitochondrial structures have been observed in a variety of neuromuscular disorders, indicating the nonspecificity of this change. However, they are present in large numbers in association with PEO and, although not pathognomonic, they are suggestive of this disorder.

OCULOPHARYNGEAL MUSCULAR DYSTROPHY

A form of progressive external ophthalmoplegia with dysphagia was given the name of oculopharyngeal muscular dystrophy by Victor et al. in 1962 (58). In addition to external ophthalmoplegia and face, neck, and limb weakness, these patients have considerable difficulty swallowing. A review of the subject by Bray et al. (3) suggested that oculopharyngeal muscular dystrophy has a later onset, more frequent facial weakness, and a higher familial incidence than ocular muscular dystrophy. Myopathic changes similar to those seen in other dystrophies have been reported in skeletal muscle. Dubowitz and Brooke (10) described a series of patients with oculopharyngeal dystrophy in which limb muscles showed variation in fiber size, small angular fibers, moth-eaten and whorled fibers, and occasional internal nuclei. In addition, a distinct change, frequent rimmed vacuoles, was a common link in these cases. By electron microscopy these vacuoles were found to be autophagic in nature (H. E. Neville, *personal communication*).

CONGENITAL MYOPATHIES

Since the description of central core disease in 1956, a group of new disorders has been described and labeled congenital myopathies. The majority of patients with these disorders have symptoms early in life, usually as floppy infants. However, detectable weakness may not develop until later in life. In general, these disorders are nonprogressive or slowly progressive. In a few instances a more rapidly progressive course has occurred, leading to death. These disorders have been defined and named on the basis of specific structural alterations in muscle fibers. The major congenital myopathies are: (a) central core disease, (b) nemaline (rod body) myopathy, (c) centronuclear (myotubular) myopathy, (d) mitochondrial myopathies, and (e) congenital fiber type disproportion. The grouping does not take into consideration the congenital muscular dystrophies, glycogen storage disorders, or myotonic disorders of early onset.

Central Core Disease

In 1956 Shy and Magee (51) initially described central core disease with five cases of a nonprogressive myopathy. After this a number of cases of central core disease were reported. It is inherited in an autosomal dominant pattern and usually causes moderate proximal limb weakness. Muscle biopsy reveals fibers with a central zone of amorphous material surrounded by normal myofibrils. These central zones are deficient in or completely lacking oxidative or glycolytic enzyme activity (Fig. 13). The cores occur primarily in type 1 fibers and may be central or eccentric.

By electron microscopy, cores consist of a disrupted sarcoplasmic pattern with smearing, widening, fragmentation or loss of the Z-band, and degeneration of the myofibrils (Fig. 14). Mitochondria, sarcoplasmic reticulum, glycogen, and the T-system are diminished or absent in cores. Recently, cores have been separated into structured and unstructured cores (45). In the former, ATPase activity is retained, the banding pattern is intact, the core is contracted, and mitochondria are sparse. In the latter, ATPase activity and the banding pattern are lost, myofibrils are degenerated, and mitochondria are absent. Recently, Engel et al. (16) described multicore disease in which multiple small, core-like structures with decreased mitochondria were present in single muscle fibers.

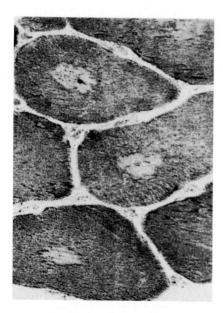

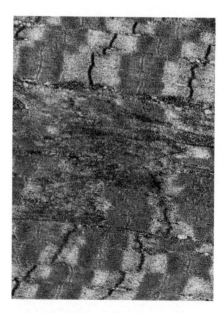

FIG. 13. Central core disease. Cores characterized by loss of enzyme activity in central portion of fibers. NADH-TR; ×260.

FIG. 14. Central core disease. Electron micrograph showing central core of disrupted sarcoplasmic pattern and loss of Z-band. ×14,200.

At the ultrastructural level, unstructured cores have some similarities to target fibers seen in denervation (44). In addition, central cores have been described in association with rod bodies in experimental animals (50) and in human nemaline myopathy (1).

Nemaline (Rod Body) Myopathy

Nemaline myopathy was first described by Shy et al. (52) in 1963 in a 4-year-old child who had been a floppy infant. Subsequently, sporadic and dominant and recessive patterns have been described in this disorder. In addition to presenting as floppy infants or with a mild proximal myopathy early in life, an occasional case has had a malignant course and has been fatal (28,49). Skeletal deformities are common in this disorder.

By light microscopy, variable numbers of dark-staining ovoid or elongated rods are found in any region of the fiber, although they most often accumulate in subsarcolemmal zones. Rods are not easily seen with the hematoxylin and eosin stain, but they are readily seen with the modified Gomori trichrome method (Fig. 15). They are not demonstrated with the usual histochemical enzyme reactions. They have been reported to involve selectively both major fiber types or to lack selectivity. The number of fibers with rods varies from case to case. A variation in fiber size has been described in some cases.

Electron microscopy has revealed rods to be moderately electron-dense, filamentous structures with periodic lines parallel and perpendicular to

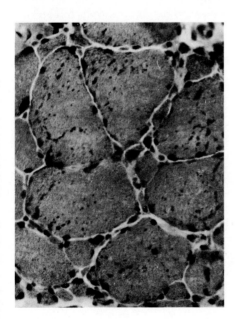

FIG. 15. Scapuloperoneal syndrome. Light micrograph showing fibers containing numerous dark, irregularly shaped rods. Trichrome; ×180.

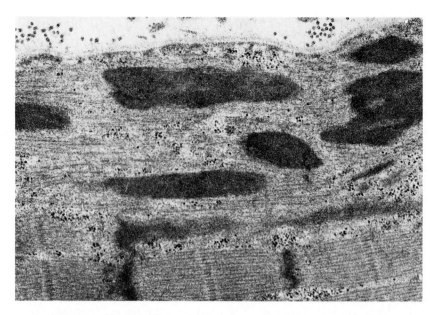

FIG. 16. Scapuloperoneal syndrome. Electron micrograph showing multiple rods in subsarcolemmal location. ×27,500.

their long axis (Fig. 16). Their lattice-like appearance on cross section and continuity with the Z-band (15,24) have led to the concept that they arise from the Z-band. Although rods seem to indicate a relatively specific childhood congenital myopathy in the setting described above, they have also been observed in a wide variety of dissimilar clinical settings. They have been described in normal muscle, muscular dystrophy, polymyositis, and denervation (35); collagen vascular diseases (47); central core disease (1,44); schizophrenia (39); late-onset myopathy (13,18); and a variety of other disorders. Recently, we have observed large numbers of rods in a patient with the scapuloperoneal syndrome (Figs. 15 and 16). These reports have led to the concept that rod formation is a nonspecific alteration of the Z-band that can occur in a variety of disorders and possibly from a variety of causes.

Centronuclear (Myotubular) Myopathy

In 1966 Spiro et al. (54) first described centronuclear myopathy in a 12-year-old child with early-onset weakness, ptosis, ophthalmoplegia, and facial weakness. Subsequently, a number of cases have been recorded with a variety of clinical manifestations. Although most reported cases have been in childhood, a few have occurred in adults. Several different inheritance patterns have been described. The typical microscopic picture of centronuclear myopathy is the presence of one or more nuclei occupying the

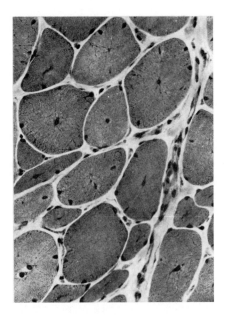

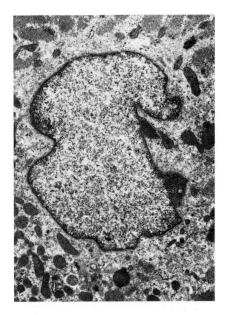

FIG 17. Centronuclear myopathy. Light micrograph showing one or multiple nuclei in central portion of fibers. Trichrome; ×180.

FIG. 18. Electron micrograph showing details of central nucleus of centronuclear myopathy. Note granular material and mitochondria around nucleus. ×9,300.

central portion of the fiber (Fig. 17). With the ATPase reaction there is no activity in the central region of the fiber. Electron microscopy shows normal-appearing nuclei in the center of fibers (Fig. 18). Surrounding the nucleus there is often an absence of myofibrils, numerous mitochondria, glycogen accumulation, and occasional vacuoles (Fig. 18). Opinions are divided over whether these structures represent true myotubes, but the majority of authors suggest this is not the case. Cases in which central nuclei are associated with atrophy of type 1 fibers (2,20,32) have been reported, and it has been suggested that this is a clinically distinct entity.

Cogenital Fiber Type Disproportion

Brooke and Engel (5) described a case in which the only histologic abnormality was a decrease in the size and predominance of type 1 fibers. Subsequently, a series of 12 children with congenital weakness with this histologic picture was described (4). Clinically, these patients are floppy infants and many have contractures of hand and feet muscles, congenital dislocations of the hips, high arch palates, kyphoscoliosis, and feet deformities. In general their weakness improves with age. Muscle biopsy shows small type 1 fibers, relatively large type 2 fibers, and type 1 fiber predominance. Ultrastructurally, Neville (44) demonstrated ring fibers, zigzag alterations in the Z-band, and smearing and distortion of the Z-band in congenital fiber type disproportion. Lenard and Goebel (33) showed sarcomeric disarray and a preferential loss of thick myofilaments in this disorder.

Mitochondrial Myopathies

Mitochondrial alterations in muscle were initially described by Luft et al. (34) in a biopsy from a patient with a nonthyroidal hypermetabolic disorder. Subsequently, Shy et al. (53) described two children with congenital myopathies, one which contained extremely large mitochondria with inclusions in muscle, termed megaconial myopathy, and the other which had an excess of mitochondria, termed pleoconial myopathy. Since that time there has been an abundance of reports in a wide spectrum of neuromuscular diseases in which alterations in mitochondria were a prominent pathological finding. Although an excess of oxidative enzyme activity by light microscopy is suggestive of mitochondrial abnormalities, electron microscopic studies are required to define these changes. Some of the ultrastructural alterations in mitochondria include enlarged mitochondria, abnormally shaped mitochondria, proliferation and abnormal orientation of cristae, increased number of mitochondria, and mitochondrial inclusions. The reader is referred to the work of others (17,35,44) for more detailed discussion of mitochondrial morphological abnormalities.

A variety of inclusions have been described in muscle mitochondria, the most interesting of which is the crystalline or paracrystalline inclusion (Fig. 12). This type of inclusion has been described in a wide variety of neuromuscular disorders, suggesting that it might represent a nonspecific reaction of mitochondria.

Classification of the different disorders with abnormal mitochondria is difficult because of our lack of basic understanding of these changes. Because of the presence of these changes in diverse neuromuscular disorders and their absence in cases with documented biochemical defects of mitochondria, DiMauro et al. (7) emphasize that morphological studies alone are not sufficient for the diagnosis of mitochondrial myopathy. They point out that such a diagnosis should be based on a combination of clinical, morphological, and biochemical information. Perhaps a better understanding of the biochemistry of some of these disorders will allow the classification of mitochondrial myopathies to be placed on a more sound basis.

Lipid Myopathy

Recently, a number of cases of accumulation of excess lipid in muscle fibers have been reported. These patients have shown varied clinical manifestations in a wide range of ages. Several patients were initially diagnosed as having muscular dystrophy. From this heterogeneous group, several patients with a deficiency of carnitine have been identified. Carnitine (gamma-trimethyl amino-beta-hydroxybutyrate) is present in high concentrations in muscle and facilitates long-chain fatty acid transport from the cytoplasm into mitochondria, where they undergo beta-oxidation.

Engel and Angelini (14) initially described carnitine deficiency in a 24-year-old woman, first suspected of having polymyositis. We have studied two patients with carnitine deficiency in muscle, both of whom had normal serum carnitine (37,56). One of these, an 8-year-old boy with early onset of proximal muscle weakness and waddling gait, was initially diagnosed as having Duchenne dystrophy (56). In another case, a 61-year-old woman had experienced proximal muscle weakness for 38 years, and early in her course she was thought to have limb-girdle dystrophy. Subsequently, she developed distal weakness and other clinical and electrophysiologic evidence of a neuropathy (37). Karpati et al. (29) also described carnitine deficiency in a patient with recurrent episodes of hepatic and cerebral dysfunction, under-developed muscles, and weakness.

Histopathologically, all of these cases have demonstrated an excess lipid accumulation in muscle fibers. Lipid vacuoles may not be appreciated in

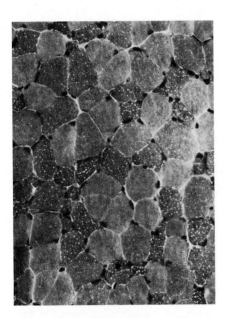

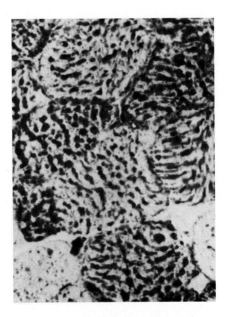

FIG. 19. Carnitine deficiency myopathy. Multiple vacuoles diffusely scattered in fibers. Trichrome; ×200.

FIG. 20. Carnitine deficiency myopathy. Multiple lipid droplets in muscle fibers. Oil Red O stain; ×550.

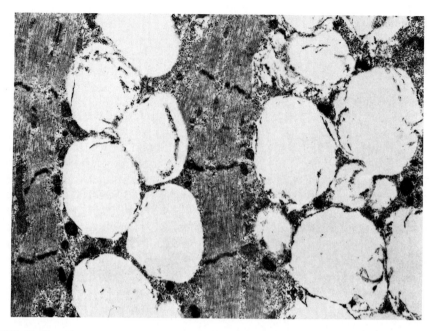

FIG. 21. Carnitine deficiency myopathy. Electron micrograph showing multiple vacuoles replacing myofibrils. Note numerous small mitochondria adjacent to vacuoles. ×16,625.

paraffin-embedded material but can be easily seen in fresh-frozen sections. The vacuoles can be recognized easily with the modified Gomori trichrome method (Fig. 19), and their true nature can be demonstrated with the Oil Red O stain (Fig. 20). They are most pronounced in type 1 fibers in most cases. By electron microscopy, muscle fibers contain variable-sized vacuoles, often in parallel rows (Fig. 21) or in large groups. In some instances, a major portion of the fiber is replaced by lipid vacuoles. Vacuoles were often adjacent to mitochondria. Mitochondria with concentric crystae and numerous tiny mitochondria were present in one of our cases (37). It is of interest that this case also showed many similar vacuoles in Schwann cells and leukocytes, suggesting a generalized disorder of carnitine metabolism. It should be emphasized that all cases in which excess lipid is stored in muscle are not associated with a deficiency of carnitine (27).

ACKNOWLEDGMENTS

The author wishes to thank Drs. Robert Griggs and Jerry Mendell for sharing biopsy material for study. The technical assistance of Ms. Miranda Broyles and Katherine Stintz and the secretarial work of Mrs. Debbie Weber are appreciated.

REFERENCES

1. Afifi, A. K., Smith, J. W., and Zellweger, H. (1965): Cogenital nonprogressive myopathy. Central core disease and nemaline myopathy in one family. *Neurology (Minneap.),* 15:371–381.
2. Bethlem, J., van Wijngaarden, G. K., Meijer, A. E. F. H., et al. (1969): Neuromuscular disease with type I fibre atrophy. Central nuclei and myotube-like structure. *Neurology (Minneap.),* 19:705–710.
3. Bray, G. M., Kaarsoo, M., and Ross, R. T. (1965): Ocular myopathy with dysphagia. *Neurology (Minneap.),* 15:678–684.
4. Brooke, M. H. (1971): A neuromuscular disease characterized by fibre types disproportion. In: *Proceedings of the Second International Congress of Muscle Disorders,* edited by B. A. Kakulas. Excerpta Medica, Amsterdam.
5. Brooke, M. H., and Engel, W. K. (1969): The histographic analysis of human muscle biopsies with regard to fiber types. Four children's biopsies. *Neurology (Minneap.),* 19:591–605.
6. Cullen, M. J., and Fulthorpe, J. J. (1975): Stages in fibre breakdown in Duchenne muscular dystrophy. *J. Neurol. Sci.,* 24:179–200.
7. DiMauro, S., Schotland, D. L., Bonalla, E., et al. (1974): Mitochondrial myopathies: Which and how many? In: *Exploratory Concepts in Muscular Dystrophy II. Proceedings of an International Conference.* Excerpta Medica, Amsterdam.
8. Drachman, D. A. (1968): Ophthalmoplegia plus. The neurodegenerative disorders associated with progressive external ophthalmoplegia. *Arch. Neurol.,* 18:654–674.
9. Dubowitz, V. (1975): Neuromuscular disorders in childhood. *Arch. Dis. Child.,* 50:335–346.
10. Dubowitz, V., and Brooke, M. (1973): *Muscle Biopsy: A Modern Approach.* W. B. Saunders Co., Philadelphia.
11. Duchenne, G. G. (1861): *De l'Electrisation Localisce et son Application a la Pathologie et a la Therapeutique, 2nd Ed.* Bailliere, Paris.
12. Duchenne, G. (1868): Recherches sur le paralysie musculaire pseudohypertrophique ou paralysie myosderosique. *Arch. Gen. Med.,* 11:532–573.
13. Engel, A. G. (1966): Late onset rod myopathy (a new syndrome?): Light and electron microscopic observation in two cases. *Mayo Clin. Proc.,* 41:713–741.
14. Engel, A. G., and Angelini, C. (1973): Carnitine deficiency of human muscle with associated lipid storage myopathy: A new syndrome. *Science,* 179:899–902.
15. Engel, A. G., and Gomez, M. R. (1967): Nemaline (Z disk) myopathy; observations on the origin, structure and solubility properties of the nemaline structures. *J. Neuropathol. Exp. Neurol.,* 26:601–619.
16. Engel, A. G., Gomez, M. R., and Groover, R. V. (1971): Multicore disease. *Mayo Clin. Proc.,* 46:666–681.
17. Engel, A. G., and Macdonald, R. D. (1969): Ultrastructural reactions in muscle disease and their light-microscopic correlates. In: *Proceedings of the International Congress of Muscle Diseases,* edited by J. N. Walton, N. Coral, and G. Scarlato. Excerpta Medica, Milan.
18. Engel, W. K. (1967): A critique of congenital myopathies and other disorders. In: *Exploratory Concepts in Muscular Dystrophy and Related Disorders,* edited by A. T. Milhorat. Excerpta Medica, Amsterdam.
19. Engel, W. K. (1973): Duchenne muscular dystrophy: A histologically based ischemic hypothesis and comparison with experimental ischemia myopathy. In: *The Striated Muscle,* edited by C. M. Pearson and F. K. Mostofi. Williams & Wilkins, Baltimore.
20. Engel, W. K., Gold, G. N., and Karpati, G. (1968): Type I fiber hypotrophy and central nuclei. *Arch. Neurol.,* 18:435–444.
21. Erb, W. H. (1891): Dystrophia muscularis progressiva. Klinische und pathologieanatomische studien. *Dtsch. Z. Nervenheilkunde,* 1:13–94.
22. Fardeau, M. (1970): Ultrastructural lesions in progressive muscular dystrophy. A critical study of their specificity. In: *Muscle Diseases,* edited by N. Coral, G. Scarlato, and J. N. Walton. Excerpta Medica, Amsterdam.
23. Gardner-Medwin, D., and Walton, J. N. (1969): A classification of the neuromuscular

disorder and a note on the clinical examinations of the voluntary muscles. In: *Disorders of the Voluntary Muscle,* edited by J. N. Walton. Little, Brown and Co., Boston.

24. Gonatas, N. K. (1966): The fine structure of the rod-like bodies in nemaline myopathy and their relation to the Z-discs. *J. Neuropathol. Exp. Neurol.,* 25:409–421.
25. Griesinger, W. (1865): Uber muskelhypertrophie. *Arch. Heilkunde,* 6:1–13.
26. Iannaccone, S. T., Griggs, R. C., Markesbery, W. R., and Joynt, R. J. (1974): Familial progressive external ophthalmoplegia and ragged-red fibers. *Neurology (Minneap.),* 24:1033–1038.
27. Jerusalem, F., Spiess, H., and Baumgartner, G. (1975): Lipid storage myopathy with normal carnitine levels. *J. Neurol. Sci.,* 24:273–282.
28. Karpati, G., Carpenter, S., and Andermann, F. (1971): A new concept of childhood nemaline myopathy. *Arch. Neurol.,* 24:291–304.
29. Karpati, G., Carpenter, S., Engel, A. G., et al. (1974): The syndrome of systemic carnitine deficiency. *Neurology (Minneap.),* 25:16–24.
30. Kearns, T. P., and Sayre, G. P. (1958): Retinitis pigmentosa, external ophthalmoplegia and complete heart block. *Arch. Ophthalmol.,* 60:280–289.
31. Kiloh, L. G., and Nevin, S. (1951): Progressive dystrophy of the external ocular muscle (ocular myopathy). *Brain,* 74:115–143.
32. Kinoshita, M., Satoyoski, E., and Matsuo, N. (1975): Myotubular myopathy and type I fiber atrophy in a family. *J. Neurol. Sci.,* 26:575–582.
33. Lenard, H. G., and Goebel, H. H. (1975): Congenital fibre type disproportion. *Neuropaediatrie,* 6:220–231.
34. Luft, R., Ikkos, D., Palmieri, G., et al. (1962): A case of severe hypermetabolism of nonthyroid origin with a defect in maintenances of mitochondrial respiratory control: A correlated clinical, biochemical and morphological study. *J. Clin. Invest.,* 41:1776–1804.
35. Mair, W. G. P., and Tome, F. M. S. (1972): *Atlas of the Ultrastructure of Diseased Human Muscle.* Williams & Wilkins, Baltimore.
36. Markesbery, W. R., Griggs, R. C., Leach, R. P., et al. (1974): Late onset hereditary distal myopathy. *Neurology (Minneap.),* 24:127–134.
37. Markesbery, W. R., McQuillen, M. P., Procopis, P. G., et al. (1974): Muscle carnitine deficiency associated with lipid myopathy, vacuolar neuropathy and vacuolated leucocytes. *Arch. Neurol.,* 31:320–324.
38. Mastaglia, F. L., Papdimitriou, J. M., and Kakulas, B. A. (1969): Restricted forms of muscular dystrophy: A study of 11 cases. *Proc. Aust. Assoc. Neurol.,* 6:107–121.
39. Meltzer, H., McBride, E., and Poppei, R. W. (1973): Rod (nemaline) bodies in the skeletal muscle of an acute schizophrenic patient. *Neurology (Minneap.),* 23:769–780.
40. Meryon, E. (1852): On granular and fatty degeneration of voluntary muscles. *Med. Chir. Trans.,* 35:73–84.
41. Milhorat, A. T., Shafiq, S. A., and Goldstone, L. (1966): Changes in muscle structure in dystrophic patients, carriers, and normal siblings seen by electron microscopy; correlation with levels of serum creatine phosphokinase (CPK). *Ann. N.Y. Acad. Sci.,* 138:246–292.
42. Mokri, B., and Engel, A. G. (1975): Duchenne dystrophy. Electron microscopic findings pointing to a basic or early abnormality in the plasma membrane of the muscle fiber. *Neurology (Minneap.),* 25:1111–1120.
43. Munsat, T. L., Piper, D., Cancilla, P., et al. (1972): Inflammatory myopathy with facioscapulo-humeral distribution. *Neurology (Minneap.),* 22:335–347.
44. Neville, H. E. (1973): Ultrastructural change in muscle disease. In: *Muscle Biopsy: A Modern Approach,* edited by V. Dubowitz and M. Brooke. W. B. Saunders Co., Philadelphia.
45. Neville, H. E., and Brooke, M. H. (1971): Central core fibers: Structured and unstructured. In: *Second International Congress on Muscle Diseases.* Excerpta Medica, Perth.
46. Olson, W., Engel, W. K., Walsh, G. O., et al. (1972): Oculocraniosomatic neuromuscular disease with "ragged-red" fibers. *Arch. Neurol.,* 26:193–211.
47. Rewcastle, N. B., and Humphrey, J. G. (1965): Vacuolar myopathy: Clinical, histochemical and microscopic study. *Arch. Neruol.,* 12:570–582.
48. Santa, T. (1969): Fine structures of the human skeletal muscle in myopathy. *Arch. Neurol.,* 21:479–489.

49. Shafiq, S. A., Dubowitz, V., Peterson, J., et al. (1967): Nemaline myopathy: report of a fatal case with histochemical and electron microscopic studies. *Brain,* 90:817–828.
50. Shafiq, S. A., Goryck, M. A., Asiedu, S. A., et al. (1969): Tenotomy. Effect in the fine structure of the soleus of the rat. *Arch. Neurol.,* 20:625–633.
51. Shy, G. M., and Magee, K. R. (1956): A new congenital non-progressive myopathy. *Brain,* 79:610–621.
52. Shy, G. M., Engel, W. K., Somers, J. E., et al. (1963): Nemaline myopathy. A new congenital myopathy. *Brain,* 86:793–810.
53. Shy, G. M., Gonatas, N. K., and Perez, M. (1966): Childhood myopathies with abnormal mitochondria. I. Megaconial myopathy. II. Pleoconial myopathy. *Brain,* 89:133–158.
54. Spiro, A. J., Shy, G. M., and Gonatas, N. K. (1966): Myotubular myopathy. *Arch. Neurol.,* 14:1–14.
55. Van Breeman, V. L. (1960): Ultrastructure of human muscle II. Observations on dystrophic muscle fibers. *Am. J. Pathol.,* 37:333–341.
56. Vandyke, D. J., Griggs, R. C., Markesbery, W. R., and DiMauro, S. (1975): Hereditary carnitine deficiency of muscle. *Neurology (Minneap.),* 25:154–159.
57. van Wijngaarden, G. K., and Bethlem, J. (1971): The facioscapulohumeral syndrome. In: *Proceedings of the Second International Congress on Muscle Disease,* edited by B. A. Kakulas. Excerpta Medica, Amsterdam.
58. Victor, M., Hayes, R., and Adams, R. D. (1962): Oculopharyngeal muscular dystrophy. *N. Engl. J. Med.,* 267:1267–1272.
59. Walton, J. N. (1973): Progressive muscular dystrophy: Structural alterations in various stages and in carriers of Duchenne dystrophy. In: *The Striated Muscle,* edited by C. M. Pearson and F. K. Mostofi. Williams & Wilkins, Baltimore.
60. Welander, L. (1951): Myopathia distalis tarda hereditaria. *Acta Med. Scand. [Suppl. 265],* 141:1–124.

Advances in Neurology, Vol. 17, edited by
R. C. Griggs and R. T. Moxley, III. Raven Press,
New York © 1977.

Investigative Approach to the Muscular Dystrophies

W. King Engel

National Institutes of Health, Bethesda, Maryland 20014

INTRODUCTION

What are "the muscular dystrophies"? They are a heterogenous group of disorders comprised of a few of the inherited myopathies (myopathies = nonneurogenic neuromuscular disorders). Because the term "muscular dystrophy" is applied to only a few diseases on a historical basis, it has no logical definition. Furthermore, not all diseases in the literature bearing the name "muscular dystrophy" are inherited—for example, vitamin E deficiency dystrophy in animals is clearly an exogenous deficiency disorder. Conversely, clearly inherited but metabolically delineated diseases of muscle, such as phosphorylase deficiency, acid maltase deficiency, and phosphofructokinase deficiency, do not bear the name "dystrophy" but perhaps they should, especially acid maltase deficiency which is associated with progressive muscle weakness and wasting. Therefore, we use the term "muscular dystrophies" not as a categorical one but only as a nonlogical historic term related to a certain few diseases. And, of course, there is not *a* muscular dystrophy, but *a number of* dystrophies. None of the inherited human diseases formally bearing the name "dystrophy" is of known cause, and thus none has yet been proved to be primary in the muscle cell (note acid maltase deficiency, below). We have postulated that some of them, e.g., Duchenne dystrophy and myotonic atrophy, may not be (see below). There is no proof that any animal inherited myopathy (in chickens, mice, hamsters, or turkeys) is a specific model of any human disease. Such a connection must remain to be established—the chances of their being of similar pathogenesis seems unlikely. Anyone suggesting an analogy between an animal hereditary myopathy and a human "muscular dystrophy" is obliged to state of which one of the human dystrophies is the animal disease a proposed model, because the few human diseases bearing the name "muscular dystrophy" are very different each from the other clinically, histologically, and in pattern of genetic inheritance.

This chapter reviews some of our investigative approaches to certain muscular dystrophies and other neuromuscular diseases. The application of histochemistry and ultrastructure has been reviewed elsewhere. The biochemical approach generates various reports reflecting various degrees of quality, insight, and prudence. We have suggested (75) that cautious interpretation of biochemical findings necessitates that for each biochemical abnormality reported the author be obliged to state his estimation of: (a) its specificity for disease, and (b) its importance to pathogenesis of the disease. That would generate the use not only of normal controls but also of the even more important but often neglected disease controls. For example, in studies of Duchenne muscular dystrophy muscle biopsies one must have disease controls with comparable numbers of regenerating, regenerating-degenerating (regen-degen) (59), and degenerating fibers in the biopsy. In studies of erythrocytes in Duchenne dystrophy patients, other diseases with chronic prominent elevation in the serum of muscle leakage products, e.g., "muscle enzymes" and myoglobin, must be disease controls, because it is hypothetically possible that chronic elevation of some of them could induce certain changes in blood cell membrane structure or function or in other factors. In studying the muscle tissue biochemically seeking the cause of a muscle degeneration disease, one often presumes that the cause lies within muscle as an organ. If the cause is imposed on the muscle cells from outside themselves, e.g., in the form of a circulating toxin or deficiency or a local vascular abnormality, that approach probably would be fruitless. For example, would the grind-and-find biochemical approach applied to study the spinal cord in subacute combined degeneration ever have led to the understanding that the disease is due to malabsorption of vitamin B_{12} because of lack of intrinsic factor from the stomach? A tissue culture approach to human muscle diseases will be referred to below in regard to muscle phosphorylase deficiency, acid maltase deficiency, diseases with ragged-red fibers, and certain vacuolar myopathies (8,9,157). Tissue culture methods, in conjunction with enhancing agents, might also be used to bring out either viral antigen or viral particles in various human neuromuscular diseases of unknown cause, especially inflammatory and dysimmune ones. For example, tissue culture potentially could be used to seek a virus in cultures of muscle cells from dermatomyositis/polymyositis patients or of thymus cells from myasthenia gravis patients. A possible model was the showing of a large amount of C-particles and viral antigen in "normal" chick muscle in tissue culture and their increased detectability after the provoking agent dinitrophenol (6,68).

Clinical electromyography (EMG) can be of considerable value in identifying the presence of disease. There are some limitations to the identification of the nature of the disease process in terms of lower motor neuron disease versus muscle disease. Loss of whole motor units as identified by ordinary EMG is fairly reliable evidence of neuropathy, as are very enlarged units (presumably based on collateral sprouting and foster innervation of orphaned muscle fibers) (54,85). However, the presence of a brief-duration, small-amplitude, overly abundant motor unit action potential (BSAP) EMG pattern is not, in our opinion, conclusive evidence of a myopathy, contrary to what has been said in the past—on theoretical grounds it can also be seen in any neurogenic disorder causing fractionation of the motor unit by direct involvement of a portion of the axonal twigs in each axonal tree or as a partial-unit expression of a total-motor neuron disease (60,61,85). Thus the concept of a "myopathic EMG" is wrong—there is none-such animal. Some investigators (J. Goodgold and N. Spielholtz, *personal communication*) support this concept although others (23,87,101,162) are still encumbered with the old concept.

Single-fiber electromyography is a refinement of clinical EMG (45,176, 177). This is useful for identifying "jitter" and "blocking," prolongation of the motor-unit potential in a form of small-spike polyphasia that would be missed by ordinary EMG, and densification of the motor unit. Although the last is seen most strikingly in neurogenic disease, presumably based on collateral sprouting and foster innervation of neurogenously orphaned muscle fibers, it is present to some extent in Duchenne dystrophy (E. Stål-berg, *personal communication*). We have therefore reviewed our Duchenne dystrophy biopsies and found the presumed histochemical parallel, "tiny type-grouping." We have also noted (*unpublished observations*) tiny type-grouping in experimental ischemic myopathy (130,131,174,175), as have others (106), and in chronic or recovering stages of dermatomyositis/poly-myositis (*unpublished observations*). We consider tiny type-groupings (and slight electrical densification of some motor units) in these myopathic disorders to be based on collateral sprouting and reinnervation of myogenously deinnervated muscle fibers. Motor and sensory nerve conduction times and distal latency measurements can be used to identify the presence of nerve involvement and show something of its nature, but normal values do not exclude neural involvement. The incrementing-stimulation technique, introduced supposedly to count the total number of motor units in a muscle by electromyographic examination (120), is controversial (14,85,146,147). The original author (120) finds a decreased total number of whole motor units in every neuromuscular disease studied. We doubt the validity of the technique for reasons detailed elsewhere and so dismiss all conclusions and hypotheses based on it (63,85).

Our new concept of "myogenous deinnervation" should be explained. We propose that lower motor neuron (LMN) influence on muscle fibers (resulting in "malinnervated fibers") can be abnormal for the following basic reasons [with real (A_1, B_1, C_1) and hypothetical (A_2, B_2) examples]: A_1—neurogenous deinnervation (axon transection); A_2—neurogenous dysinnervation (partially faulty delivery of LMN influence to muscle fiber); B_1—myogenous deinnervation (separation of a remaining viable portion of a muscle fiber from the original portion containing the neuromuscular junction, as by longitudinal splitting or transverse focal lesion); B_2—myogenous dysinnervation (partially faulty reception or translation of the LMN influence by the muscle fiber); C_1—primary noninnervation (pre-innervated state of generating muscle fibers in embryogenesis, regeneration *in vivo*, regeneration in tissue culture). A_1, B_1, and C_1 result in the identical appearance of diffuse plasmalemmal ("extrajunctional") acetylcholine receptors (8,10,11,154–156). Hypothetically, A_2 and B_2 might or might not, depending on the qualitative and quantitative aspects of the abnormality.

In this brief chapter will be given examples of our investigative approaches to some of the myopathies and some of the diseases that are of yet unproven pathogenesis regarding myopathic versus neuropathic, but the definite neuropathies will not be discussed.

BIOCHEMICALLY DISTINCT MYOPATHIES

Muscle Phosphorylase Deficiency

Muscle phosphorylase deficiency is discussed by Dr. DiMauro (*this volume*). From our own work we would emphasize that clinically there is not only the well-known juvenile form but also an adult-onset form (in regard to clinical expression), which we have seen in four cases of three families (73; W. K. Engel, *unpublished observations*). In all types of cases, phosphorylase has been shown to become rejuvenated in regenerating muscle fibers, as seen both *in vivo* and after a spontaneous attack or after direct injury of muscle (157; W. K. Engel, R. Brumback, and R. W. Kula, *unpublished observations*), and in tissue-cultured muscle from the patients (8,157). The phosphorylase of the muscle in tissue culture from these patients is like that of cultured normal muscle having both muscle-type and brain-type isozymes (40). It is known that liver phosphorylase is functionally normal (per response to glucagon) in this disease complex, and leukocyte phosphorylase and vascular smooth muscle phosphorylase are measurably normal (73). However, the status of phosphorylase in motor neurons is not known. Because motor neurons normally have a large amount of phosphorylase (26–28,53), at least hypothetically they too could have a deficiency of the enzyme, although there is nearly no evidence of malfunction of the motor neurons from the clinical, electromyographic, or histochemical point of view—there are only rare small, angular NADH-TR-dark, i.e., denervated-looking, muscle fibers in such patients (W. K. Engel, *unpublished observations*).

Acid Maltase Deficiency

In biopsies of six acid maltase deficiency patients, four chronic infantile and two adult-onset cases, the biochemical and morphologic (glycogen-laden lysosomes) defects have been shown to be reincarnated in muscle fibers grown *de novo* in tissue culture from the patients' muscle biopsy (8,9). That was the first demonstration that a biochemical defect exists primarily in muscle cells, as evidenced by its reincarnability in culture away from other bodily environmental influences such as the blood, the nervous system, and "use." Having the living muscle cells with the actual identified defect available in culture provides a potential test object for therapeutic trials *in vitro*.

UNUSUAL NEUROMUSCULAR CONDITIONS

Here we will discuss four groups of disorders that are of uncertain pathogenesis regarding whether they are myopathic or neuropathic.

Rod Disease

Rod disease is usually manifest in the form of a congenital, very slowly progressive disorder (66,83,172,173), but there is also an adult-onset form (48,80,81). Small rods accumulate in the cytoplasm of many muscle fibers. They have a characteristic morphologic appearance of approximately 180 Å periodicity and appear to develop as lateral aggrandizementing of the Z-discs. Rods therefore appear to represent excessive formation of Z-disc structures. Since the Z-discs are composed of actin and α-actinin, it is likely that the rods are also. We consider that the rods, like normal Z-discs, are actin filaments "decorated" with osmiophilic material at least part of which is α-actinin and cross-linked in a three-dimensional grid pattern. Antibody against α-actinin has been shown to react with rods as it does with normal Z-discs (78,167). The congenital cases typically have marked "type II fiber paucity" (the designation preferred to the equally descriptive "type I fiber predominance because it probably more correctly suggests the pathokinetic mechanism), and therefore a major or minor neurogenic element remains a possibility (54,66,85). Rods can be produced experimentally by tenotomy (70,153). They also have been found in rhabdomyosarcomas, some cases of dermatomyositis, and sometimes at the neuromuscular junction in otherwise normal biopsies (51,66) — each of these occurrences is harmonious with our suggestion that the rods may result, at least partly, from an abnormality of tension on the muscle fiber (66,80). Recently, rods have been found in a number of muscle nuclei in two patients with late-onset rod disease (66,80). The rods were histochemically and ultrastructurally identical to those in the cytoplasm. It is a question whether they represent intranuclear formation of the rod structure or transport of subunit precursors of it into the nucleus through the nuclear pores from the cytoplasm. The latter general mechanism is favored since nuclei are not sites of significant protein synthesis. The nuclear pores are known to admit molecules to up to approximately 50,000 to 60,000 M.W. Possible subunits of the rods which could be transported include subunits of actin (as G-actin, 43,000 to 47,000 M.W.) and tropomyosin B (33,000 M.W.) (43,44,108,124,

180); α-actinin has not yet been considered to be smaller than 95,000 (107,180), but it is possible that subunits will be found. Such a "transnuclear pore" mechanism would represent a new type of pathogenic mechanism. Recently two patients with dermatomyositis have been found to have a few nuclei with histochemically similar rods by light microscopy (W. K. Engel, *unpublished observations*). A transnuclear pore transport of subunits might underlie their formation too. Previously, it has been shown that an occasional patient with dermatomyositis can have some fibers with abundant cytoplasmic rods (51). To date, rods have not been reincarnated in muscle fibers tissue-cultured from any type of patient.

Central Core Disease

Central core disease is not yet resolved regarding a neurogenic versus myopathic origin. We favor the former (54,62,85) on the basis of: (a) histochemical and electron microscopic similarity of the core lesions to target fibers of ordinary denervation; (b) marked type II fiber paucity (I fiber predominance); (c) the presence of cores in certain type-grouped fibers in chronic peripheral neuropathy (peroneal muscular atrophy) patients; (d) experimental production of core-like lesions by total denervation of cat muscle (70), and their similarity to the target-like lesions recently produced by partial denervation of cat muscle (29); and (e) absence of any definitely myopathic features in the biopsy. The marked type I fiber predominance in the central core disease patients as demonstrable with the regular myofibrillar ATPase reaction was, in two of our patients, shown by the single-fiber EMG technique not to represent increased motor unit density (E. Stålberg, T. Bertorini, and W. K. Engel, *unpublished observations*) – histochemistry showed that there was rather even distribution and intermixture of type I fiber subtypes, as defined previously (7), in the large areas of type I fiber predominance (W. K. Engel and T. Bertorini, *unpublished observations*). This demonstrates that the regular ATPase for identifying the two primary muscle fiber types is sufficient to exclude type-grouping and type-predominance if a normal pattern is seen, but it is not sufficient to identify the presence of these changes positively unless subtype-grouping or predominance of subtypes is seen. It also supports the previous suggestion (54,55,84,85) that muscle fiber subtypes are determined by hypothetical corresponding subtypes of lower motor neurons. In central core disease the apparently normal distribution of the muscle fibers of the motor units that are there and the type-paucity support the previous suggestion (61,62) that the disorder is due, on a neuronal basis, to a congenital paucity of entire type II units – during either primary formation of motor units or perhaps early loss of type II units during early fetogenesis – but it is not acquired at a stage when neuronal loss would provoke collateral sprouting of axonal twigs from surviving motor neurons to innervate formed muscle fibers which had become denervated. The principle and necessity of evaluating subtype-grouping was further emphasized in another patient, one with atypical neuromuscular disease who had marked type I fiber predominance —she had an even distribution of type I fiber subtypes, correlated with no increased density of muscle fibers in motor units by the single-fiber EMG technique.

Benign Congenital Hypotonia

Benign congenital hypotonia with type II fiber paucity (type I fiber predominance) (62,69) is one kind of disorder within the general category of "benign congenital hypotonia syndrome." The type II fiber paucity, as well as a BAP pattern on EMG and the clinical presentation and course, is like that of central core disease, which led to our proposing that both disorders are caused by a similar pathogenic mechanism, namely, marked nondevelopment and/or hypoplasia of a number of type II motor units and slight nondevelopment and/or hypoplasia of a few type I units (61,62). Some of those II fiber paucity BCH patients, like central core disease patients, have an occasional small angular NADH-TR-dark fiber as do central core patients, suggesting a minimal smouldering neuronal failure (62,69).

Malignant Hyperthermia Rigidity Syndrome

In three families with central core disease, the malignant hyperthermia rigidity (MHR) syndrome has now been associated. We have studied two (47; W. K. Engel, *unpublished observations*): one was from Australia (37), and one from South Africa (100). Because both conditions are rare, this association must be considered more than chance. The MHR syndrome is a severe reaction provoked by the events of general anesthesia, usually attributed to the effects of halothane and/or succinylcholine, but a number of other agents have occasionally been provocative (47,92). The hyperthermia is usually associated with generalized severe muscle rigidity, although either can occur alone. Muscle fiber plasmalemmal breakdown occurs, leading to outpouring of muscle fiber contents, e.g., creatine phosphokinase (CPK), myoglobin, and potassium from the breached muscle fibers; and presumably serum contents, e.g., calcium and proteins, pour in (see below). Although some have postulated that the defect is of sarcoplasmic reticulum (SR) and its inability to take up and hold calcium, we propose (47,67) that the disorder is based to a large extent on a particular susceptibility of the muscle fiber plasmalemmal membrane to the provoking agents (with a possible additional susceptibility of the sarcoplasmic reticulum). Quite harmonious are the following: (a) Halothane induction of contracture in human MH muscle *in vitro* is not possible when extracellular calcium (in the bath) is removed but returns again when calcium is readded

(139). (b) Procaine, a treatment for MH (see below), not only reduces loss of Ca^{2+} from the SR (18,181,188) but also stabilizes the plasmalemma (169) and antagonizes calcium influx (18). [Marcaine, another local anesthetic, causes acute muscle necrosis (94), probably by a toxicity to the plasmalemma.] (c) Dantrolene sodium, a treatment for MH (see below), not only reduces loss of Ca^{2+} from the SR but, because it is a hydantoin, might also have a plasmalemmal-stabilizing effect on pathologic plasmalemma. It is known that diphenylhydantoin hyperpolarizes and stabilizes the plasmalemma and increases the sodium gradient, which could increase calcium efflux since that occurs by an exchange with extracellular sodium (18). (d) Succinylcholine in normal patients often causes detectable myoglobinemia. This toxic effect on the muscle fiber, presumably its plasmalemma, is seen in at least 20% of pediatric patients (13,164), the age-group susceptible to MH, but not in adults. (e) A major increase ($2\times$) of total calcium was found in the muscle biopsy in a patient 4 days after an MH episode. The intracellular effects of increased calcium causing the hyperthermia and rigidity are detailed below under Duchenne muscular dystrophy.

A rather close model of the MHR syndrome is present in some strains of pig (1,96,110), the clinical attack being provokable by halothane, succinylcholine, or even extreme excitement. Patients with the MHR syndrome often have some type of neuromuscular disease, but in most it is not a well-characterized one. Moreover, the MHR syndrome is not associated with the clinically pathologically well-defined neuromuscular diseases, other than its presumptive association with central core disease. For example, it has not yet been reported in association with Duchenne muscular dystrophy, myotonic atrophy, facioscapular humeral dystrophy, infantile and juvenile proximal spinal muscular atrophy, amyotrophic lateral sclerosis, chronic peripheral neuropathies, or myasthenia gravis. It has been associated in patients with extraocular movement disorder ("squint") and various "orthopedic abnormalities." The exact sort of underlying neuromuscular disease in each of these cases was not clarified by special studies. MHR syndrome is not one specific disease—it is a pathophysiological response, like coma, footdrop, or jaundice, and is not to be considered a single entity. Thus, one cannot speak of the inheritance of MHR. In some families there is a dominantly inherited propensity to develop MHR (22,37,111), and occasionally it is associated with mild persistent elevation of serum CPK values. If central core disease is indeed neurogenic as postulated, perhaps in other patients with the MHR response the muscles are also predisposed on the basis of atypical neuropathic mechanism. Whether the predisposition to develop MHR is usually neuropathic or myopathic is not known.

Abnormalities of the acute attack of MHR and the urgent treatment they require are hyperthermia—cooling externally and by gastric, rectal, and peritoneal lavage; metabolic acidosis—bicarbonate; hyperkalemia—glucose and insulin; hypocalcemia—calcium gluconate; and rigidity—procaine or procainamide (avoiding lidocaine) and possibly dantrolene (1,16,21,24, 95,96,117,138,139,143), when it becomes available for parenteral use in humans. (It may be important to correct the acidosis before giving procaine or procainamide.) (95,97,98.) The anesthesia should be ceased as rapidly as possible. Prevention includes obtaining a careful history for any such reaction in a patient to be operated on or in any other members of the family, avoidance of the more provocative drugs, and careful monitoring of the patient's temperature throughout the anesthesia. We suggest that loading with oral dantrolene before the anesthesia may be helpful since parenteral dantrolene (not yet available for human use) prevents and reverses the MHR syndrome in susceptible pigs (1,96), and oral loading can completely prevent it in those pigs (96). Dantrolene is considered to lessen the release of calcium from the SR (46,136). Whether this is its only effect on muscle is not known – it is a hydantoin and conceivably could affect the plasmalemma like other hydantoins do. Screening of all patients prior to general anesthesia by obtaining their CPK values has been suggested. That would be of limited value because a number of patients who develop MHR do not have elevated basal CPKs, and most of those with mildly or prominently elevated CPKs do not develop MHR (e.g., Duchenne dystrophy patients).

CLINICALLY AND/OR GENETICALLY "DISTINCT" NEUROMUSCULAR DISORDERS

The first two discussed are specific diseases and the other two are mixed syndromes.

Myotonic Atrophy

Myotonic atrophy previously was called myotonic dystrophy. The former term is preferred because it indicates the typical pathology of the early-affected muscle, demonstrable especially well in the biceps brachialis muscle. The muscle fibers atrophy, usually with a preference for type I fibers to atrophy (50,54,71,85). A number of the atrophic fibers (71,85) have the histochemical characteristics of denervated fibers (71,85). These progress on to pyknotic nuclear clumps, resembling those of ordinary denervation. Occasionally a target fiber is seen. From these histochemical findings we have suggested that the disease might be neurogenic (54,56,85). Abnormalities of motor axonal endings have been shown by others (33,121). The muscle EMG findings of myotonic atrophy are not in disagreement with a neurogenic pathogenesis because the BSAP pattern could reflect fractionation of the motor unit on the basis either of a neuropathic partial-unit disease or of a partial-unit expression of a total-unit neuronal disease (56, 61,85).

Another possibility, which we consider somewhat less likely, is that the muscle fiber is abnormal because it cannot properly receive or translate the neural influence on it, i.e., a "myogenous dysinnervation" mechanism (56,85; W. K. Engel, *unpublished observations*). We emphasize that our hypothesis is not one of loss of total motor units, contrary to what we consider the erroneous view of others (120). Some recent electrical findings of neural tissue abnormality are in harmony with our dysneural hypothesis (25,148). Bizarre high-frequency (pseudomyotonic) potentials and even true myotonia can be seen in occasional frankly neurogenic diseases, and so do not necessarily reflect a primary muscle plasmalemmal defect, contrary to what is often stated.

Two rather special metabolic defects offer potential avenues toward the primary metabolic defect in myotonic atrophy. One is hypercatabolism of immunoglobulin G (78,79,189). The other is the marked elevation of plasma insulin in response to glucose tolerance test with normal responsivity to exogenous insulin (91,99). The cause of this is not known, but it has recently been suggested to be increased sensitivity of the pancreatic β-cell to a variety of stimuli (15,103,104).

The occasional congenitally manifest cases of myotonic atrophy have been emphasized recently (42,107). They are "floppy babies," usually with more severe mental retardation than cases becoming clinically apparent in later childhood or adulthood. In all congenitally manifest cases of myotonic atrophy, the mother transmitted the abnormal gene; therefore, it is possible that an intrauterine environmental harmful influence transmitted from the abnormal mother's serum transplacentally is additive with the genetic defect in some of the babies inheriting the autosomal dominant disease from the mother. This provokes the research possibility of looking for a transmittable toxic or deficiency influence in the serum of myotonic atrophy patients; since the ovum contributes most of the cytoplasm to the embryo, cytoplasmic inheritance factors (as in coiling determinants in snails) can also be considered.

The more severe "childhood-onset" cases of myotonic atrophy are also usually transmitted via the mother, suggesting an intrauterine defect having affected them too—and the frequent presence of a very high palate, presumably a developmental defect, in them further suggests an intrauterine onset of the clinical disease. It is also possible that a harmful intrauterine environment (or cytoplasmic inheritance factors) may play a role in the increasing severity of disease in successive generations often noted when the genetic transmission is through the mother (W. K. Engel, *unpublished observations*). Some of the congenitally manifest myotonic atrophy patients on muscle biopsy have type I fiber hypotrophy with central nuclei (W. K. Engel, *unpublished observations*), indistinguishable from the same pathology (54,65,74,77,85) in congenitally weak infants, or siblings, who do not in themselves or in their family have any other stigma of myotonic atrophy.

This latter disorder, type I fiber hypotrophy with central nuclei, like myotonic atrophy, has been proposed as possibly of neurogenic pathogenesis (54,65,74,77,85).

Duchenne Muscular Dystrophy

The cause of Duchenne muscular dystrophy remains unknown. No hypothesis has been proved correct and with each there are unresolved problems. A primary plasmalemmal defect has been suggested by some investigators. Because we have reservations about this proposal, it will be discussed under the subheading of "Holes in the Membrane Hypothesis."

In Duchenne muscle biopsies there was a lesser activation of adenyl cyclase (Ac) by fluoride and epinephrine in comparison to normal muscle (128). However, since the same change was also found in biopsies of facioscapulohumeral myopathies, its lack of specificity was not inspiring. Subsequently, the same finding was reported in muscle cultured from Duchenne patients in contrast to that cultured from other myopathy patients, suggesting to the authors greater disease specificity (127). However, since elevation of basal levels of Ac and less enhancement of it by fluoride are characteristics of immature muscle cells, especially those prior to fusion (183,191), an alternative explanation is that in the cultured Duchenne muscle there may be a larger percentage of less-mature muscle cells than in the disease controls.

Another concern is that the authors assumed that in both the muscle biopsy homogenates and in the cultures one was studying only muscle cells. However, in a biopsy certainly there are other muscle-as-a-mixed-organ tissues, e.g., blood vessels and connective tissue cells, and in a culture from primary explants there are not only muscle cells but presumably fibroblasts as well as epithelial cells and smooth muscle cells from the blood vessels. The heterogeneity of the muscle biopsies and cultures is of potential importance in view of the findings from our histochemical technique recently developed (W. K. Engel and R. W. Kula, *unpublished observations*) to show adenyl cyclase activity using an artificial substrate adenylyl-imidodiphosphate (AMP-PNP). (41) The various controls suggested that the histochemical activity demonstrated is adenyl cyclase (and not ATPase, 5-nucleotidase, or alkaline phosphatase). If that histochemical activity is indeed Ac, it should be pointed out that in normal muscle with short incubation times the blood vessels, particularly the arterial vessels but also the capillaries and venous vessels, were very strongly stained, whereas the normal muscle fibers were only slightly stained. Within the normal fibers, the stain by light microscopy was mainly in the plasmalemma with short incubation times; somewhat longer incubations showed staining in a smooth intermyofibrillar network pattern presumably reflecting t-tubules and/or sarcoplasmic reticulum. In Duchenne dystrophy muscle, as well as in muscle affected by other myopathies, the obviously regenerating fibers were darkly stained with this Ac reaction (in contrast to lightly stained normal fibers). In Duchenne dystrophy, apparently more so than in other diseases, not only were the obviously regenerating fibers very dark but many additional fibers which by other staining techniques appeared to be normal were moderately dark.

Therefore, in Duchenne dystrophy many fibers appear to be in a state of slight regenerative activity, or perhaps in the dual state of regeneration-degeneration ("regen-degen") (59). (This may be related to, and perhaps preceded by, histochemically and autoradiographically evident increase of calcium in some light microscopically intact fibers, as noted below.) Therefore, in Duchenne dystrophy one cannot necessarily conclude that the bio-chemically determined abnormality of adenyl cyclase activity is primary, or disease specific, or even important in the pathogenesis of the disease. If that abnormal Ac activity is in the muscle fibers, it may simply reflect a nonspecific change of the regenerating aspects of the fibers. Since the blood vessels are normally the richest possessors of the histochemical "Ac" activity, the intriguing alternative possibility is that the abnormal Ac activity could be related to cells of the blood vessels in the Duchenne muscle and not the muscle fibers themselves. That could have a bearing on the ischemia hypothesis of Duchenne dystrophy (see below).

The erythrocytes in Duchenne disease have been reported as being abnormal in the form of "echinocytes" (126). However, that was not disease specific, having been reported also in facioscapulohumeral dystrophy and limb-girdle dystrophy and even in mouse "muscular dystrophy" subjects (137). Furthermore, a repeat blinded control study showed no abnormality of erythrocytes detectable in Duchenne patients compared with control patients of the same age (125). More recently, a different kind of erythrocyte abnormality has been proposed in Duchenne disease, namely cup-shaped erythrocytes ("stomatocytes") (133,159). This finding has yet to be confirmed in another laboratory, and in the original study disease controls consisting of patients with chronic high elevations of serum CPK and other soluble muscle cell components were not used. This may be important because it is conceivable that some external factor in the erythrocyte environment is affecting the membrane, if indeed the stomatocyte defect is found by others. Recent studies of configuration responses of normal erythrocytes show that there are two general classes of agents, one causing crenation (which is similar in principle to echinocytosis or to acanthocytosis), and the other causing cupping. Crenating agents are usually anionic and cupping agents usually cationic (38,170,171). The former include free fatty acids, barbiturates, bilirubin, and salicylates, and the latter include local anesthetics, phenothiazine derivatives, antihistamines, colchicine, vinblastine, and reserpine (38,171). Depletion of ATP supply leads to crenation (170). Therefore, the study of morphology of erythrocytes needs to be carefully controlled to determine whether the changes are found reproducibly in Duchenne disease, whether they are exclusively there, and, if so, whether they are related to a factor exogenous to the erythrocytes or to an intrinsic erythrocyte abnormality. If a configurational defect would be found to be intrinsic in the erythrocyte, it would not necessarily be caused by a primary membrane defect. It could be secondary to an energy supply from within the erythrocyte—for example, it is known that an enzyme defect related to energy supply, namely, pyruvate kinase deficiency, is associated with acanthocytosis.

Recently, a plasmalemmal biochemical defect of erythrocytes has been proposed in Duchenne disease, namely, one related to protein kinase activity (161). By a series of analogies, it was speculated that the muscle equivalent of this yet unconfirmed defect may be related to the myosin molecule and not to the plasmalemma (159). Therefore, even a purported erythrocyte plasmalemmal defect is not, strangely, proposed to be an indication of a muscle cell plasmalemmal defect. Myosin itself has been studied in a number of ways in many laboratories and has been found to have no consistent abnormality in Duchenne dystrophy (151,163).

A biochemical defect in Duchenne dystrophy patients and carriers in the form of elevation of serum hemopexin was discovered a few years ago (2–4,12) and recently confirmed (34,35). Further studies are needed to determine whether it is qualitatively disease specific or only quantitatively typical caused by the quantitatively greater and more prolonged chronic myoglobin leakage from muscle cells. Even if not absolutely disease specific, the test may have importance in identifying the presence of muscle disease in Duchenne carrier suspects and perhaps in other patients with chronic muscle cell leakage when their CPK values are border line or normal.

A platelet defect has been found in Duchenne dystrophy, namely, decreased uptake of 5-hydroxytryptamine (serotonin) (141). It too needs to be further evaluated in non-Duchenne dystrophy patients with chronically elevated muscle leakage products. If proved to be significant, a definite pathogenic role of this platelet abnormality in relation to the muscle fiber degeneration would need to be sought. One possible formulation has been proposed in relation to blood vessels (57,59,141). Conceivably, their cells may also have a defect in serotonin uptake. A major mechanism of inactivating serotonin is known to be uptake by the target cells, such as smooth muscle cells. Thus, with defective uptake there would be persistence of serotonin acting on smooth muscle cell surface receptors of blood vessels, for example, vessels within muscle. Serotonin is known to be a potent vasoconstrictor of blood vessels within muscle (39,130), more so than in blood vessels of some other tissues, at least in experimental animals (39). Conceivably, a hypothetical defective uptake of serotonin by smooth muscle cells in blood vessels might preferentially involve intramuscular vessels in some muscles more so than in others, e.g., more so in proximal muscles as a basis of the greater degeneration of proximal muscles characteristic of Duchenne dystrophy. Another possible explanation is that muscle blood vessels in Duchenne dystrophy patients may be especially sensitive to slight amounts of locally excessive serotonin present because of defective platelet uptake. No matter what hypothesis is proposed in Duchenne disease, it must explain the relative sparing of most of the distal muscles and the eye muscles, the greater proximal muscle involvement, and also the involvement of the heart and the minimal and perhaps nonprogressive involvement of the brain. Selective abnormality of blood vessels in those areas could explain these events.

The vascular hypothesis regarding transient functional ischemias as a cause of muscle degeneration in Duchenne disease has been reviewed in detail (67), arguments against it were presented (19,20,49,102,149,150) and rebuttals to those counterarguments given (67). In summary, none of the criticism of the hypothesis appears overwhelming. However, in the actual patient with Duchenne disease an ischemia mechanism or an abnormal reactivity of some intramuscular blood vessels of the arterial tree has yet to be demonstrated—that is the most important next clinicoinvestigative step in following the ischemia hypothesis.

Looking at the effect of known ischemia on human limb muscle as evidenced in limbs amputated for peripheral vascular occlusive disease (76), we have demonstrated that there were group lesions like those seen in Duchenne disease and in the experimental ischemic myopathy model, and in minimally affected areas there were scattered necrotic or regenerating fibers like one sees in known carriers of Duchenne disease and in minimally affected areas of Duchenne muscle and experimental ischemic myopathy.

The animal model employed for studying functional ischemia in muscles has entailed combining two subthreshold lesions in the rat, aorta ligation and a small dose of vasoconstrictor (serotonin or norepinephrine, usually the former). Applying new techniques to the experimental ischemic myopathy (EIM) model has provided more detailed information about the damage of muscle fibers in general. In the damaged muscle, large amounts of the calcium-seeking agent ^{99m}Tc-diphosphonate accumulate (174,175). That the ^{99m}Tc-diphosphonate was demonstrating increase of calcium in the damaged tissue was shown by its close correlation with calcium increases measured directly by atomic absorption (175). The ^{99m}Tc-diphosphonate accumulation in the muscle was closely correlated with the rise of muscle CPK in the plasma of the various rats and with loss of potassium from their damaged muscles (174,175). Thus the ^{99m}Tc-diphosphonate accumulation was an approximately quantitative index of muscle damage. In the EIM animals it showed greater damage in the proximal quadriceps than in the distal gastrocnemius, which was paralleled by tissue histochemical results (174,175)—when the amount of ^{99m}Tc-diphosphonate in the unaffected forelimb triceps was considered as the unitary value, there was a 17 to 30-fold increase of ^{99m}Tc-diphosphonate accumulated in the quadriceps muscle and only a 5- to 10-fold increase in the gastrocnemius.

The increased calcium in the EIM muscle was demonstrated histochemically by light microscopy with the alizarin red stain. There was increased staining of muscle fibers throughout the ischemic infarct zones with a marked increase in fibers at the border (175), forming a "ring" or "doughnut" pattern of increased calcium localization in these infarcts histologically comparable to the ring patterns identified by the radioisotope pyrophosphate or tetracycline localizations in myocardial infarcts by clinical scanning. The "ring" (actually a section of a sphere geometrically) is thought to arise because the increased calcium in the muscle cells comes from the blood supply which continues in the marginal zone but not within the center of the infarct. In the excessively stained fibers the calcium is in the form of small dots suggesting loaded mitochondria or perhaps clumps of loaded sarcoplasmic reticulum. Identical calcium-burdened muscle fibers were seen occasionally in various human myopathies including Duchenne disease, dermatomyositis/polymyotitis, and ischemic myopathy from peripheral vascular disease, more so in the patients with greater elevations of serum CPK; calcium-burdened fibers were numerous in idiopathic and in phosphorylase-deficient rhabdomyolyses during attacks (W. K. Engel and G. G. Cunningham, *unpublished observations*).

In the EIM animals the amount of accumulation of ^{99m}Tc-diphosphonate in the damaged muscle was directly correlated with the accumulation of ^{3}H-diphosphonate (175). Therefore, it appeared valid to use the ^{3}H-diphosphonate in autoradiographic studies for identifying increased calcium in damaged muscle fibers. In the clearly abnormal muscle fibers there was marked increase of autoradiographically demonstrable grains of the ^{3}H-diphosphonate, signifying a large accumulation of calcium (R. W. Kula and W. K. Engel, *unpublished observations*). Moreover, there was also moderate to high increase in some muscle fibers that were normal appearing by modified trichrome or hematoxylin-eosin stains of frozen sections, indicating a type of minimal muscle damage below the level detectable by ordinary light microscopy. Presumably, similar changes are occurring in human myopathies such as Duchenne dystrophy. At the electron microscopic level the increased calcium in damaged muscle fibers has been localized in cell components with potassium pyroantimonate staining (144). The calcium was markedly increased in mitochondria, highly increased in sarcoplasmic reticulum, and slightly increased in myofibrils. There was also increased staining of the nuclei in their nucleolar and heterochromatin regions. These localizations were the same in all mildly or more significantly damaged muscle fibers in experimentally injured animal muscle and in various human diseases such as Duchenne dystrophy and dermatomyositis/polymyositis. Moreover, the identical localization of increased calcium occurred in normal animal muscle soaked in high (136 mM) calcium concentrations (which may also have damaged the plasmalemma).

Our proposed explanation is as follows. Normally, extracellular calcium contentration is 10,000 to 20,000 times greater than that of intracellular calcium. This high gradient is maintained by an ATP-requiring extrusion process of the plasmalemma associated with its sodium-potassium ATPase function, pumping out (by an exchange for sodium) the small amount of calcium that enters the cell with each action potential (93,113,168). Probably any mild or severe pathologic breach of the plasmalemma (from any cause, traumatic or metabolic, extrinsic or intrinsic to the muscle fiber) allows calcium to flow into the aqueous sarcoplasm just as plasma proteins (e.g., albumin and immunoglobulins) and other molecules normally barriered from entry are known to leak into damaged muscle fibers (184,185). A large amount of creatine phosphokinase, transaminases, lactate dehydrogenase, aldolase, potassium, and other soluble intracellular barriered molecules are known to leak out of the fiber and appear in the plasma (130,131).

In such damaged muscle fibers, various organelles continue to function (just as the SR, mitochondria, myofibrils, and nuclei function *in vitro* even after the cells are completely broken and fractionated by various techniques, a persistent functioning which is the basis of virtually all biochemical studies of muscle and other cells). Thus the excessive calcium in the aqueous sarcoplasm would be taken up by those organelles having the propensity to accumulate calcium. The SR can accumulate calcium avidly, down to a concentration outside of the SR of the 0.1 μM (123,129). Mitochondria can also accumulate calcium down to an external concentration of 4 μM and, although more slowly than SR, can accumulate very large amounts (114–116). (Those organelles continue to function at least initially after plasmalemmal breakdown, just as they do in homogenated cell fractions in *in vitro* studies.) Myofibrils are known to bind some calcium, as are the nucleoli and heterochromatin. Increase of calcium in the aqueous sarcoplasm is known to promote interaction of thick and thin myofilaments, and we propose it is responsible for the contractures we usually see at the cut ends of normal fibers and in the pathologic fibers containing excess calcium. It is likely that large amounts of calcium within organelles directly or indirectly damage their function and perhaps their structure.

High calcium in the aqueous sarcoplasm provokes uptake of calcium into mitochondria and SR by "pump" processes known to consume ATP (18, 119,135,168,190). As mitochondria take up excess calcium their oxidative phosphorylation (ATP synthesis) is obligatorily diminished as they use high-energy intermediates from oxidation directly and preferentially for calcium uptake processes (18,30,31,114–116). The resultant cellular ATP depletion may be presumed to (a) further impair plasmalemmal barrier function as well as SR and mitochondrial transport and various molecular synthesis, and (b) cause exhaustion of cellular glycogen in "last-gasp" anaerobic glycolysis (which is also enhanced by calcium-promoted activation of phosphorylase kinase). The increased aqueous sarcoplasmic calcium concurrently would activate catalytic enzymes of lysosomes, SR, and aqueous sarcoplasm, a known effect (89,152,158). Calcium saturation of calcium-binding groups on protein and phospholipid molecules would not only impair their function but also sensitize them to breakdown by hydrolysis (174), as does ATP depletion (88). The high cellular calcium might also further damage the plasmalemma by depolymerizing its microtubule cytoskeleton (142) just as it does neurotubules in axons (97,165,166).

In nuclei the precipitates of excess calcium (144) were concentrated in the nucleoli and the heterochromatin. At these sites the large amounts of RNA and DNA account for high concentrations of phosphate groups (32, 36), with which calcium is probably affiliating. Although under normal conditions, it has been suggested that calcium may help to stabilize the structure of the complex three-dimensional DNA molecules (36), in cell-free systems Ca^{2+} lowers the melting point of the thermoresistant fraction of DNA (36). Large increases of calcium could be detrimental to nuclear molecular functions. Thus we have proposed that excess calcium within muscle (or other) cells may be the "ultimate molecular assassin," pushing damaged muscle fibers past their point of no return (64,67,82).

We have postulated that the malignant hyperthermia rigidity syndrome is due mainly to a pharmacologically provoked (usually by succinylcholine and/or halothane) plasmalemmal leakage of calcium into the muscle fiber in susceptible persons (see above). The increased aqueous-sarcoplasmic calcium would cause muscle fiber contractures (clinical rigidity). The attempts of the cell to expel calcium or sequester it in mitochondria and SR would consume large amounts of ATP—to make this, and because of oxidative phosphorylation uncoupling effects of calcium, and to replace ATP consumed by the contractures would result in greatly enhanced oxidation and heat production (clinical hyperthermia). It is possible that the rigidity is a phenomenon mainly of type II fibers and the hyperthermia of type I fibers. Patients having more of one than the other may have preferential involvement of one fiber type. Since a massive calcium influx into all the skeletal muscle fibers would probably result in rapid inactivation of their function, we postulate a lesser but continuous leak, at least in the type I fibers if they continue to oxidize and produce heat.

Also relevant is the electrically silent contracture produced in phosphorylase deficiency patients by ischemic exercise. When the deficiency is severe, the muscle is focally rigid and hot, like a focal MHR phenomenon. We have shown by clinical ^{99m}Tc-diphosphonate scanning, by cellular autoradiography with that agent, and by calcium histochemistry that muscle fibers in the contracture contain excess calcium (113). This not only explains the nature of the electrically silent contracture but also establishes a model for the MHR syndrome — in this situation, though, the plasmalemmal defect is secondary to a defect of ATP supply caused by a defect of anaerobic glycolysis made manifest by the ischemic exercise. (Perhaps in the MHR syndrome one could also wonder whether a plasmalemmal defect is consequent to defective ATP supply, but we prefer a direct effect of the drug on the plasmalemma.)

In contrast to the lethal cascade of events proposed to result from unrestricted or marked calcium ingress, if the increase of intracellular calcium is only slight, it could conceivably be relatively benign and not impair recovery of minimally damaged muscle fibers. Moreover, it might be beneficial. We suggest that the slightly increased intracellular calcium may be the spark for repair or hypertrophy of muscle fibers through activation (depression) of DNA-RNA transcription and RNA-protein translation systems, perhaps by displacing histones or other suppressor proteins in cells destined to survive. This would lead to messenger and ribosomal RNA synthesis, which results in increased protein synthesis and cellular repair/regeneration. Increased calcium may also be the spark for cellular proliferation through activation (depression) of DNA-replicating systems in minimally injured resting satellite cells (myoblasts), the cells destined to repopulate the tissue with myoblasts for reconstitution of muscle fibers. These activating effects of calcium can be inferred from results in other cell systems (86,105,179,186).

Recently, other investigators have reported in muscle fibers of Duchenne dystrophy patients the appearance of small focal wedge-shaped zones of contraction and wedged and rounded zones of peroxidase infusion into the edges of muscle fibers, and major breaks of the plasmalemma in similar regions evident by electron microscopy. These lesions were considered to be specific and evidence of a primary plasmalemmal defect in Duchenne disease (134). However, we consider that these findings are not disease specific and in most instances are artifacts. With alizarin red staining for calcium, we have found small focal rounded or wedge-shaped accumulations in the periphery of some fibers or throughout some fibers (W. K. Engel and G. G. Cunningham, *unpublished observations*). They are more common in Duchenne disease than in other myopathies, although a number are seen in dermatomyositis/polymyositis biopsies.

Most of these fibers appear in serial sections to be the so-called dark fibers [dark with the modified trichrome, NADH-TR, myofibrillar ATPase (pH 9.4), nonspecific esterase, and most other histochemical stain preparations]. In these peripheral foci the increased calcium staining is in the form of small dots suggesting loaded mitochondria. The dot appearance resembles that seen throughout some severely or mildly abnormal fibers in various animal and human myopathies (see above) and at the cut ends of normal fibers (W. K. Engel and G. G. Cunningham, *unpublished observations*). The increased calcium at the cut ends of normal fibers is probably from calcium ingress through the plasmalemmal breach and probably explains the contraction artifact always seen there because of calcium's causing myofibrillar shortening. We conclude that fibers showing the peripheral foci of increased calcium staining and overcontraction, particularly the ones with the wedge-shaped regions in the study by others (134), reflect focal contraction artifacts because of muscle fiber damage suffered at the time of biopsy or subsequently.

Even though the foci may be artifactual, we propose that their greater number in Duchenne dystrophy reflects a predisposing fragilized state of the muscle fiber plasmalemma *in vivo,* making them more susceptible to injury. However, in Duchenne dystrophy our proposed fragilized state of the muscle fiber plasmalemma does not necessarily imply a defect primary in the plasmalemma. We suggest it may be a fragility imposed by defective energy supply to maintain the integrity of the plasmalemma—defective supply from within the fiber (noting that the defective energy supply because of phosphorylase deficiency causes widespread breakdown of plasmalemmal integrity during ischemic contraction, which results in calcium-burdened damaged muscle fibers evident by clinical ^{99m}Tc-diphosphonate scanning and histochemical staining) (R. W. Kula, W. K. Engel, and R. A. Brumback, *unpublished observations*) or from outside (e.g., a vascular problem; see above).

The electron microscopic changes of significant gaps in the plasmalemma shown by others (134) in Duchenne dystrophy we consider nonspecific artifact and not a reflection of a persistent *in vivo* state because certainly such a fiber would quickly become loaded with calcium and probably not survive; it could, though, be an artifact more common in that disease for reasons of preexisting fragility as noted above. In minimally damaged fibers into which there is (according to our hypothesis) slight calcium infusion promoting reversible, repairable damage, the breaches of plasmalemmal integrity must be transient and very minor, perhaps even beyond the level of the resolution of the electron microscope. Fibers having a diffuse dispersion of the increased calcium, in a dot pattern, we interpret as having been fragilized and actually breached *in vivo.* Some are overcontracted "dark fibers" and others not overcontracted—the former are interpreted as recently and/or severely damaged and the latter as not-so-recently and/or mildly injured fibers which are beginning to recover (W. K. Engel and G. G. Cunningham, *unpublished observations*).

Finding accumulation of calcium in damaged muscle fibers led us to try total-patient scanning with ^{99m}Tc-diphosphonate as a way of identifying damaged muscle clinically by its increased calcium content (113). There was a moderate increase of uptake into the limb "soft tissue" compartment (non-bone tissue, comprised of muscle, subcutaneous tissue, skin, and fat) in Duchenne patients, and in patients with the dermatomyositis/polymyositis (DM/PM) complex there was a large increase in soft tissue ^{99m}Tc-diphosphonate. However, in the group of Duchenne patients there was comparatively a much greater elevation of serum CPK, indicating a larger amount of leakage from muscle fibers than in the group of DM/PM patients studied and giving reverse proportions of the CPK:disphosphonate accumulation ratios in the two diseases (113). Results of the alizarin red histochemical staining for calcium in the muscle biopsies from the two types of patients offered an explanation (W. K. Engel and G. G. Cunningham, *unpublished observations*). Of the fibers which presumably accumulated larger amounts of calcium *in vivo* (ones with small round dots throughout), there did not appear to be a major difference in number. The fibers considered to have been fragilized with the trauma of the biopsy procedure (fibers having, in portions not obviously near a biopsy cut region, peripheral wedge-shaped or rounded foci of calcium in small dots and being "dark" with all other histochemical reactions) are more frequent in Duchenne disease. [Both kinds of abnormal fibers may have been, in the patient, leaking CPK and other contents out and small amounts of calcium in, the latter provoking a slight regenerative state in many Duchenne patient fibers, comparable to those seen with the adenyl cyclase histochemical reaction (see above)].

The greatest difference, though, was with other tissue elements. In the myositis patients there were a number of collections, sometimes large, of calcium in the regions between muscle fibers, particularly in the regions of mononuclear inflammatory cell reactions (perhaps those calcium collections were always in relation to current or previous mononuclear inflammatory cell reactions). It is probable that the between-muscle-fiber calcium is also being localized by the ^{99m}Tc-diphosphonate, and that may be what makes the soft tissue scans so much more positive in the DM/PM patients. Because very positive soft tissue scans in DM/PM can be reduced to normal as the patient improves with treatment (R. W. Kula, B. R. Line, and W. K. Engel, *unpublished observations*), it seems that the extracellular calcium sometimes, although probably not always, can be mobilized. Our DM/PM patients just mentioned did not have the obvious gross subcutaneous and cutaneous calcification, termed calcinosis universalis, sometimes seen in children with dermatomyositis, which is also clearly seen in ^{99m}Tc-diphosphonate scans (R. W. Kula, B. R. Line, and W. K. Engel, *unpublished observations*). Nevertheless, minor increases of subcutaneous calcium in children and adults could be additive in producing the very positive soft tissue in ^{99m}Tc-diphosphonate scans in myositis.

The site of a diagnostic muscle biopsy, which contains some surgically traumatized tissue, provides a muscle lesion of known time of onset. It is positive maximally beginning approximately 2 to 3 days after the biopsy, and its initial detectability lasts until about 10 to 12 days. The slight delay in maximal positivity may in some way be correlated with the gradual accumulation of inflammatory cells. Light microscopically, the excess calcium is in damaged muscles and in the inflammatory cell reactions (R. W. Kula, W. K. Engel, and R. A. Brumback, *unpublished observations*).

Facioscapulohumeral and Scapuloperoneal Syndromes

These two constellations of clinical findings are both slowly progressive, may or may not show evidence of inheritance in a given case, and are associated with different types of muscle pathology (neuropathic or myopathic or mixed) in various cases. Each constellation therefore appears to be a mixed syndrome, not one disease (52). Some patients, even some familial cases, with the facioscapulohumeral syndrome can have significant mononuclear inflammatory cell response in their muscle biopsies (140; R. B. Rosenbaum and W. K. Engel, *unpublished observations*), but its significance is not known because the patients with it do not show clinical improvement of the weakness with prednisone treatment. Underlying causes of the facioscapulohumeral and the scapuloperoneal syndromes are not known.

NEUROMUSCULAR DISEASES NOT CLEARLY INHERITED

It is important to emphasize that in two conditions sometimes misdiagnosed as "muscular dystrophy" (sic) the patient can be significantly helped. One is the *dermatomyositis/polymyositis complex,* usually treatable with high single-dose alternate-day (or initial single-dose daily) prednisone (69) or azathioprine (122; W. K. Engel and R. W. Kula, *unpublished observations*) or other immunosuppressants (132). The other is *pentazocine (Talwin®) fibrosing neuromyopathy* producing the *"levitated arms"* and *"levitated legs" syndromes* (112,118). Stopping the injections of pentazocine (or sometimes another sclerosing drug) halts progression of the fibrosis; and selective cutting of fibrosed shortened muscles relieves the postural distortion and its resultant pain.

Ragged-red fibers (and the very similar *rugged-red fibers*) are prevalent in biopsies of certain rare patients. Ragged-red and rugged-red fibers have their bright red color on modified trichrome staining (72) because of abnormal mitochondria identifiable with the succinate dehydrogenase and cytochrome oxidase reactions light microscopically and demonstrated electron microscopically to be too numerous, too large, with distorted cristae, and to contain crystal-like inclusions. Unusual as they are, such mitochondria do not identify a uniform clinicopathologic syndrome (17,58, 145,182,187,188).

However, there is one group of children with a characteristic syndrome of oculocraniosomatic neuromuscular weakness and ragged-red fibers accompanied by cardiac conduction defect, short stature, neural hearing defects, ataxia, elevated spinal protein, sometimes mild mental impairment, atypical retinal pigmentation, and developing diabetes mellitus as the disease progresses (58,109,145). Because nearly all of these children lack a family history of such disease, the possibility arises of this being an acquired disease in many cases. It is certainly a multitissue disease. It is not established whether the ragged-red muscle fibers and their abnormal mitochondria represent an ongoing self-perpetuating defect within the muscle cell (regardless of what was the initial triggering mechanism) or one continuously imposed on it from another cell or fluid. The fact that some but not all aspects of the mitochondrial morphologic abnormalities have been reincarnated in muscle fibers newly grown in tissue cultures of biopsies from some of these patients indicates an ongoing intrinsic and transmittable mechanism for at least some of the mitochondrial changes (5,8). It could, hypothetically, be an intrinsic biochemical defect or an infectious agent transmitted in culture vertically or horizontally at the cellular level. Because 2,4-dinitrophenol added to cultured "normal" chick embryo muscle can induce some mitochondrial changes reminiscent of some of the changes in human ragged-red fibers (5,8) and at the same time enhance the viral content of those muscle fibers newly grown in culture (6,68), the possibility has been raised that there may be occult viruses within the mitochondria of ragged-red fibers which could be termed "mitochondriophages" (6,68). If so, reincarnation of some of the ragged-red mitochondrial changes in culture might represent at least partial transmission of a responsible virus from the originally explanted muscle fibers to those newly grown in culture.

Vacuolar cabbage myopathy is another disease not yet known to be hereditary because we have seen only three isolated cases, one studied in culture as well as in biopsy. (In the muscle biopsy there is an accompanying minor neuropathic component.) The disease affects proximal and distal muscles with equal severity—for example, forearm wasting can be prominant. The vacuolar cabbage myopathy consists of muscle fibers with vacuoles containing membranous whorls that often resemble cross-sectioned cabbages (8). These apparently are lysosomes containing whorls of undigested membranous material. Because the vacuolar and cabbage changes have been reincarnated in the patient's muscle (8) fibers newly grown in tissue culture, this appears to be an intrinsic defect of the muscle cell, but whether it is a biochemical defect or an infectious mechanism transmitted in culture is not known.

SUMMARY

The above described findings from our studies are not complete descriptions of all the current investigations nor of the current status of any of the diseases mentioned. They may, however, be provocative for further research of these diseases.

REFERENCES

1. Anderson, I. L., and Jones, E. W. (1976): Porcine malignant hyperthermia: Effect of dantrolene sodium on in-vitro halothane-induced contraction of susceptible muscle. *Anesthesiology,* 44:57–61.
2. Askanas, V. (1966): Identification of the agent responsible for the abnormal immuno-electrophoretic pattern of serum in Duchenne's progressive muscular dystrophy. *Life Sci.,* 5:1767–1773.
3. Askanas, V. (1967a): Immunoelectrophoretic investigations of blood serum in muscular disease. *J. Neurol. Neurosurg. Psychiatry,* 30:43–46.
4. Askanas, V. (1967b): Immunoelectrophoretic study of sera of patients with Duchenne's progressive muscular dystrophy. *Neurol. Neurochir. Pol.,* 1:141–146.
5. Askanas, V., and Engel, W. K. (1974): Contribution of human muscle tissue culture (TC) in elucidating pathogeneses of neuromuscular disorders: mitochondria of "ragged red" fibers from biopsied and cultured muscles. In: *Proceedings of the III International Congress on Muscle Disease,* International Congress Series No. 334, p. 14. Excerpta Medica, Amsterdam.
6. Askanas, V., and Engel, W. K. (1975a): Chick muscle in tissue culture: The ubiquity of viral infection. *Acta Neuropathol. (Berl.),* 32:271–279.
7. Askanas, V., and Engel, W. K. (1975b): Distinct subtypes of type I fibers of human skeletal muscle. *Neurology (Minneap.),* 25:879–887.
8. Askanas, V., and Engel, W. K. (1976): Diseased human muscle tissue culture. Presented at Muscular Dystrophy Association's 5th International Scientific Conference, Durango, Colorado, June 21–26.
9. Askanas, V., Engel, W. K., DiMauro, S., et al. (1976): Adult-onset acid maltase deficiency. *N. Engl. J. Med.,* 294:573–578.
10. Askanas, V., Engel, W. K., Ringel, S. P., et al. (1976a): Acetylcholine receptors in aneurally cultured human and animal skeletal muscle fibers. *Neurology (Minneap.)* (*in press*).
11. Askanas, V., Engel, W. K., Ringel, S. P., et al. (1976b): Acetylcholine receptors in aneurally cultured human and animal skeletal muscle fibers. *Neurology (Minneap.),* 26:348.
12. Askanas, V., and Mazurczak, J. (1966): The serum immunoelectrophoretic test in patients with Duchenne's progressive muscular dystrophy. *Life Sci.,* 5:247–251.
13. Auerbach, V. H., DiGeorge, A. M., Mayer, B. W., Hayden, M., et al. (1973): Rhabdomyolysis and hyperpyrexia in children after administration of succinylcholine. In: *International Symposium on Malignant Hyperthermia,* edited by R. A. Gordon, B. A. Britt, and W. Kalow, pp. 30–51. Charles C. Thomas, Springfield, Ill.
14. Ballantyne, J. P., and Hanson, S. (1975): Computer method for the analysis of evoked motor unit potentials: II. Duchenne, limb-girdle, facioscapulohumeral and myotonic muscular dystrophies. *J. Neurol. Neurosurg. Psychiatry,* 38:417–428.
15. Barbosa, J. (1976): Letter: Insulin action in myotonic dystrophy and acanthosis nigricans. *N. Engl. J. Med.,* 295:107.
16. Beldars, J., Small, V., Cooper, D. A., et al. (1971): Postoperative malignant hyperthermia: A case report. *Can. Anaesth. Soc. J.,* 18:202–212.
17. Bender, A. N., and Engel, W. K. (1976): Light-cored dense particles in mitochondria of a patient with skeletal muscle and myocardial disease. *J. Neuropathol. Exp. Neurol.,* 35:46–52.
18. Bianchi, C. P. (1973): Cell calcium and malignant hyperthermia. In: *Malignant Hyperthermia,* edited by R. A. Gordon, B. A. Britt, and W. Kalow, pp. 147–151. Charles C. Thomas, Springfield, Ill.
19. Boysun, G., and Engel, A. G. (1975): Effects of microembolization on the skeletal muscle blood flow. *Acta Neurol. Scand.,* 52:71–80.
20. Bradley, W. G., O'Brien, M. D., Walder, D. N., et al. (1975): Failure to confirm a vascular cause of muscular dystrophy. *Arch. Neurol.,* 32:466–473.
21. Brebner, J., and Jozefowicz, J. A. (1974): Procainamide therapy of malignant hyperthermia: Case report. *Can. Anaesth. Soc. J.,* 21:96–105.
22. Britt, B. A., and Kalow, W. (1970): Malignant hyperthermia: A statistical review. *Can. Anaesth. Soc. J.,* 17:293–315.

23. Buchthal, F. (1976): Diagnostic significance of "myopathic" EMG. Presented at Muscular Dystrophy Association 5th International Scientific Conference, Durango, Colorado, June 21–26.

24. Bull, A. B., and Harrison, G. G. (1973): Recent advances in the understanding of anesthetic-induced malignant hyperpyrexia. *Acta Anaesthesiol. Belg.*, 24:97–108.

25. Caccia, M. R., Negri, S., Boriardi, A., et al. (1972): Study of the dispersion of motor nerve conduction velocity in Charcot-Marie-Tooth-Hoffman disease and Steinert's syndrome. *Z. Neurol.*, 201:211–217.

26. Campa, J. F., and Engel, W. K. (1970): Histochemistry of motor neurons and interneurons in the cat lumbar spinal cord. *Neurology (Minneap.)*, 20:559–568.

27. Campa, J. F., and Engel, W. K. (1971): Histochemical and functional correlations in anterior horn neurons of the cat spinal cord. *Science*, 171:198–199.

28. Campa, J. F., and Engel, W. K. (1973): Histochemistry of motoneurons innervating slow and fast motor units. In: *New Developments in EMG and Clinical Neurophysiology*, edited by J. E. Desmedt, pp. 178–185. Karger, Basel.

29. Campa, J. F., Singer, P. A., and Engel, W. K. (1974): The histochemical pathology of partially denervated cat muscles: sequential changes during denervation and reinnervation. In: *Proceedings of the III International Congress on Muscle Diseases*. International Congress Series No. 334, p. 77. Excerpta Medica, Amsterdam.

30. Carafoli, E. (1973): The transport of Ca^{2+} by mitochondria. Problems and perspectives. *Biochemie*, 55:755–762.

31. Carafoli, E., Patriarca, P., and Rossi, C. S. (1969): A comparative study of the role of mitochondria and the SR in the uptake and release of Ca^{2+} by the rat diaphragm. *J. Cell Physiol.*, 74:17–30.

32. Clark, M., and Ackerman, G. A. (1971): A histochemical evaluation of pyroantimonate-osmium reaction. *J. Histochem. Cytochem.*, 19:727–737.

33. Cöers, C., and Woolf, A. L. (1959): *Innervation of Muscle — a Biopsy Study*. Blackwell, Oxford.

34. Danieli, G. A., and Angelini, C. (1976a): Duchenne carrier detection. *Lancet*, 2:90.

35. Danieli, G. A., and Angelini, C. (1976b): Duchenne carrier detection. *Lancet*, 2:415.

36. Darzynkiewicz, Z., Traganos, F., Sharpless, T., et al. (1976): DNA denaturation *in situ*. *J. Cell Biol.*, 68:1–10.

37. Denborough, M. A., Dennett, X., and Anderson, R. McD. (1973): Central-core disease and malignant hyperpyrexia. *Br. Med. J.*, 1:272–273.

38. Deutick, B. (1968): Transformation and restoration of biconcave shape of human erythrocytes induced by amphiphilic agents and changes of ionic environment. *Biochim. Biophys. Acta*, 63:494–500.

39. DiSalvo, J., and Schmidt, C. (1976): Contractile responses to epinephrine, serotonin, and potassium in arterial smooth muscle. *Proc. Soc. Exp. Biol. Med.*, 151:478–483.

40. Dreyfus, J. C., Askanas, V., and Engel, W. K.: *Unpublished observations*.

41. Dubrovsky, A. L., and Engel, W. K. (1976): New histochemical technique for demonstrating adenyl cyclase in nervous system and muscle. *Arch. Neurol.*, 33:386.

42. Dyken, P. R., and Harper, P. S. (1973): Congenital dystrophica myotonica. *Neurology (Minneap.)*, 24:465–473.

43. Ebashi, S. (1973): Structural proteins of muscle. In: *Basic Research in Myology*, edited by B. A. Kakulas, pp. 145–154. American Elsevier Co., New York.

44. Ebashi, S., Ohtsuki, I., and Mihashi, K. (1972): Regulatory proteins of muscle with special reference to troponin. *Cold Spring Harbor Symp.*, 37:215–223.

45. Ekstedt, J., and Stålberg, E. (1973): Single fibre electromyography for the study of the microphysiology of the human muscle. In: *New Developments in Electromyography and Clinical Neurophysiology, Vol. I*, edited by J. E. Desmedt, pp. 89–112. Karger, Basel.

46. Ellis, K. O., and Carpenter, J. F. (1974): Mechanisms of control of skeletal muscle contraction by Dantrolene sodium. *Arch. Phys. Med. Rehabil.*, 55:362–369.

47. Eng, G., Epstein, R., and Engel, W. K. (1976): Malignant hyperthermia. *Arch. Neurol.*, (*in press*).

48. Engel, A. G. (1966): Later onset rod myopathy (a new syndrome?): Light and electron microscopic observations in two cases. *Mayo Clin. Proc.*, 41:713–741.

49. Engel, A. G., Jerusalem, F., Tsujihata, M., et al. (1975): The neuromuscular junction in myopathies. A quantitative ultrastructural study. In: *Recent Advances in Myology*,

edited by W. G. Bradley, D. Gardner-Medwin, and J. N. Walton, pp. 132–143. Excerpta Medica, Amsterdam.

50. Engel, W. K. (1965): Histochemistry of neuromuscular disease — significance of muscle fiber types. "Neuromuscular diseases." In: *Proceedings of the VIII International Congress of Neurology, Vol. II,* International Congress Series, Excerpta Medica, pp. 67–101, Amsterdam.

51. Engel, W. K. (1967*a*): A critique of congenital myopathies and other disorders. In: *Exploratory Concepts in Muscular Dystrophy and Related Disorders,* edited by A. T. Milhorat, pp. 27–40. Excerpta Medica, Amsterdam.

52. Engel, W. K. (1967*b*): Muscle biopsies in neuromuscular diseases. *Pediatr. Clin. North Am.,* 14:963–995.

53. Engel, W. K. (1969): Motor neuron histochemistry in ALS and infantile spinal muscular atrophy. In: *Motor Neuron Diseases,* edited by F. H. Norris, Jr., and L. T. Kurland, pp. 218–234. Grune & Stratton, New York.

54. Engel, W. K. (1970): Selective and nonselective susceptibility of muscle fiber types. A new approach to human neuromuscular diseases. *Arch. Neurol.,* 22:97–117.

55. Engel, W. K. (1971*a*): Classification of neuromuscular disorders. *Birth Defects,* 7(2): 18–37.

56. Engel, W. K. (1971*b*): Myotonia — a different point of view. *Calif. Med.,* 114:32–37.

57. Engel, W. K. (1971*c*): Nouvelle hypothese sur la pathogenie de la dystrophie musculaire pseudo-hypertrophique. *Rev. Neurol.* (Paris), 124:291–298.

58. Engel, W. K. (1971*d*): "Ragged-red fibers" in ophthalmoplegia syndromes and their differential diagnosis. *II International Congress on Muscle Diseases.* International Congress Series No. 237, Excerpta Medica, Amsterdam.

59. Engel, W. K. (1973*a*): Duchenne muscular dystrophy: A histologically based ischemia hypothesis and comparison with experimental ischemia myopathy. In: *The Striated Muscle,* International Academy of Pathology Monograph No. 12, edited by C. M. Pearson and F. K. Mustofi. Williams & Wilkins Co., Baltimore.

60. Engel, W. K. (1973*b*): "Myopathic EMG" — nonesuch animal. *N. Engl. J. Med.,* 289: 485–486.

61. Engel, W. K. (1975): Brief, small, abundant motor-unit action potentials. *Neurology (Minneap.),* 25:173–176.

62. Engel, W. K. (1976*a*): Central core disease and focal loss of cross-striations. In: *The Cellular and Molecular Basis of Neurologic Disease,* edited by G. M. Shy, E. S. Goldensohn, and S. H. Appel. Lea & Febiger, Philadelphia (*in press*).

63. Engel, W. K. (1976*b*): Introduction to diseases of the lower motor neuron. In: *The Cellular and Molecular Basis of Neurologic Disease,* edited by G. M. Shy, E. S. Goldensohn, and S. H. Appel. Lea & Febiger, Philadelphia (*in press*).

64. Engel, W. K. (1976*c*): Introduction to the myopathies. In: *The Cellular and Molecular Basis of Neurologic Disease,* edited by G. M. Shy, E. S. Goldensohn, and S. H. Appel. Lea & Febiger, Philadelphia (*in press*).

65. Engel, W. K. (1976*d*): Muscle fiber hypotrophy with central nuclei. In: *The Cellular and Molecular Basis of Neurologic Disease,* edited by G. M. Shy, E. S. Goldensohn, and S. H. Appel. Lea & Febiger, Philadelphia (*in press*).

66. Engel, W. K. (1976*e*): Rod (nemaline) disease. In: *The Cellular and Molecular Basis of Neurologic Disease,* edited by G. M. Shy, E. S. Goldensohn, and S. H. Appel. Lea & Febiger, Philadelphia (*in press*).

67. Engel, W. K. (1976*b*): Workshop on the aetiology of Duchenne muscular dystrophy. In: *Recent Advances in Myology,* edited by W. G. Bradley, D. Gardner-Medwin, and J. N. Walton, pp. 166–177. Excerpta Medica, Amsterdam.

68. Engel, W. K., and Askanas, V. (1976): Overlooked avian oncornavirus in cultured muscle — functionally significant? *Science,* 192:1252–1253.

69. Engel, W. K., Borenstein, A., DeVivo, D., et al. (1972): High-single-dose alternate-day prednisone (HSDAD-PRED) in the treatment of the dermatomyositis/polymyositis complex. *Trans. Am. Neurol. Assoc.* pp. 272–275. (*Abstract*).

70. Engel, W. K., Brooke, M. H., and Nelson, P. G. (1966): Histochemical studies of denervated or tenotomized cat muscle. Illustrating difficulties in relating experimental animal conditions to human neuromuscular diseases. *Ann. N.Y. Acad. Sci.,* 138:160–185.

71. Engel, W. K., and Brooke, M. J. (1966): Histochemistry of the myotonic disorders. In: *Progressive Muskeldystrophie, Myotonie, Myasthenie,* edited by E. Kuhn, pp. 203–222. Springer-Verlag, Heidelberg.
72. Engel, W. K., and Cunningham, G. G. (1963): Rapid examination of muscle tissue – an improved trichrome method for rapid diagnosis of muscle biopsy fresh-frozen sections. *Neurology (Minneap.),* 13:919–923.
73. Engel, W. K., Eyerman, E. J., and Williams, H. E. (1963): Late-onset type of skeletal muscle phosphorylase deficiency: a new familial variety of completely and partially affected subjects. *N. Engl. J. Med.,* 268:135–137.
74. Engel, W. K., Gold, G. N., and Karpati, G. (1968): Type I fiber hypotrophy and central nuclei – a rare congenital muscle abnormality with a possible experimental model. *Arch. Neurol.,* 18:435–444.
75. Engel, W. K., and Hatcher, M. A. (1968): Evaluating significance of biochemical abnormalities in inherited neuromuscular disorders. In: *Progress in Neuro-Genetics,* edited by A. Barbeau and J. R. Brunette, pp. 17–22. Excerpta Medica, Amsterdam.
76. Engel, W. K., and Hawley, R. J. (1976): Focal lesions of muscle in peripheral vascular disease. *Neurology (Minneap.) (in press).*
77. Engel, W. K., and Karpati, G. (1968): Impaired skeletal muscle maturation fcllowing neonatal neurectomy. *Dev. Biol.,* 18:713–723.
78. Engel, W. K., McFarlin, D. E., Drews, G., et al. (1966*a*): Protein abnormalities in neuromuscular diseases – Part 1. JAMA, 195:754–760.
79. Engel, W. K., McFarlin, D. E., Drews, G., et al. (1966*b*): Protein abnormalities in neuromuscular diseases – Part 2. JAMA, 195:837–842.
80. Engel, W. K., and Oberc, M. A. (1975): Abundant nuclear rods in adult-onset rod disease. *J. Neuropathol. Exp. Neurol.,* 34:119–132.
81. Engel, W. K., and Resnick, J. S. (1966): Late-onset rod myopathy – a newly recognized and progressive disease. *Neurology (Minneap.),* 16:308.
82. Engel, W. K., Siegel, B. A., Kula, Roger W., et al.: To be published.
83. Engel, W. K., Wanko, T., and Fenichel, G. M. (1964): Nemaline myopathy, a second case. *Arch. Neurol.,* 11:22–39.
84. Engel, W. K., and Warmolts, J. R. (1971): New concepts on the possible role of motoneuron abnormalities in neuromuscular disorders not usually considered neurogenic. In: *Advances in Neuromuscular Diseases,* edited by G. Serratrice and H. Roux. L'expansion Scientifique Francais, Paris.
85. Engel, W. K., and Warmolts, J. R. (1973): The motor unit: Diseases affecting it *in toto* or *in portio.* In: *New Developments in EMG and Clinical Neurophysiology,* edited by J. E. Desmedt. Karger, Basel.
86. Freedman, M. H., Roff, M. C., and Gomperts, B. (1975): Induction of increased calcium uptake in mouse T lymphocytes by concanavalin A and its modulation by cyclic nucleotides. *Nature,* 255:378–382.
87. Fuglsang-Frederiksen, A., Scheel, U., and Buchthal, F. (1976): Diagnostic yield of analysis of the pattern of electrical activity and of individual motor unit potentials in myopathy. *J. Neurol. Neurosurg. Psychiatry,* 39:742–750.
88. Gazitt, Y., Ohad, J., and Layter, A. (1975): Changes in phospholipid susceptibility toward phospholypases in ATP depletion in avian and amphibian erythrocyte membranes. *Biochim. Biophys. Acta,* 382:65–72.
89. Gilbert, D. S., Newby, B. J., and Anderton, B. H. (1975): Neurofilament disguise, destruction and discipline. *Nature,* 256:586.
90. Goodman, L. S., and Gilman, A. (1975): *The Pharmacological Basis of Therapeutics.* Macmillan, New York.
91. Gordon, P., Griggs, R. C., Nissley, S. P., et al. (1969): Studies of plasma insulin in myotonic dystrophy. *J. Clin. Endocrinol. Metab.,* 29:684–690.
92. Gordon, R. A., Britt, B. A., and Kalow, W. (1973): *Malignant Hyperthermia.* Charles C. Thomas, Springfield, Ill.
93. Hadju, S., and Leonard, E. J. (1975): A calcium transport system for mammalian cells. *Life Sci.,* 17:1527–1534.
94. Hall-Craggs, E. C. B. (1974): Rapid regeneration of a whole skeletal muscle following treatment with bupivacaine. *Exp. Neurol.,* 43:349–358.

95. Harrison, G. G. (1971): Anesthetic-induced malignant hyperpyrexia: A suggested method of treatment. *Br. Med. J.*, 3:454–456.
96. Harrison, G. G. (1975): Control of the malignant hyperpyrexic syndrome in MHS swine by dantrolene sodium. *Br. J. Anaesth.*, 47:62–65.
97. Hinkley, R. E., and Green, L. S. (1971): Effects of halothane and colchicine on microtubules and electrical activity of rabbit vagus nerves. *J. Neurobiol.*, 2:97.
98. Howik, B., and Stovner, J. (1975): Procaine and malignant hyperthermia. *Lancet*, 2:185.
99. Huff, T. A., Horton, E. S., and Lebovitz, H. E. (1967): Abnormal insulin secretion in myotonic dystrophy. *N. Engl. J. Med.*, 277:837–841.
100. Isaacs, H., and Barlow, M. B. (1974): Central core disease associated with elevated creatine phosphokinase levels. Two members of a family known to be susceptible to malignant hyperthermia. *S. Afr. Med. J.*, 48:640.
101. Jerusalem, F., Angelini, C., Engel, A. G., et al. (1973): Mitochrondria-lipid-glycogen (MLG) disease of muscle. A morphologically regressive congenital myopathy. *Arch. Neurol.*, 29:162–169.
102. Jerusalem, F., Engel, A. G., and Gomez, M. R. (1974): Duchenne dystrophy: Morphometric study of the muscle microvasculature. *Brain*, 97:115.
103. Kahn, C. R., Archer, J. A., Bar, R. S., et al. (1976): The syndromes of insulin resistance and acanthosis nigricans. *N. Engl. J. Med.*, 294:739–745.
104. Kahn, C. R., Bar, R. S., Flier, J. S., et al. (1976): Letter: Insulin action in myotonic dystrophy and acanthosis nigricans. *N. Engl. J. Med.*, 296:107.
105. Kaplan, E., and Richman, H. G. (1976): Effect of calcium on RNA and protein synthesis in the hypertrophied myocardium. *Proc. Soc. Exp. Biol. Med.*, 152:24–28.
106. Karpati, G., and Carpenter, S. M. (1974): Experimental ischemic myopathy. *J. Neurol. Sci.*, 23:129–161.
107. Karpati, G., Carpenter, S., Watters, G. V., et al. (1973): Infantile myotonic dystrophy. Histochemical and electron microscopic features in skeletal muscle. *Neurology (Minneap.)*, 23:1066–1077.
108. Katz, A. M. (1972): Contractile proteins in normal and failing myocardium. *Hosp. Prac.*, 7:57–59.
109. Kearns, T. P. (1965): External ophthalmoplegia, pigmentary degeneration of the retina and cardiomyopathy: A newly recognized syndrome. *Trans. Am. Ophthalmol. Soc.*, 63:559–625.
110. Kerr, D. D., Winegard, D. W., and Gatz, E. E. (1975): Prevention of porcine malignant hyperthermia by epidural block. *Anesthesiology*, 42:307–311.
111. King, J. O., and Denborough, R. A. (1973): Malignant hyperpyrexia in Australia and New Zealand. *Med. J. Aust.*, 1:525–528.
112. Konkel, K. F., and Lucas, G. L. (1974): Abduction contracture of the shoulder. *Clin. Orthop.*, 104:224–227.
113. Kula, R. W., Line, B. R., Siegel, B. A., et al. (1976): ^{99m}Tc-diphosphonate scanning of soft-tissue in neuromuscular diseases. *Neurology (Minneap.)*, 26:370.
113a. Langer, A. (1976): Events at the cardiac sarcolemma location and movement of contractile-dependent calcium. *Fed. Proc.*, 35:1274–1278.
114. Lehninger, A. (1966): Dynamics and mechanisms of active ion transport across the mitochondrial membrane. *Ann. N.Y. Acad. Sci.*, 137:700–736.
115. Lehninger, A. (1970): Mitochondria and Ca^{2+} ion transport. *Biochem. J.*, 119:129–138.
116. Lehninger, A., Carafoli, E., and Rossi, C. (1967): Energy linked ion movements in mitochondrial systems. *Adv. Enzymol.*, 29:259–320.
117. Leigh, M. D., Lewis, G. B., and Scott, E. B. (1971): Successful treatment of malignant hyperthermia. *Anesth. Analg. (Cleve.)*, 50:39–42.
118. Levin, B. E., and Engel, W. K. (1975): Iatrogenic muscle fibrosis – arm levitation as an initial sign. *J.A.M.A.*, 234:621.
119. Maclennan, D. H., and Holland, P. C. C. (1975): Calcium transport in sarcoplasmic reticulum. *Ann. Rev. Biophys. Bioeng.*, 4:377–404.
120. McComas, A. J., and Sica, R. E. P. (1973): Single motor unit twitches in man. In: *New Developments in Electromyography and Neurophysiology, Vol. I*, edited by J. E. Desmedt, pp. 55–68. Karger, Basel.

121. McDermot, V. (1970): The changes in the motor endplate in myasthenia gravis. *Brain,* 83:24–39.
122. McFarlin, D. E., and Griggs, R. C. (1968): Treatment of inflammatory myopathies with azathioprine. *Trans. Am. Neurol. Assoc.,* 93:244–246.
123. Makinose, M. (1973): Possible functional states of the enzyme of the sarcoplasmic calcium pump. *FEBS Lett.,* 39:140–143.
124. Maruyama, K., and Ebashi, S. (1970): Regulatory proteins of muscle. In: *The Physiology and Biochemistry of Muscle as a Food, Vol. 2,* edited by E. J. Briskey, R. G. Cassens, and B. B. Marsh, pp. 373–381. University of Wisconsin Press, Madison.
125. Matheson, D. E., Engel, W. K., and Derrer, E. C. (1976): Erythrocyte shape in Duchenne muscular dystrophy. *Neurology (Minneap.),* 26:1182–1183.
126. Matheson, D. W., and Howland, J. L. (1974): Erythrocyte deformation in human muscular dystrophy. *Science,* 184:165–166.
127. Mawatari, S., quoted in Rowland, L. P. (1976): Pathogenesis of muscular dystrophies. *Arch. Neurol.,* 33:315–321.
128. Mawatari, S., Takagi, A., and Rowland, L. P. (1974): Adenyl cyclase in normal and pathologic human muscle. *Arch. Neurol.,* 30:96–102.
129. Meissner, G. (1973): ATP and Ca^{++} binding by the Ca^{++} pump protein of sarcoplasmic reticulum. *Biochim. Biphys. Acta,* 298:906–926.
130. Mendell, J. R., Engel, W. K., and Derrer, E. C. (1971): Duchenne muscular dystrophy: functional ischemia reproduces its characteristic lesions. *Science,* 172:1143–1145.
131. Mendell, J. R., Engel, W. K., and Derrer, E. C. (1972): Increased plasma enzyme concentrations in rats with functional ischaemia of muscle provide a possible model of Duchenne muscular dystrophy. *Nature,* 239:522–524.
132. Metzger, A. L., Bohan, A., Goldberg, L. S., et al. (1974): Polymyositis and dermatomyositis: Combined methotrexate and corticosteroid therapy. *Ann. Intern. Med.,* 81:182–189.
133. Miller, S. E., Roses, A. D., and Appel, S. H. (1976): Scanning electron microscopy studies in muscular dystrophy. *Arch. Neurol.,* 33:172–174.
134. Mokri, B., and Engel, A. G. (1975): Duchenne dystrophy: electron microscopic findings pointing to a basic or early abnormality in the plasma membrane of the muscle fiber. *Neurology (Minneap.),* 25:1111–1120.
135. Moore, L., Chen, T., Knapp, H. R., et al. (1975): Energy-dependent calcium sequestration activity in rat liver microsomes. *J. Biol. Chem.,* 250:4562–4568.
136. Morgan, K. G., and Bryant, S. H. (1975): The mechanism of action of dantrolene sodium on skeletal muscle. *Fed. Proc.* 100:290 (Abs.).
137. Morse, P. F., and Howland, J. L. (1973): Erythrocytes from animals with genetic muscular dystrophy. *Nature,* 245:156–157.
138. Moulds, R. F., and Denborough, M. A. (1972): Procaine in malignant hyperpyrexia. *Br. Med. J.,* 4:526–528.
139. Moulds, R. F. W., and Denborough, M. A. (1974): Biochemical basis of malignant hyperpyrexia. *Br. Med. J.,* 2:241–244.
140. Munsat, T. L., Piper, D., Cancilla, P., and Mednick, J. (1972): Inflammatory myopathy with facioscapulohumeral distribution. *Neurology (Minneap.),* 22:335–347.
141. Murphy, D. L., Mendell, J. R., and Engel, W. K. (1973): Serotonin and platelet function in Duchenne muscular dystrophy. *Arch. Neurol.,* 28:239–242.
142. Nicolson, G., and Paste, G. (1976): The cancer cell: Dynamic aspects and modifications in cell-surface organization. *N. Engl. J. Med.,* 295:197–203.
143. Noble, W. H., McKee, D., and Gates, B. (1975): Malignant hyperthermia with rigidity successfully treated with procainamide. *Anesthesiology,* 39:450–451.
144. Oberc, M. A., and Engel, W. K. (1976): To be published.
145. Olson, W., Engel, W. K., Walsh, G. O., et al. (1972): Oculocraniosomatic neuromuscular disease with "ragged-red" fibers. *Arch. Neurol.,* 26:193–211.
146. Panayiotopoulos, C. P. (1974): Electrophysiological estimation of motor units in Duchenne muscular dystrophy. *J. Neurol. Sci.,* 23:89–98.
147. Panayiotopoulos, C. P., and Scarpalezos, S. (1975): Electrophysiological estimation of motor units in limb-girdle muscular dystrophy and chronic spinal muscular atrophy. *J. Neurol. Sci.,* 24:95–107.

148. Panayiotopoulos, C. P., and Scarpalezos, S. (1975): Neural and muscular involvement in dystrophia myotonica. *Lancet,* 2:329.
149. Paulson, O. B. (1975): Workshop on the aetiology of Duchenne muscular dystrophy. In: *Recent Advances in Myology,* edited by W. G. Bradley, D. Gardner-Medwin, and J. N. Walton, pp. 148–188. Excerpta Medica, Amsterdam.
150. Paulson, O. B., Engel, A. G., and Gomez, M. R. (1974): Muscle blood flow in Duchenne type muscular dystrophy, limb-girdle dystrophy, polymyositis and in normal controls. *J. Neurol. Neurosurg. Psychiatry,* 37:685.
151. Penn, A. S., Cloak, R. A., and Rowland, L. P. (1972): Myosin from normal and dystrophic human muscle: Immunochemical and electrophoretic study. *Arch. Neurol.,* 27:159–174.
152. Reddy, M. K., Etlinger, J. D., Rabinowitz, M., et al. (1975): Removal of Z-lines and α-actinin from isolated myofibrils by a calcium-activated neutral protease. *J. Biol. Chem.,* 250:4278–4284.
153. Resnick, J. S., Engel, W. K., and Nelson, P. G. (1968): Changes in the Z-disk of skeletal muscle induced by tenotomy. *Neurology (Minneap.),* 18:737–740.
154. Ringel, S. P., Bender, A. N., and Engel, W. K. (1975): A sequential study of denervation-ultrastructural immunoperoxidase localization of alpha-bungarotoxin. *Trans. Am. Neurol. Assoc.,* 100:52–56.
155. Ringel, S. P., Bender, A. N., and Engel, W. K. (1976): Alterations of acetylcholine receptors in human and experimental neuromuscular diseases. *Arch. Neurol. (in press).*
156. Ringel, S. P., Engel, W. K., and Bender, A. N. (1976): Extrajunctional acetylcholine receptors on myogenously de-innervated muscle fibers. *J. Histochem. Cytochem.,* 24:1033–1034.
157. Roelofs, R. I., Engel, W. K., and Chauvin, P. B. (1972): Histochemical phosphorylase activity in regenerating muscle fibers from myophosphorylase-deficient patients. *Science,* 177:795–797.
158. Roobel, A., and Alleyne, G. A. O. (1972): A study of stabilization of gluconeogenic activity in rat liver slices by calcium and manganese ions. *Biochem. J.,* 129:231–239.
159. Roses, A. D. (1976): Erythrocytes in dystrophy. Presented at Muscular Dystrophy Association 5th International Scientific Conference, Durango, Colorado, June 21–26.
160. Roses, A. D., and Appel, S. F. (1974): Muscular dystrophies. *Lancet,* 2:1400.
161. Roses, A. D., Herbstreith, N. H., and Appel, S. H. (1975): Membrane protein kinase alteration in Duchenne muscular dystrophy. *Nature* 254:350–351.
162. Rowland, L. P. (1974): Are the muscular dystrophies neurogenic? *Ann. N.Y. Acad. Sci.,* 228:244–260.
163. Rowland, L. P. (1976): Pathogenesis of the muscular dystrophies. *Arch. Neurol.,* 33:315–321.
164. Ryan, J. F. (1973): The early treatment of malignant hyperthermia. In: *International Symposium on Malignant Hyperthermia,* edited by R. A. Gordon, B. A. Britt, and W. Kalow, pp. 430–440. Charles C. Thomas, Springfield, Ill.
165. Samson, F. E., and Hinkley, R. E. (1972): Neuronal microtubular systems (editorial views). *Anesthesiology,* 36:417.
166. Schlaepfer, W., and Bingg, R. (1973): High Ca^{++} solution needed for Wallerian degeneration. *J. Cell Biol.,* 59:456.
167. Schollmeyer, J. E., Gol, D. E., Robson, R. M., et al. (1973): Localization of alpha-actinin and tropomyosin in different muscles. *J. Cell Biol.,* 59:306a.
168. Schwartz, A. (1976): Cell membrane Na^+, K^+-ATPase and SR: Possible regulators of intracellular ion activity. *Fed. Proc.,* 35:1279–1282.
169. Shanes, A. M. (1958): Electrochemical aspects of physiological and pharmacological action in excitable cells. *Pharmacol. Rev.,* 10:59–273.
170. Sheetz, M. P., Painter, R. G., and Singer, S. (1976): Biological membranes as bilayer couples. III. Compensatory shape changes induced in membranes. *J. Cell Biol.,* 70:193–203.
171. Sheetz, M. P., and Singer, S. J. (1976): Equilibrium and kinetic effects of drugs on the shapes of human erythrocytes. *J. Cell Biol.,* 70:247–251.
172. Shy, G. M., Engel, W. K., Somers, J. E., and Wanko, T. (1963): Nemaline myopathy – a new congenital myopathy. *Brain,* 86:793–810.

173. Shy, G. M., Engel, W. K., and Wanko, T. (1962): Central core disease: A myofibrillary and mitochonrial abnormality of muscle. *Ann. Intern. Med.,* 56:511–520.
174. Siegel, B. A., Engel, W. K., and Derrer, E. C. (1975): ^{99m}Tc-diphosphonate uptake in skeletal muscle: A quantitative index of acute damage. *Neurology (Minneap.),* 25:1055–1058.
175. Siegel, B. A., Engel, W. K., and Derrer, E. C. (1976): Localization of ^{99m}Tc-diphosphonate in acutely injured muscle: Relationship to muscle calcium deposition. *Neurology (Minneap.) (in press).*
176. Stålberg, E., and Ekstedt, J. (1973): Single fibre EMG and microphysiology of the motor unit in normal and diseased human muscle. In: *New Developments in Electromyography and Clinical Neurophysiology, Vol. I,* edited by J. E. Desmedt, pp. 113–129. Karger, Basel.
177. Stålberg, E., and Theile, B. (1973): Discharge pattern of motoneurons in humans. In: *New Developments in Electromyography and Neurophysiology, Vol. III,* edited by J. E. Desmedt, pp. 234–241. Karger, Basel.
178. Sugita, H., Masaki, T., Ebashi, S., et al. (1974): Staining of the nemaline rod by fluorescent antibody against 10S-actinin. *Proc. Jap. Acad.,* 50:237–240.
179. Swierenga, S. H. H., McManus, J. P., and Whitfield, J. F. (1976): Regulation of calcium of the proliferation of heart cells from young adult rats. *In Vitro,* 12:31–36.
180. Taylor, E. W. (1972): Chemistry of muscle contraction. In: *Ann. Rev. Biochem.,* 42:196–203.
181. Thorpe, W., and Seeman, P. (1973): Drug-induced contracture of muscle. In: *International Symposium on Malignant Hyperthermia,* edited by R. A. Gordon, B. A. Britt, and W. Kalow, pp. 152–162. Charles C. Thomas, Springfield, Ill.
182. Tsairis, P., Engel, W. K., and Kark, P. (1973): Familial epilepsy syndrome associated with skeletal muscle mitochondrial abnormalities. *Neurology (Minneap.),* 23:408.
183. Wahrmann, J. B., Luzzati, D., and Winand, R. (1973): Changes in adenylcyclase specific activity during differentiation of an established myogenic cell line. *Biochem. Biophys. Res. Commun.,* 52:576–581.
184. Whitaker, J. N., and Engel, W. K. (1971): Vascular deposits of immunoglobulin and complement in idiopathic inflammatory myopathy. *N. Engl. J. Med.,* 286:333–339.
185. Whitaker, J. N., and Engel, W. K. (1973): Mechanisms of muscle injury in idiopathic inflammatory myopathy. *N. Engl. J. Med.,* 289:107–108.
186. Whitfield, J. F., MacManus, J. P., Rixan, R. H., et al. (1973): The calcium-independent stimulation of thymic lymphoblast DNA synthesis by low cyclic GMP concentrations. *Proc. Soc. Exp. Biol. Med.,* 144:808–812.
187. Wijngaarden, P. K., Bethlem, J., Meijer, A. E. F. H., et al. (1967): Skeletal muscle disease with abnormal mitochondria. *Brain,* 90:577–592.
188. Wilcox, W. D., and Fuchs, F. (1969): The effect of some local anesthetic compounds on sarcotubular calcium transport. *Biochem. Biophys. Acta,* 180:210–212.
189. Wochner, R. D., Drews, G., Strober, W., et al. (1966): Accelerated breakdown of immunoglobulin G (IgG) in myotonic dystrophy: A hereditary error of immunoglobulin catabolism. *J. Clin. Invest.,* 45:321–329.
190. Yu, B. P., Masoro, E. J., and Morley, T. F. (1976): Analysis of the arrangement of protein components in the sarcoplasmic reticulum of rat skeletal muscle. *J. Biol. Chem.,* 251:2037–2043.
191. Zalin, R. J., and Montague, W. (1975): Changes in cyclic AMP, adenylate cyclase and protein kinase levels during the development of embryonic chick skeletal muscle. *Exp. Cell Res.,* 93:55–62.

Advances in Neurology, Vol. 17, edited by
R. C. Griggs and R. T. Moxley, III. Raven Press,
New York © 1977.

Genetic Considerations in Neuromuscular Diseases

Peter T. Rowley

Departments of Medicine, Pediatrics, and Genetics, University of Rochester Medical Center, 601 Elmwood Avenue, Rochester, New York 14642

CLASSIFICATION BY INHERITANCE PATTERN

Neuromuscular diseases inherited as mendelian traits may be classified as autosomal dominant, autosomal recessive, and X-linked recessive conditions (Table 1).

In *autosomal dominant* inheritance an individual need have only one gene of a given type to be affected. An affected individual has an affected parent except in the case of a new mutation or incomplete penetrance. An affected individual's offspring is equally likely to be affected and to be normal.

In *autosomal recessive* inheritance an affected individual has the given gene in double dose. Relatives at risk are generally siblings. For the offspring of two carriers the probability is $1/4$ for being affected and $1/2$ for being a carrier. In the case of rare recessives there is an increased probability of parental consanguinity.

In *X-linked recessive* inheritance an affected individual has no normal X chromosome. The great majority of affected individuals are males. Affected individuals of the same family are related through females. A female carrier married to a normal male has in any given pregnancy an equal chance of producing an affected male, a normal male, a carrier female, and a normal female.

PROBLEMS IN THE DETERMINATION OF GENOTYPE

Variable Expression

A single gene may be variously expressed in different members of the same family. In the case of most traits the cause for this variability is not known. Myotonic dystrophy is a condition with marked variation in expression in the same family. Some individuals have primarily muscular weakness or myotonia, some have myocardial disease, others have cataracts, and still others have all of these plus retarded mental development.

227

TABLE 1. *Neuromuscular diseases inherited as mendelian traits*

Autosomal dominant
  Facioscapulohumeral neuromuscular disease (15890)[a]
  Oculopharyngeal muscular dystrophy (16430)
  Central core disease of muscle (11700)
  Nemaline myopathy (16180)
  Myotonic dystrophy (16090)
  Myotonia congenita (16080)[b]
  Paramyotonia congenita (16830)
  Familial periodic paralysis
      Hypokalemic type (17040)
      Hyperkalemic type (17050)
      Normokalemic type (17060)
  Familial hypertrophic polyneuritis (14590)
  Amyloidosis, Andrade or Portuguese type (10480)
  Hereditary sensory radicular neuropathy (16240)
  Acute intermittent porphyria (17600)
Autosomal recessive
  Limb-girdle muscular dystrophy (25360)
  Glycogen storage disease of muscle
      Type 5, phosphorylase deficiency (23260)
      Type 7, phosphofructokinase deficiency (23280)
  Werdnig-Hoffmann's disease (25330)
  Kugelberg-Welander's disease (25340)
  Refsum's disease (26650)
X-linked recessive
  X-linked muscular dystrophy
      Duchenne type (31020)
      Becker type (31010)

---

[a] The number after each disease refers to the listing in McKusick (1), which provides citations to the genetic literature.
[b] A recessively inherited form of myotonia congenita has been described (2).

The age of onset is also variable, some individuals being affected in infancy and others asymptomatic until middle life. Subjects with infantile onset are generally the products of affected mothers. This finding suggests that infantile onset requires both that the fetus and the mother have the myotonic dystrophy gene and that the mother's genotype adversely affects the development of the fetus (3).

Carrier Diagnosis

In recessive conditions it is advantageous to be able to identify carriers or heterozygotes. In neuromuscular diseases this problem is especially critical with regard to the female relatives of patients with Duchenne muscular dystrophy. The mother or sister of a Duchenne patient may wish to know the likelihood of carrier status in order to predict the likelihood of bearing affected sons. A proven carrier has a $\frac{1}{4}$ chance that any given

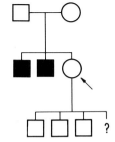

FIG. 1. Pedigree of family with Duchenne muscular dystrophy.

pregnancy will result in an affected male. The problem then is to determine the likelihood that a specific female relative is a carrier. The patient's mother is not necessarily a carrier for the patient might be the result of a new mutation. With two affected sons, or one affected brother and one affected son, she can be considered definitely a carrier. A woman with only one affected son and an otherwise negative family history may represent a carrier or not. Such a woman can be considered probably a carrier if her serum creatine phosphokinase is elevated on more than one occasion or if her muscle is abnormal on biopsy.

In estimating the probability of carrier status in the case of a female relative of a Duchenne patient, it is important to take into account all of the information provided by normal male relatives. In Fig. 1, the woman with an affected brother and two affected sons must be a carrier. Her daughter has a 50% chance of inheriting the Duchenne gene from her mother. The chance that the son of a definite carrier is normal is $\frac{1}{2}$, therefore the chance that a definite carrier would have three normal sons out of three is $(\frac{1}{2})^3$, or $\frac{1}{8}$. The chance that a definite carrier has a normal serum creatine phosphokinase is approximately 70% (4,5). Thus the chance that the daughter shown in Fig. 1 is a carrier is not simply $\frac{1}{2}$ as might be inferred from just the information that her mother is a known carrier. A calculation of probability should also take into account the fact that if the daughter were a definite carrier, the chance of her having three normal sons out of three would be only $\frac{1}{8}$. Such analysis which takes into account the relative risks because of alternative possibilities is called bayesian analysis. Risks of carrier status based on positive family history information only may be too high. Taking into account normal males generally reduces the risk to a more correct figure. A detailed discussion of the application of bayesian analysis to the estimation of probability of carrier status in female relatives of Duchenne patients is given by Murphy and Chase (6).

PRENATAL DIAGNOSIS

Prenatal diagnosis is possible because amniotic fluid can be removed from the 14th week of pregnancy onward and because the cells cultured from amniotic fluid are fetal in origin. Such cultures provide material for cytologic or biochemical analysis. An example of neuromuscular disease which could be diagnosed *in utero* by biochemical analysis is Refsum's disease, in which phytanic acid oxidation is defective. The phenotype can be recognized in culture of skin fibroblasts (7). It is therefore reasonable to expect that prenatal diagnosis will be also possible from cultured amniotic fluid cells.

With X-linked traits determination of fetal sex by chromosome analysis may be useful. In the case of a serious X-linked condition such as Duchenne muscular dystrophy, the couple at risk may wish to consider aborting all male children in order to avoid having an affected male.

A third type of analysis applied to fetal material in amniotic fluid is genetic linkage. To say that two loci are linked means that they are on the same chromosome close enough to each other so that alleles on the same chromosome in one individual tend to be transmitted together to offspring. In some couples in which one partner has myotonic dystrophy, genetic linkage permits an estimation of the likelihood that the fetus has inherited the myotonic dystrophy gene (8–10). This possibility rests on the fact that the locus for myotonic dystrophy is genetically linked to the locus for secretor (Fig. 2).

An individual is called a secretor if he secretes ABH blood group substances into his body secretions. For example, an individual who is blood group A according to a test of his red cells is called a secretor if A substance is also demonstrable in his saliva. The ability to secrete ABH substances into body fluids is dictated by the genotype at the locus called secretor. The two alleles at this locus are called *Se* and $\overline{se}$. Secretors must have at least one *Se* gene and therefore are of two types, *Se/Se* and *Se/$\overline{se}$*. Nonsecretors have no *Se* gene and are therefore *se/se*.

Three genetic requirements must be fulfilled before prenatal diagnosis of myotonic dystrophy based on linkage of its locus and the secretor locus can be offered to a couple in which one partner has myotonic dystrophy. The first requirement is that the propositus must be type *Se/$\overline{se}$*, i.e., a heterozygote for secretor. If the saliva of the propositus contains no ABH substances, he is a nonsecretor and no prenatal diagnosis will be possible using the secretor linkage. If he is a secretor, then relatives should be tested in an attempt to establish that he is a heterozygote. In the family shown in Fig. 3 the propositus is a secretor. He must be a secretor heterozygote

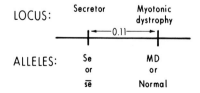

FIG. 2. Genetic map showing linkage relationship of the loci for myotonic dystrophy and for secretor status.

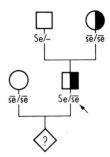

FIG. 3. Pedigree of family with myotonic dystrophy seeking prenatal diagnosis.

since his mother is a nonsecretor and therefore could give him only a nonsecretor gene.

The second requirement is that the phase of linkage must be known, i.e., it must be established whether the gene for myotonic dystrophy in the propositus is located on the chromosome with the *Se* gene or on the chromosome with the *se* gene. In the family in Fig. 3, the myotonic dystrophy gene must be located on the same chromosome as the *se* gene since the propositus' affected mother has no *Se* gene.

The third requirement is that the propositus' spouse must not be *Se/Se*. If the propositus' spouse has this genotype, the fetus can inherit only an *Se* gene from the normal parent and thus will be a secretor; hence the fetal secretor type will be independent of whether or not the fetus has inherited the myotonic dystrophy gene. In the family shown in Fig. 3, the propositus' spouse is a nonsecretor and thus fulfills the criterion.

In the family shown in Fig. 3, if amniotic fluid shows no ABH substances it can be concluded that the fetus is a nonsecretor. In this case the fetus has probably inherited the myotonic dystrophy gene because it was on the same chromosome with the *se* gene in the father. If on the other hand the fetus is a secretor, it must have inherited the *Se* gene from the affected parent since the normal parent does not have it and therefore it has probably *not* inherited the myotonic dystrophy gene. The reason for these predictions being probable rather than certain is that recombination is always possible between separate genetic loci. The likeliest probability of recombination between the locus for myotonic dystrophy and the locus for secretor is 0.11 or 11% (8). Thus these predictions just described have a probability of 100% − 11%, or 89%.

If the spouse of the propositus in Fig. 3 had been a secretor, then one would have tried to determine if the spouse was a heterozygote. One way of doing this would be to show that one of the spouse's parents is a nonsecretor. In such a case, if the fetus were a nonsecretor, then it probably would have inherited the muscular dystrophy gene as in the first example. However, if it were a secretor, one could not tell whether it had inherited the *Se* gene from the affected parent or from the unaffected parent, and therefore no

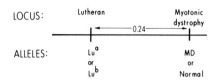

FIG. 4. Genetic map showing linkage relationship of loci for myotonic dystrophy and for Lutheran blood group.

information relative to myotonic dystrophy would have been provided by amniocentesis.

Myotonic dystrophy is linked not only to the secretor locus but also to the Lutheran locus (Fig. 4). The Lutheran locus determines if red cells have on their surface Lu^a or Lu^b antigens. In order to type the fetus for Lutheran, one would have to obtain fetal red cells. A method for sampling fetal red cells is not generally available at present. Predicting the inheritance of myotonic dystrophy using the linkage of the myotonic dystrophy locus to the Lutheran locus is at present useful only postnatally. The postnatal determination of the likelihood of inheritance of the myotonic dystrophy gene might be helpful with regard to certain practical decisions that the subject at risk faces such as choice of occupation. The likeliest recombination frequency between the locus for myotonic dystrophy and the Lutheran locus is 0.24 or 24% (8). Therefore, predictions based on this linkage have a probability of 100% − 24%, or 76%. Thus for postnatal analysis, linkage to either the secretor or the Lutheran locus may be useful.

The percentage of couples who can profit from prenatal diagnosis is theoretically 37.5%, based on the incidence of blood groups in U.S. populations. However, the percentage of couples who can actually be helped is smaller because in some cases the necessary relatives may not be available for determination of heterozygosity or phase of linkage, lowering the fraction of couples who can actually be helped to 10 to 20%. Nevertheless, the principle of prenatal detection of disease through genetic linkage will be increasingly important in the future since the number of known genetic markers and knowledge of their location on chromosomes in relationship to human disease loci are increasing rapidly.

IMPACT OF GENETIC COUNSELING

Do recurrence risk figures actually influence family planning decisions? Hutton and Thompson (11) have studied 105 female relatives of patients with Duchenne muscular dystrophy in an attempt to answer this question. The female relatives were classified as high risk, moderate risk, or low risk according to their family history and serum creatine phosphokinase values. Deterrence was judged by answers to a questionnaire. Of 42 females at high risk, 81% were deterred. Of 40 individuals with moderate risk, 35% were deterred. Of 23 females with low risk, 5% were deterred. Scored alternately by sterilization of the woman or her spouse, incidence in the high-risk group was 55%, in the moderate-risk group 12%, and in the low-risk group 13%. Thus risk of carrier status did correlate with deterrence as judged by statement of reproductive decision or by sterilization of one marriage partner.

Hutton and Thompson also asked if there is a correlation between the actual number of liveborns and information received about probability of carrier status. In the high-risk group 67% were deterred, in the moderate-risk group 40% were deterred, and in the low-risk group 24% were deterred.

One measure of success of genetic counseling is the decline in the incidence of positive family history in new cases of Duchenne muscular dystrophy. The Toronto group categorized their experience for each year from 1965 to 1974 in terms of the numbers of new cases in which the mother is aware of a positive family history before the conception of the propositus. In 1965 this figure was 42%, whereas in 1973 and 1974 it was 7% and 9%, respectively.

The authors concluded that not only reproductive intent but also reproductive performance is highly correlated with the risk information provided.

Since there is evidence that reproductive behavior is significantly influenced by risk figures, the physician has a serious responsibility to provide the most accurate genetic information available.

REFERENCES

1. McKusick, V. A. (1975): *Mendelian Inheritance in Man. Catalog of Autosomal Dominant, Autosomal Recessive, and X-Linked Phenotypes, 4th Ed.* Johns Hopkins University Press, Baltimore.
2. Harper, P. S., and Johnstone, D. M. (1972): Recessively inherited myotonia congenita. *J. Med. Genet.,* 9:213–215.
3. Harper, P. S., and Dyken, P. R. (1972): Early-onset dystrophia myotonica. Evidence supporting a maternal environmental factor. *Lancet,* 2:53.
4. Thompson, M. W., Murphy, E. G., and McAlpine, P. J. (1967): An assessment of the creatine kinase test in the detection of carriers of Duchenne muscular dystrophy. *J. Pediatr.,* 71:82–93.
5. Emery, A. E. H. (1967): The use of serum creatine kinase for detecting carriers of Duchenne muscular dystrophy. In: *Exploratory Concepts in Muscular Dystrophy and Related Disorders,* pp. 90–97. International Congress Series No. 147, Excerpta Medica, New York.
6. Murphy, E. A., and Chase, G. A. (1975): *Principles of Genetic Counseling.* Year Book Medical Publishers, Chicago.
7. Herndon, J. H., Steinberg, D., Uhlendorf, B. W., and Fales, H. M. (1969): Refsum's disease: Characterization of the enzyme defect in cell culture. *J. Clin. Invest.,* 48:1017–1032.
8. Harper, P. S., Rivas, M. L., Bias, W. B., et al. (1972): Genetic linkage confirmed between the locus for myotonic dystrophy and the ABH-secretion and Lutheran blood group loci. *Am. J. Hum. Genet.,* 24:310–316.
9. Schrott, H. G., Karp, L., and Omenn, G. S. (1973): Prenatal prediction in myotonic dystrophy: Guidelines for genetic counseling. *Clin. Genet.,* 4:38–45.
10. Schrott, H. G., and Omenn, G. S. (1975): Myotonic dystrophy: Opportunities for prenatal prediction. *Neurology (Minneap.),* 25:789–791.
11. Hutton, E., and Thompson, M. (1976): The application of carrier detection to genetic counseling in Duchenne muscular dystrophy: A ten year review. *Can. Med. Assoc. J.* (*in press*).

Advances in Neurology, Vol. 17, edited by
R. C. Griggs and R. T. Moxley, III. Raven Press,
New York © 1977.

Treatable Neuropathies

Mark J. Brown

*Department of Neurology, Hospital of the University of Pennsylvania,
Philadelphia, Pennsylvania 19104*

The investigation and treatment of peripheral nerve disorders has become one of the most exciting and gratifying endeavors in clinical neurology. Two recently published compendia (16,44) and a new monograph (3) chronicle advances in understanding the pathogenesis and pathophysiology of neuropathies. Most neuropathies are now amenable to classification, with the assistance of biochemical studies, electromyography, and nerve biopsy. A specific etiology can be found in the majority of neuropathies throughout the world, most prevalent being leprosy, vitamin deficiency, and diabetes. In nontropical countries, where neuropathies are less common, obscure cases are relatively more frequent. Even so, an etiologic diagnosis can be found in more than half the patients who require hospital admission for evaluation (34). When the cause is known, as in leprosy and deficiency disorders, therapy can be direct and effective. When the diagnosis is elusive or when specific treatments are not available, supportive measures can reduce the morbidity and mortality associated with nerve disease.

Diagnosis of a patient's neuropathy is facilitated by use of formal classification systems, a number of which are listed in Table 1. The most helpful for the would-be therapist is based on underlying cause (3,16,19), although this is often the last thing learned about a new patient with neuropathy. In some cases, historical details at the outset do suggest the etiology. Previously known metabolic or systemic disorders could be causing neuropathy. Recognized exposure to nerve toxins may have occurred at home or work. Past habitation in areas of Asia, Africa, or the southwestern United States increases the likelihood of leprosy as the cause. A patient with familial neuropathy might be aware of gait or motor disturbance in a relative. Occasionally, epidemiological detective work can uncover the etiological culprit:

The uniformed guard in Fig. 1 is overlooking three Viet Cong prisoners who suffered from paresthesias in their legs and could not rise from a squatting position unaided. They were the most severely affected among 70 prisoners in their camp. Symptoms appeared approximately 7 months after capture and transfer to a new, clean, well-equipped Army of Republic of Viet Nam prison. In an attempt to make living conditions as humane as possible, American advisors arranged to import most of the prisoners' food, including daily rations of polished

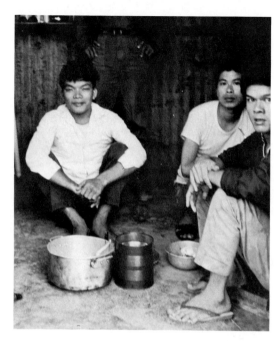

FIG. 1 Three prisoners of war (seated), in excellent health aside from severe sensorimotor neuropathy, caused by a thiamine-deficient polished rice diet.

white rice. Beriberi was diagnosed when the association between the neuropathy and the thiamine-deficient rice was recognized. The prisoners improved slowly with supplemental vitamin B_1.

Clinical features must be used to construct a differential diagnosis (Table 1) when the etiology is not apparent. It is helpful to consider the age at onset. Neuropathies in the newborn period are often traumatic; those in infancy and childhood, genetic or inflammatory; and those in adults, primarily metabolic, toxic, or inflammatory. Ascertaining the anatomical distribution of nerve lesions is also valuable. In most cases, mapping the sensory and motor loss will quickly point to a pattern that involves one nerve (mononeuropathy), multiple single nerves (mononeuropathy multiplex), or all nerves in a distal, symmetric fashion (polyneuropathy). Differentiation is not always easy. The drawing in Fig. 2 (*left*) is the sensory map of a patient with moderately severe sensorimotor polyneuropathy. Areas hypesthetic to pinprick are shaded. Arrows represent the distance from the level of lost sensibility to the dorsal root ganglion of that dermatome. The length of functioning nerve that remains is roughly equal in the arms and legs, a point emphasized by Dr. T. Sabin. The center patient (Fig. 2) also has polyneuropathy, but in this case limited to his feet. The length of viable nerve is great enough so that hands should not yet be affected. Sensory loss in his hands is

TABLE 1. *Systems for classification of neuropathies*

Etiology
  Metabolic, toxic, infectious, inflammatory, vascular, traumatic, neoplastic, genetic, idiopathic, others
Clinical features
  A. Age of onset:
    Newborn, infant, child, young adult, adult
  B. Length of progressive phase:
    Acute (up to 3 weeks), subacute (weeks to months), chronic (years), and relapsing
  C. Distribution of symptoms and signs:
    Mononeuropathy, mononeuropathy multiplex, plexopathy, and polyneuropathy (predominantly sensory, motor, autonomic, or mixed)
Nerve electrophysiology
  A. Anatomical pattern (mononeuropathy, polyneuropathy, mixed)
  B. Pathological response (axonal degeneration, segmental demyelination)
Spinal fluid protein
  Normal, elevated
Nerve pathology
  A. Neural elements (myelinated and unmyelinated fiber degeneration, segmental demyelination, regeneration, mixed, others)
  B. Nonneural elements (Schwann cells, fibroblasts, collagen, vessels, inflammatory cells, microorganisms, stored material, others)

deceptive and results from an ulnar neuropathy on the right and a median neuropathy on the left. Both are due to superimposed focal compressive lesions and are not part of the polyneuropathy. The sensory map on the right also appears to represent a distal symmetric neuropathy. However, certain distal areas such as the forearms and right hand are entirely spared, and some proximal regions such as the ears are severely affected. This is a "superficial neuropathy," characteristic of the temperature-dependent

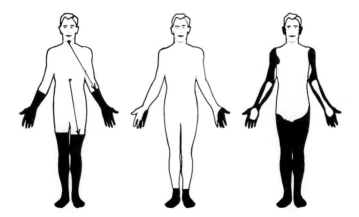

FIG. 2. Sensory maps of hypalgesia for 3 patients with neuropathy. **Left:** Distal, symmetric polyneuropathy. **Center:** Mild distal neuropathy with right ulnar and left median nerve compression. **Right:** temperature-dependent superficial neuropathy (from a patient of Dr. T. Swift).

TABLE 2. *Causes of mononeuropathy and mononeuropathy multiplex*

Vascular
  Connective tissue diseases, diabetes mellitus, coagulation disorders, sickle cell anemia, amphetamine angiitis
Traumatic
  Local injury, occupational trauma, minor trauma with underlying neuropathy, hereditary liability to pressure palsies
Infectious
  Herpes zoster, leprosy
Neoplastic
  Benign and malignant tumor, hematoma
Other
  Myxedema, amyloidosis, mucopolysaccharidosis, serum sickness, post-immunization, brachial neuritis

---

lesions of leprosy. Determining the pattern of a neuropathy thus may suggest a diagnosis or limit the diagnostic possibilities. Table 2 lists disorders associated with patterns of mononeuropathy and mononeuropathy multiplex, whereas Tables 3 and 4 include disorders associated with polyneuropathy.

Findings in the physical examination may point to a correct diagnosis. Curly hair in a straight-hair family is associated with giant axonal neuropathy. A tick on the scalp or skin can cause toxic paralysis. Alopecia follows thallium intoxication. Mee's lines (Fig. 3), transverse white ridges on fingernails, indicate chronic arsenic intoxication, as do hyperkeratotic palms and soles. Hyperpigmentation of sun-exposed areas of skin is characteristic of pellagra. Malar flush of systemic lupus erythematosus, xanthomas of hyperlipemia, jaundice of hepatic failure, ichthyosis of Refsum disease, purple macules of Fabry disease, and hemorrhages of coagulation disorders are additional skin signs that may be associated with neuropathy. Argyll-Robertson pupils may be seen with familial neuropathies and diabetes, as well as with tabes dorsalis. Pigmentary retinal degeneration is a sign of Refsum disease. Lack of tears is part of dysautonomia. Pigmented dental-gingival margin is seen in lead- or bismuth-intoxicated patients with poor

TABLE 3. *Causes of acute polyneuropathy*

Inflammatory polyneuritis
  Acute idiopathic, post-infectious, post-surgical
  Associated with hepatitis, mumps, mononucleosis, lymphoma, other neoplasms
  Relapsing
Porphyria
Diphtheria
Tick paralysis[a]
Some toxic neuropathies

---

[a] Tick paralysis appears to result from distal neuropathy and not a myoneural junction defect (43).

TABLE 4. *Causes of subacute and chronic polyneuropathy by clinical distribution*

Predominantly sensory
  A. Large-fiber modalities most affected:
     Tabes dorsalis, remote effect of carcinoma, genetic (hereditary sensory neuro-pathy type 2, a-betalipoproteinemia, spinocerebellar degeneration)
  B. Small-fiber modalities most affected:
     Leprosy, amyloidosis, diabetes, genetic (hereditary sensory neuropathy type 1, Fabry disease, a-alphalipoproteinemia)
Predominantly motor
  Inflammatory polyneuritis, lead, dapsone, hypoglycemia, insulinoma, porphyria, genetic (peroneal muscular atrophies, others), anterior horn cell diseases
Predominantly autonomic
  Diabetes, amyloidosis, acute pandysautonomia, Riley-Day syndrome
Mixed sensory-motor-autonomic
  A. Systemic disorders
    1. Endocrine (diabetes, hypothyroidism, hyperthyroidism, acromegaly)
    2. Connective tissue (systemic lupus erythematosus, scleroderma, rheumatoid arthritis, polyarteritis, others)
    3. Dysproteinemia (myeloma, cryoglobulinemia, amyloidosis, macroglobulinemia)
    4. Carcinoma and sarcoma (direct infiltration and remote effect)
    5. Others (uremia, porphyria, hepatic failure, hyperlipemia, sarcoid, pulmonary disease, others)
  B. Deficiency disorders
     Malnutrition with multiple deficiencies, malabsorption syndromes, deficiency of vitamins B_1, B_6, B_{12}, and other water-soluble vitamins
  C. Therapeutic agents
    1. Antibiotics and antimicrobials (amphotericin B, chloramphenicol, chloroquine, clioquinol, ethambutal, isoniazid, nitrofurantoin, streptomycin, sulfonamides, others)
    2. Sedatives and hypnotics (amitriptylene, ethylchlorovinyl, glutethimide, imipra-mine, meprobamate, methaqualone, monoamine oxidase inhibitors, thalidomide, others)
    3. Anticancer agents (vincristine, vinblastine, nitrogen mustards)
    4. Others [carbamazepine (?), disulfiram, ergotamine, hydralazine, insulin, pheny-toin, others]
  D. Environmental hazards
    1. Metals (antimony, arsenic, bismuth, copper, lead, mercury, thallium, zinc)
    2. Solvents [carbon disulfide, glue (*n*-hexane), methyl *n*-butyl ketone, others]
    3. Others (carbon monoxide, 2,4 D, hexachlorophene, Lathyrus peas, methyl bromide, tri-orthocresyl phosphate, vibration, cold, others)
  E. Genetic disorders
     Refsum disease, Krabbe disease, metachromatic leukodystrophy, others

dental hygiene. Stomatitis can occur with deficiency of B vitamins. Patchy white pharyngitis may herald the onset of diphtheritic neuropathy by several weeks. Enlarged lipid-filled tonsils are found in patients with α-alphalipo-proteinemia. Chronic respiratory insufficiency has been linked with neurop-athy. Abdominal tenderness and "surgical abdomen" may be part of por-phyria. Lymphadenopathy or splenomegaly may follow mononucleosis or lymphoma, both associated with neuropathy. Bone tenderness with neuropathy suggests myeloma. Scoliosis and pes cavus are skeletal de-formities that may result from neuropathy at an early age. Finally, superficial cutaneous nerves may be palpably thickened and visibly enlarged, indicating

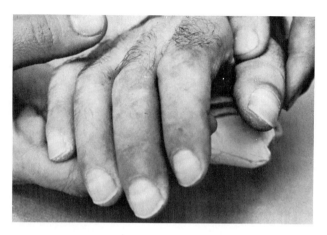

FIG. 3. Mee's lines in fingernails after unsuspected chronic arsenic ingestion (courtesy of Dr. R. Porter).

intraneural scarring with leprosy (Fig. 4), a hypertrophic form of peroneal muscular atrophy, or Refsum disease.

Elucidation of the course of a neuropathy, that is, the length of its progressive phase, can be of diagnostic help. Table 3 list disorders that can cause acute or rapidly progressive neuropathy. These conditions produce primarily

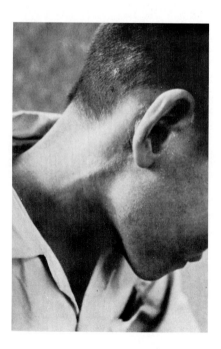

FIG. 4. Thickened great auricular nerve of a boy with lepromatous leprosy.

motor symptoms, and so they must be distinguished from myoneural junction disorders such as myasthenia gravis and botulism, and from anterior horn cell diseases such as poliomyelitis.

The bulk of neuropathies occur in adults and progress with a subacute or chronic course. Careful attention to clinical details may reveal distinguishing features within this large, apparently homogenous group. In some cases the physiological deficit in affected nerves may appear restricted to sensory, motor, or autonomic fibers (Table 4). Sensory neuropathies may involve primarily large fibers, with reduced perception of vibration and position, decreased tactile discrimination, and absent tendon reflexes. If small fibers are affected, reduced pain and temperature sensibility may predominate. Motor neuropathies may have minimal sensory disturbances, and isolated autonomic neuropathies are well recognized. For the most part, however, chronic neuropathies produce a stereotypic mixture of sensory, motor, and autonomic deficits.

Further work-up of a chronic neuropathy requires performance of laboratory studies to search for an underlying disorder (Table 4). These studies include complete blood cell count; of sedimentation rate, creatinine, glutamic oxaloacetic transaminase, bilirubin, serologic test for syphilis, serum protein electrophoresis; antinuclear antibody, rheumatoid factor, thyroxine, porphobilinogen, measurement of heavy metals in urine, chest X-ray, and check of urine and stool for blood. Elevated spinal fluid protein is found with inflammatory polyneuritis, myxedema, paraproteinemia, malignancy, tabes dorsalis, Dejerine-Sottas disease, Refsum disease, and childhood leukodystrophies. Nerve conduction studies can confirm the clinically suspected anatomical distribution of nerve lesions and occasionally reveal unexpected areas of focal nerve compression. Conduction velocities usually will be at least 30% slower than normal when segmental demyelination is the primary pathological process (6,20,27), and the amplitudes of nerve action potentials will be reduced, with minimal conduction slowing, when the process is primarily axonal. Demyelination predominates in neuropathies of inflammatory polyneuritis, hypothyroidism, diphtheria, Refsum disease, leukodystrophies, hypertrophic forms of peroneal muscular atrophy, and some cases of carcinoma; most other neuropathies are mixed or axonal.

Cutaneous nerve biopsy may yield evidence about the chronicity of a neuropathy at the site sampled, and the degree of axonal destruction and demyelination. Certain features, if present, can suggest or establish a clinical diagnosis. *Mycobacterium leprae* are seen in leprous Schwann cells. Vasonecrosis with inflammatory cell infiltrates is diagnostic of necrotizing vasculitis. Mononuclear elements may indicate a paraproteinemia. Onion bulbs signify repeated segmental demyelination and remyelination. Amyloid fibrils or metachromatic sulfatide may be identified with special stains.

Having correctly diagnosed a neuropathy, one would like a specific treatment to remove the underlying disorder. If the cause relents, symptoms and signs due exclusively to segmental demyelination will improve quickly over weeks, whereas those from axonal degeneration will reverse much more slowly, over months, at a rate of 1 to 2 mm a day. Extent of repair will be limited to some degree by the amount of collagen and fibroblast proliferation that appears in the diseased nerve, presumably impeding the progress of regenerating sprouts. In leprosy, perhaps the major cause of neuropathy in the world, the underlying cause can be eliminated. Treatment with dapsone (diaminodiphenylsulfone), sometimes in conjunction with other antimicrobial agents, can render a patient free of *Mycobacterium leprae.* Similarly, exposure to an agent causing toxic neuropathy can be terminated. (see Table 4).

In many instances our knowledge of pathogenesis is insufficient to reverse the basic disorder. Still, therapeutic measures can be effective. Hormonal replacement is of proven value in hypothyroidism, where evidence of recovery is found 6 weeks after administration of the thyroid hormone (11,14). Similarly, insulin replacement has been associated with reduction of diabetic neuropathy (22), although the correlation between degree of hyperglycemic control and improvement in nerve conduction velocity is not always good (47). The neuropathies of B_{12}, pyridoxine, and thiamine deficiency respond to vitamin supplementation. Isoniazid and hydralazine neuropathies, which result from relative pyridoxine deficiency (37), improve with replacement of vitamin B_6.

Uremic neuropathy usually responds favorably to hemodialysis, and nerve conduction velocity increases toward normal (33). Results with renal transplantation are even more promising (2), although there is evidence to suggest that the demyelinating component of the neuropathy improves to a greater degree than the axonal component (1). Renal transplantation also has been used in patients with Fabry disease, again with improvement of neuropathic symptoms (4). Attacks of porphyric neuropathy may cease when all precipitating drugs are discontinued. Radiation to a solitary plasmacytoma can produce long-term remission of myeloma neuropathy (12). Dietary manipulation is effective in the treatment of Refsum disease, a rare disorder of phytanic acid metabolism. Workers have shown that patients who adhere strictly to a low phytanic acid diet, eliminating chlorophyll-containing vegetables, have improved muscle strength and nerve conduction, and a fall in spinal fluid protein to normal (42).

The place of corticosteroids in the treatment of neuropathies is controversial, as it is in other areas of neurology and medicine. There is little evidence that high-dose corticosteroids affect recovery from acute inflammatory polyneuritis (Guillain-Barré syndrome) (21,28), although a 1-week trial is justifiable in quadriplegic patients who show no sign of improvement. The case for the use of corticosteroids in the treatment of chronic inflammatory polyneuritis is stronger (13,35). Some patients with chronic or relapsing polyneuritis are unquestionably responsive to prednisone, and in such cases neuropathy deteriorates with decrements in daily dose as small as 5 mg. Neuropathies occurring as a remote manifestation of carcinoma also may respond to corticosteroid therapy. To find such responsive cases, one should consider a 2- or 3-week trial of prednisone, 60 to 80 mg/day, in patients with subacute or chronic demyelinating neuropathy and elevated CSF protein. The notion that steroid therapy can aggravate rheumatoid neuropathy probably reflects the greater degree of illness in patients requiring high doses of steroids (10).

Surgery has several limited roles in the definitive therapy of peripheral nerve disorders. One is excision of a cyst or other tumor mass that produces focal compression. Another is neurolysis, reanastomosis, or graft repair of a segment of nerve damaged by trauma or an inflammatory process (41).

Many general measures can be used to a patient's advantage even when the cause of his peripheral nerve disorder is obscure, and in that sense, all neuropathies are treatable. Foremost are measures of general life support, especially for patients with acute inflammatory polyneuritis who develop quadriplegia and paralysis of respiratory muscles. Patients with rapidly advancing weakness should be followed closely for signs of respiratory insufficiency. If vital capacity falls precipitously or drops below 500 cc, elective tracheostomy may be necessary. Arterial blood gases are sometimes unreliable when following patients with impending respiratory failure, because tachypnea can compensate for decreased vital capacity until shortly before the exhausted patient slips into hypoxic coma. Sudden sometimes fatal arrhythmias occur with frequency in patients with acute polyneuritis (24), especially during endotracheal suction, and nurses should be attentive to the cardiac monitor at that time. They are also at risk for pulmonary emboli (36).

Bedfast patients with neurogenic weakness should eat a low-residue diet, supplemented with stool softeners, to avoid constipation. Acute urinary retention may be avoided by performing the Credé maneuver three times a day, although intermittent catheterization is sometimes required. Urecholine is useful with some patients who have sufficient neural control to micturate voluntarily on occasion. In any case, anticholinergic medications should be avoided in the presence of urinary hesitation.

Symptoms of autonomic dysfunction become especially annoying once the patient is ambulatory. Postural hypotension is best treated with high thigh or lower body stockings, and the patient is instructed to arise from supine gradually in stages. Fluorohydrocortisone may reduce postural hypotension by expanding blood volume. It should be used with caution in patients with congestive heart failure or low serum albumin (7). Impotence is a common but underreported symptom of autonomic neuropathy in males. When impotence occurs, all medications should be carefully screened to rule out drugs — parasympathetic and ganglionic blockers, antihistamines, and phenothiazines—that are known to cause impotence. Artificial penile implants have been considered successful by a minority of patients.

A number of measures directed at the musculoskeletal system are valuable in patients with neuropathies of any cause. Passive and when possible active physiotherapy prevents contractures across weakened distal joints, and disuse immobility at larger, more proximal joints. Splints that hold an immobile hand or foot in position of function are useful in preventing deformities that can be so troublesome if reinnervation occurs. Occupational therapists have access to ingenious devices that allow performance of fine motor tasks that otherwise would be impossible for weakened fingers. Transplanting the tendon from a strong proximal muscle to the insertion of a weakened distal one is occasionally of value in patients with paralysis from indolent chronic neuropathies.

A neuropathy may cause anesthesia sufficient to eliminate pain as the major warning signal of impending tissue injury. Other protective measures must be substituted. If the cornea is anesthetic or the orbicularis oculi muscle weak, patients should use protective eyeglasses and apply methycellulose eyedrops to keep conjunctivae moist. Paralyzed upper lids should be taped closed at night. Anesthetic hands and feet must be assiduously protected from injury, as episodes of repeated unrecognized trauma can destroy the digits. Sabin (40) demonstrated this in remarkable photographs of one man's insensitive hands over 10 years. Extensive damage to skin and bone shortened digits of his strong, active hand, whereas his weak, immobile hand remained structurally intact. Patients should check the temperature of pot handles, bath water, and other potentially hot surfaces with a portion of skin that has normal sensation. Toenails should be clipped carefully by an assistant, and shoes should be examined twice daily for pebbles or nails. Thin, dry, denervated skin should be moistened with a suitable cream. Since patients with polyneuropathies are predisposed to compression lesions (26,31), they should avoid leaning on their elbows or sitting with legs crossed for an extended period of time. The physician frequently should search for such superimposed neuropathies as these respond well to a change in the patient's habits or to surgical decompression.

Although anesthesia is a major disabling feature of neuropathy, its opposite, pain, can also be troublesome. Neuropathic pain has been explained by an imbalance input from small pain fibers and the large proprioceptive fibers that may inhibit them (30). Recent clinical studies suggest that the correlation between presence of pain and the ratio of small-to-large fibers is not good, and that other mechanisms must be operative (15,32). Pain in some neuropathies may result from spontaneous electrical discharge of regenerating sprouts (5). When drug therapy is undertaken for pain, simple analgesics such as buffered aspirin are the first choice. Aspirin with codeine, although more effective, may produce poorly tolerated constipation. The dull, aching pain that complicates chronic active neuropathies may require long-term administeration of narcotic substitutes. Therapeutic success for brief shooting, stabbing, episodic pains has been more satisfying. Phenytoin (Dilantin®), 300 to 500 mg/day, has proved effective in some cases (18,38). Before abandoning phenytoin, one should be certain that the serum level has been 15 to 20 μg/cc for several weeks. Some patients who fail to respond to phenytoin have a good response to carbamazepine (Tegretol®), 200 to 1,200 mg/day (39,46). The smallest effective dose is chosen, and initially serum white blood cell count and hepatic enzyme levels are carefully monitored. Tricyclic antidepressant drugs may have an ameliorative effect on pain, aside from their mood-elevating action. A combined regimen of antidepressants and phenothiazines has been used for the relief of chronic intractable pain. Nevertheless, chronic administration of phenytoin (17) or tricyclic antidepressants can cause neuropathy of itself.

Surgery for neurogenic pain is usually limited to the most severe cases and only in those whose prognosis for general recovery is poor. Anesthetic blocks or surgical section of nerve, root, spinal cord, or thalamic pain pathways have been variably effective in pain relief. Frontal lobotomy has given relief to terminally ill patients with otherwise unresponsive pain. Chemical or surgical sympathectomy is reserved for reflex sympathetic dystrophy (causalgia).

Counterstimulation is an effective way of ameliorating pain (23,29,45). The soothing result of rubbing an injured part or applying an ointment has been well recognized. This may be because of the aforementioned central inhibitory effect of large proprioceptive fibers on small fibers (30,45), or it may work through a peripheral mechanism of "jamming" A-delta fibers (8). The most satisfactory method for applying counterstimulation is to induce the patient to exercise his injured limb. Increasing proprioceptive input decreases subjective pain, in addition to reducing the occurrence of secondary osteoarthritic changes from immobility. Whirlpool therapy with either warm or cool water is a useful adjunct in urging reluctant patients to move a painful limb. Cutaneous electrical stimulation, applied over an injured nerve, has been said to relieve otherwise intractable pain (29). Nerves, dorsal columns, and the internal capsule have been stimulated directly. Impressive results have been claimed for acupuncture therapy (25). Symptomatic improvement with acupuncture seems to reflect an alteration in the subject's acceptance of pain, but not his physiologic threshold for noxious stimuli (9).

Peripheral neuropathies are associated with a wide variety of neurological and systemic disorders. In many cases the etiology can be found and a specific treatment instituted. Whether or not the cause is known, therapies are available to ameliorate the disabilities of all patients with neuropathy.

REFERENCES

1. Bolton, C. F. (1976): Electrophysiologic changes in uremic neuropathy after successful renal transplantation. *Neurology (Minneap.)*, 26:152–161.

2. Bolton, C. F., Baltzan, M. A., and Baltzan, R. B. (1971): Effects of renal transplantation on uremic neuropathy. A clinical and electrophysiologic study. *N. Engl. J. Med.*, 184:1170–1175.

3. Bradley, W. G. (1974): *Disorders of Peripheral Nerves.* Blackwell Scientific Publishers, Oxford.

4. Brady, R. O., and King, F. M. (1975): Fabry's disease. In: *Peripheral Neuropathy*, edited by P. J. Dyck, P. K. Thomas, and E. H. Lambert. W. B. Saunders Co., Philadelphia.

5. Brown, M. J., Martin, J. R., and Asbury, A. K. (1976): Painful diabetic neuropathy. *Arch. Neurol.*, 33:164–171.

6. Buchthal, F., Rosenfalck, A., and Behse, F. (1975): Sensory potentials of normal and diseased nerves. In: *Peripheral Neuropathy*, edited by P. J. Dyck, P. K. Thomas, and E. H. Lambert. W. B. Saunders Co., Philadelphia.

7. Campbell, I. W., Ewing, D. J., and Clarke, B. F. (1975): 9-Alpha-fluorohydrocortisone in the treatment of postural hypotension in diabetic autonomic neuropathy. *Diabetes*, 24:381–384.

8. Campbell, J. N., and Taub, A. (1973): Local analgesia from percutaneous electrical stimulation. A peripheral mechanism. *Arch. Neurol.*, 28:347–350.

9. Clark, W. C., and Yang, J. C. (1974): Acupuncture analgesia? Evaluation by signal detection theory. *Science*, 184:1096–1097.

10. Conn, D. L., and Dyck, P. J. (1975): Angiopathic neuropathy in connective tissue diseases. In: *Peripheral Neuropathy*, edited by P. J. Dyck, P. K. Thomas, and E. H. Lambert. W. B. Saunders Co., Philadelphia.

11. Crevasse, L. E., and Logue, R. B. (1959): Peripheral neuropathy in myxedema. *Ann. Intern. Med.*, 50:1433–1437.

12. Davis, L. E., and Drachman, D. B. (1972): Myeloma neuropathy. Successful treatment of two patients and review of cases. *Arch. Neurol.*, 27:507–511.

13. Dyck, P. J., Lais, A. C., Ohta, M., Bastron, J. A., Okazaki, H., and Groover, R. V. (1975): Chronic inflammatory polyradiculoneuropathy. *Mayo Clin. Proc.*, 50:621–637.

14. Dyck, P. J., and Lambert, E. H. (1970): Polyneuropathy associated with hypothyroidism. *J. Neuropathol. Exp. Neurol.*, 29:631–658.

15. Dyck, P. J., Lambert, E. H., and O'Brien, P. C. (1976): Pain in peripheral neuropathy related to rate and kind of fiber degeneration. *Neurology (Minneap.)*, 26:466–471.

16. Dyck, P. J., Thomas, P. K., and Lambert, E. H. (Eds.) (1975): *Peripheral Neuropathy.* W. B. Saunders Co., Philadelphia.

17. Eisen, A. A., Woods, J. F., and Sherwin, A. L. (1974): Peripheral nerve function in long-term therapy with diphenylhydantoin. A clinical and electrophysiologic correlation. *Neurology (Minneap.)*, 24:411–417.

18. Ellenberg, M. (1968): Treatment of diabetic neuropathy with diphenylhydantoin. *N.Y. State Med. J.*, 68:2653–2655.

19. Freemon, F. R. (1975): Causes of polyneuropathy. *Acta Neurol. Scand. [Suppl. 59]*, 51.

20. Gilliatt, R. W. (1966): Nerve conduction in human and experimental neuropathies. *Proc. R. Soc. Med.*, 59:989–992.

21. Goodall, J. A. D., Kosmidis, J. C., and Geddes, A. M. (1974): Effect of corticosteroids on course of Guillain-Barré syndrome. *Lancet*, 1:524–526.

22. Gregersen, G. (1967): Diabetic neuropathy: influence of age, sex, metabolic control, and duration of diabetes on motor nerve conduction velocity. *Neurology (Minneap.)*, 17:972–980.

23. Higgins, J. D., Tursky, B., and Schwartz, G. E. (1971): Shock-elicited pain and its reduction by concurrent tactile stimulation. *Science*, 172:866–867.

24. Lichtenfeld, P. (1971): Autonomic dysfunction in the Guillain-Barré syndrome. *Am. J. Med.*, 50:772–780.

25. Mann, F., Bowser, D., Mumford, J., Lipton, S., and Miles, J. (1973): Treatment of intractable pain by acupuncture. *Lancet*, 2:57–60.

26. Mayer, R. F. (1965): Peripheral nerve function in vitamin B_{12} deficiency. *Arch. Neurol.*, 13:355–362.

27. McLeod, J. G., Prineas, J. W., and Walsh, J. C. (1973): The relationship of conduction velocity to pathology in peripheral nerves. In: *New Developments in Electromyography and Clinical Neurophysiology*, edited by J. E. Desmedt. S. Karger, Basel.

28. McLeod, J. G., Walsh, J. C., Prineas, J. W., and Pollard, J. D. (1976): Acute idiopathic

polyneuritis. A clinical and electrophysiological follow-up study. *J. Neurol. Sci.*, 27:145–162.

29. Melzack, R. (1975): Prolonged relief of pain by brief, intense transcutaneous somatic stimulation. *Pain*, 1:357–373.
30. Melzack, R., and Wall, P. D. (1965): Pain mechanisms; a new theory. *Science*, 150:971–979.
31. Mulder, D. W., Lambert, E. H., Bastron, J. A., and Sprague, R. G. (1961): The neuropathies associated with diabetes. A clinical and electromyographic study of 103 unselected diabetic patients. *Neurology (Minneap.)*, 11:275–284.
32. Nathan, P. W. (1976): The gate-control theory of pain—a critical review. *Brain*, 99:123–158.
33. Nielson, V. K. (1974): The peripheral nerve function in chronic renal failure. A survey. *Acta Med. Scand. [Suppl. 573]*.
34. Prineas, J. (1970): Polyneuropathies of unknown cause. *Acta Neurol. Scand. [Suppl. 44]*, 46.
35. Prineas, J. W., and McLeod, J. G. (1976): Chronic relapsing polyneuritis. *J. Neurol. Sci.*, 27:427–458.
36. Raman, T. K., Blake, J. A., and Harris, T. M. (1971): Pulmonary embolism in Landry-Guillan-Barre-Strohl syndrome. *Chest*, 60:555–557.
37. Raskin, N. H., and Fishman, R. A. (1965): Pyridoxine-deficiency neuropathy due to hydralazine. *N. Engl. J. Med.*, 273:1182–1185.
38. Raskin, N. H., Levinson, S. A., Hoffman, P. M., Pickett, J. B. E., and Fields, H. L. (1974): Postsympathectomy neuralgia. Amelioration with diphenylhydantoin and carbamazepine. *Am. J. Surg.*, 128:75–78.
39. Rull, J. A., Quibrera, R., Gonzalez-Millan, H., and Lozano-Castanedo, O. (1969): Symptomatic treatment of peripheral diabetic neuropathy with carbamazepine. Double blind cross over study. *Diabetologia*, 5:215–218.
40. Sabin, T. D. (1969): Lessons from leprosy. *Am. J. Occup. Ther.*, 33:473–478.
41. Seddon, H. (1975): *Surgical Disorders of the Peripheral Nerves*. Churchill Livingstone, London.
42. Stokke, O., and Eldjarn, L. (1975): Biochemical and dietary aspects of Refsum's disease. In: *Peripheral Neuropathies*, edited by P. J. Dyck, P. K. Thomas, and E. H. Lambert. W. B. Saunders Co., Philadelphia.
43. Swift, T. R., and Ignacio, O. J. (1975): Tick paralysis: Electrophysiologic studies. *Neurology (Minneap.)*, 25:1130–1133.
44. Vinken, P. J., and Bruyn, G. W. (Eds.) (1970): *Handbook of Clinical Neurology, Vols. 7 and 8: Diseases of Nerves*. Elsevier, New York.
45. Wall, P. D., and Sweet, W. H. (1967): Temporary abolition of pain in man. *Science*, 155:108–109.
46. Wilton, T. D. (1974): Tegretol in the treatment of diabetic neuropathy. *S. Afr. Med. J.*, 48:869–872.
47. Winegrad, A. I., and Greene, D. A. (1976): Diabetic polyneuropathy: Could insulin deficiency, hyperglycemia, and alterations in myoinositol metabolism contribute to its pathogenesis? *N. Engl. J. Med.*, 295:1416–1421.

Advances in Neurology, Vol. 17, edited by
R. C. Griggs and R. T. Moxley, III. Raven Press,
New York © 1977.

Investigative Approaches: Pathologic and Morphometric Three-Dimensional Studies in Peripheral Neuropathy

Peter James Dyck

Mayo Clinic and Mayo Foundation, Rochester, Minnesota 55901

INTRODUCTION

Because peripheral neuropathies occur frequently and because they are often associated with prolonged morbidity, research directed at understanding their causes and at finding their remedies is needed. Such research should probably be directed broadly at understanding: the cell biology of the peripheral nervous system, the mechanisms resulting in the disease associated with neuropathy, the mechanism by which the disease process damages peripheral nerve cells (and at what sites), and the factors that result in symptoms.

Areas of investigation with application to an understanding of the mechanisms of development of peripheral neuropathy are many and include the following: the factors that control nerve development, differentiation, and growth; the factors that regulate and determine the peculiar symbiosis of nerve cells and Schwann cells and how these are affected by disease; the nature and mechanism of the control of the target tissue by the innervating cell, and the effect on the nerve cell of loss of the target tissue; the mechanisms that promote nerve sprouting and its direction; the metabolic events that maintain the integrity of the neuron; and the mechanism and role of axonal flow in nerve function and maintenance of integrity.

Because neuropathy is usually associated with systemic disease or the complication of such disease, it undoubtedly would be helpful to understand how the underlying disease develops. Increasingly, it has become clear that diseases such as diabetes mellitus are not simply owing to one cause: multiple factors influence their development and expression.

The mechanisms by which disease causes nerve fiber degeneration may be studied by various techniques. In human peripheral neuropathy a good place to start is to perform systematic morphometric and pathologic study at the level of the cell body, the roots, the segmental nerve, the plexus, the nerve trunks, and the terminal twigs. Such a three-dimensional study might not only provide an understanding of which populations of fibers are affected and at what sites, but it might also indicate something about the mechanism involved.

MORPHOMETRIC AND PATHOLOGIC THREE-DIMENSIONAL STUDIES OF PERIPHERAL NEUROPATHY

Previous Studies

During the early years of the development of the specialty of pathology, German and French investigators did quite extensive evaluations of the peripheral nervous system in patients with peripheral neuropathy coming to postmortem. A few examples of important insights that have come from such studies are the following: the site and pathologic characteristics of familial hypertrophic neuropathy (3,10), lead neuropathy (11,12), angiopathic neuropathy (9,14), dominantly inherited sensory neuropathy (4,13), and uremic neuropathy (2).

As conventionally done, postmortem examination provides little insight into the mechanism of the neuropathy, because tissue is inadequately sampled, control material is not used, and the histologic methods are not optimized. In the conventional postmortem examination, only fragments of peripheral nerve tissue may be taken—often only from portions available through the chest and abdominal incisions. An extensive sampling and evaluation of the peripheral nervous system is time consuming and expensive. In recent time, the value of a systematic study along the length of the peripheral nervous system has come from evaluation of the Cr III nerve palsy associated with diabetes mellitus—extraocular muscle weakness with pupillomotor sparing (1,5). In this disorder serial sections showed a central fascicular region that was demyelinated—probably from ischemic damage.

To illustrate the use of pathologic and morphometric three-dimensional studies, we will discuss our findings in angiopathic neuropathy (in which the defect is interstitial) and in Fabry's disease (in which the defect is parenchymatous).

Necrotizing Angiopathic Neuropathy: Fiber Degeneration and Sites of Occluded Vessels (7)

From a patient with rheumatoid arthritis with multiple mononeuropathy owing to a necrotizing angiitis, the limb nerves were taken from the axilla to just above the wrist and from the gluteal fold to the ankle. Fixation was in 10% neutral formalin. From proximal to distal, consecutive blocks along the length of the nerves were cut. Alternatively, the blocks of nerve were 6 to 8 mm long (even-numbered blocks) and 1 to 2 mm long (uneven-numbered blocks). Even-numbered blocks were embedded in paraffin and stained with hematoxylin and eosin to show vessel and histologic detail. Uneven-numbered blocks of tissue were additionally fixed in osmium tetroxide, embedded in paraffin, and sectioned. The latter blocks of tissue were used, without further staining, to evaluate myelinated fiber density. A few transverse sections were cut from all blocks of tissue. To identify the proximal onset of fiber degeneration or the distribution of a vascular lesion, serial sections were cut from the entire block in some cases. Using these methods, it was possible to identify and characterize vessel and fiber abnormalities along the length of the peripheral nerve trunks.

BLOOD VESSEL PATHOLOGY

The small arteries of limb nerves are usually 100 to 200 μm in diameter and lie in the epineurium between the fascicles of nerves. They usually have an internal elastic lamina and a well-developed media, usually consisting of smooth muscle but occasionally with some elastic tissue. Small arterioles ≤ 75 μm are sometimes found in the perineurium or in the endoneurium adjacent to the perineurium.

To quantitate the arterial disease along the length of nerve trunks, we used the following simple grading system: A, normal; B, perivascular inflammatory cells; C, perivascular inflammatory cells and intimal proliferation; D, changes of C and degeneration of media with or without inflammatory cells; E, changes of C and D and recent occlusion of the lumen; and F, changes of C, D, and E and hemorrhage or presence of hemosiderin.

In the sciatic nerve, occluded vessels were seen at the 6-, 7-, 10-, and 19-cm levels in the peroneal division and at the 7-, 10-, and 14-cm levels in the tibial division. In the median nerve, occlusion was seen at the 18-, 20-, 21-, and 22-cm levels. In the ulnar nerve, occlusion was seen at the 24- and 25-cm levels. Particularly in the tibial division, arteries with perivascular inflammatory cells and with proliferation were widely distributed.

NERVE FIBER PATHOLOGY

Sections from blocks that had been fixed in osmium tetroxide were examined serially from proximal to distal along the nerve trunks, so the regions with marked fiber degeneration or loss could readily be identified and differentiated from control nerves. Density of intact myelinated fibers in fascicles was graded as: A, normal numbers; B, equivocally decreased numbers; C, moderately decreased numbers; and D, greatly decreased numbers. Regions of fiber degeneration (FD) could be identified by ballooned-out myelin rings, presence of myelin balls, decrease in density of fibers, or absence of myelinated fibers. Regions of FD began at the mid-upper arm and mid-thigh levels. The relationship between the distribution of arteriolar and fiber disease is shown in Table 1 for the median nerve. The central

TABLE 1. *Arteriolar pathology and fascicle density of myelinated fibers*

Site	Condition of arterioles (frequency)						Condition of fascicles (frequency)			
	A	B	C	D	E	F	A	B	C	D
1			1				14			
2	1						17			
3	1						12	1		
4	1						11	3	2	
5	1						17	2	1	
6	1						14	2	1	
7							3		13	
8							2	1	12	
9							4	2	12	
10		1					4	1	14	
11		1								16
12		1								16
13			1							20
14		1								16
15	1									18
16	1									12
17										16
18		1			1					26
19	2									29
20	1	2			1					33
21	1	1	1		1					32
22	2	1			1					31
23	1		1							24
24	2	1								22
25		1	1							20
26	1	1								20
27	1	1								21
28	2									24
29	1									23
30	1									25

Fibers at 1-cm intervals in median nerve in a patient with rheumatoid arthritis and necrotizing angiopathy.
From ref. 7.

fascicular decrease in density of myelinated fibers which could be recognized especially in the median nerve is shown in Fig. 1. A roughly similar relationship between ubiquitous small-artery disease and focal onset of fiber disease at mid-upper arm and mid-thigh level was found for the other nerves.

That ischemia probably accounts for the fiber damage is strongly suggested by the ubiquitous necrotizing angiopathy with occlusion, the patchy and often total loss of fibers, and in some cases capillary stasis and hemorrhage in the region of fiber degeneration. A probable explanation for the onset of fiber degeneration in central fascicular locations at mid-upper arm and mid-thigh levels is that these affected regions are watershed zones of poor perfusion.

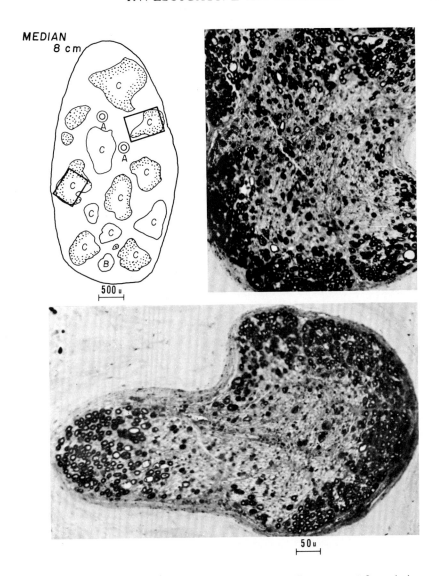

FIG. 1. Low-power tracing of fascicular pattern of median nerve at 8 cm below axilla (case 84–69). Regions of fascicles shown in accompanying photomicrographs are in rectangles on tracing. Note central fascicular degeneration of myelinated fibers, surrounded by borderline zone with increased number of degenerating fibers, which in turn is surrounded by fibers of normal density and without degenerating fibers. A-normal density of myelinated fibers, B-slight decrease in density, and C-moderate decrease in density (From ref. 7)

Since the publication of the preceding case, we have studied two other cases with similar techniques and the findings have been milder but similar.

Sections from peripheral nerve trunks in patients dying with necrotizing angiopathy have been seen by many pathologists, but the relationship just described was not recognized because systematic three-dimensional studies were not undertaken.

LOSS OF SMALL PERIPHERAL SENSORY NEURONS IN FABRY'S DISEASE (17)

In a 44-year-old man with features of Fabry's disease — typical red spots on lower abdomen and groin, attacks of shooting, lightening pains deep in the limbs, cerebellar ataxia, and death from a stroke — the peripheral sensory neurons were quantitatively analyzed at the level of the peripheral nerve (sural nerve), spinal ganglion (L-3 ganglion), and fasciculus gracilis of the spinal cord (C-1 and C-8).

The sural nerves were fixed in 2% glutaraldehyde in 0.1 M cacodylate buffer (pH 7.4) for 2 hr. A portion of the tissue was washed, additionally fixed in 1% osmium tetroxide for 2 hr, dehydrated, and embedded in epoxy. Transverse 1.5-μm sections were cut, systematically sampled sections were photographed in a phase microscope, and photographic enlargements (1,500 ×) were prepared. The frequency distributions of the diameters of the myelinated fibers in the photographic enlargements were determined using a particle-size analyzer set on the large measuring range, exponential, and frequency distribution settings. Programmed calculation and plotting were used. Another portion was prepared as teased fibers (6). Abnormalities of teased fibers were descriptively graded according to the criteria illustrated and described in Fig. 2.

Thin transverse sections were cut, stained with uranyl acetate and lead citrate, and examined under the electron microscope. For determining the frequency distribution of unmyelinated fibers per square millimeter, we prepared electron micrographs (7,600×) of all portions of endoneurial regions not covered by copper screen. Using the particle-size analyzer with settings of small measuring range and linear and frequency distribution, and using programmed calculation and plotting, we prepared number and diameter histograms of unmyelinated fibers.

The number and diameter histograms of the L-3 spinal ganglia were obtained using the method described in our laboratory by Offord and co-workers (16). In this method serially numbered transverse paraffin (or preferably celloidin sections since there is a lesser degree of shrinkage of cytoplasm from the basket cells) sections of the entire spinal ganglion are prepared. The first and last sections are identified by arbitrary criteria such as the first and last section having parts of 10 cytons. Systematically, low-power photomicrographs of the first and last and of every 50th section are prepared. The area of each section is obtained by digitizing the endoneurial area and correcting for magnification. The volume of the ganglion is then derived by determining the volumes of the sampled sections and interpolating values between sampled sections.

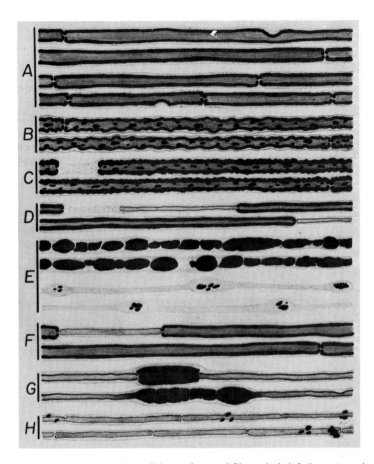

FIG. 2. Drawings of descriptive conditions of teased fibers. In brief, the categories are as follows: **A,** fiber of normal appearance; **B,** fiber with excessive irregularity of myelin; **C,** fiber with segmental demyelination and with variability of myelin thickness between internodes of less than 50% (demyelination without remyelination); **D,** fiber with segmental demyelination and variability of myelin thickness between internodes of more than 50% (demyelination and remyelination); **E,** fiber that has undergone myelin degeneration into linear ovoids and balls (wallerian and axonal degeneration); **F,** fibers with variability of myelin thickness between internodes of more than 50% (includes fibers with intercalated internodes); **G,** fibers with excessive variability of myelin thickness within internodes to form "globules" or "sausages"; **H,** fiber with myelin ovoids or balls adjacent to it (probably regenerating fiber). [From Dyck, P. J., Stevens, J. C., Mulder, D. W., and Espinosa, R. E. (1975): *Neurology,* 25:781–785.]

To determine the number of cytons in the ganglia, one must count nucleoli of sampled sections using the rectangular ocular grid of the microscope and mechanical screws to traverse the endoneurial area in *x* and *y* directions. If nucleoli would not be cleaved by the microtome knife, it would not be necessary to correct for split-cell error. Cleavage of nucleoli, however, does occur, so corrections must be made. Split-cell error depends on nucleolar size, relationship of diameter of nucleoli to diameter of cyton, and thickness of section. We have found that spurious results are obtained from relating the diameter of the nucleolus to the diameter of the cyton in one section, as the larger-diameter portion of the nucleolus may be found in the preceding or subsequent serial section. It is necessary therefore to view the preceding and subsequent sections to see which one contains the largest-diameter nucleolus, and then measurements can be made. It has been found that large cytons have larger-diameter nucleoli than do small-diameter cytons. The relationship between cyton and nucleoli diameter can be expressed as a straight-line relationship. Diameter histograms of cytons are prepared by measuring the diameter of cytons having nuceoli on photomicrographs of sampled sections. The mathematical formulas needed will not be given here, but they are found in the article by Offord and co-workers (16).

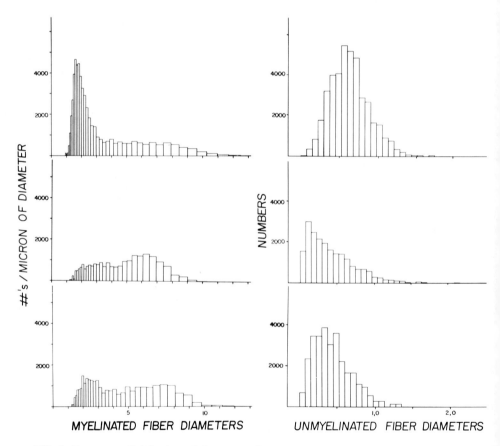

FIG. 3. Frequency distribution of diameters of myelinated (*left*) and unmyelinated (*right*) fibers of healthy sural nerves (*top*) and of sural nerves of patients 1 (*middle*) and 2 (*bottom*). Note decrease in numbers of small myelinated and unmyelinated fibers. (From ref. 17.)

The C-1 and C-8 segments of spinal cord of this patient and from a control case were removed. Under the dissecting microscope the fasciculus gracilis from the left side was excised and split into several blocks. After osmication the tissue was embedded in epoxy, and 1.5-μm transverse sections were cut.

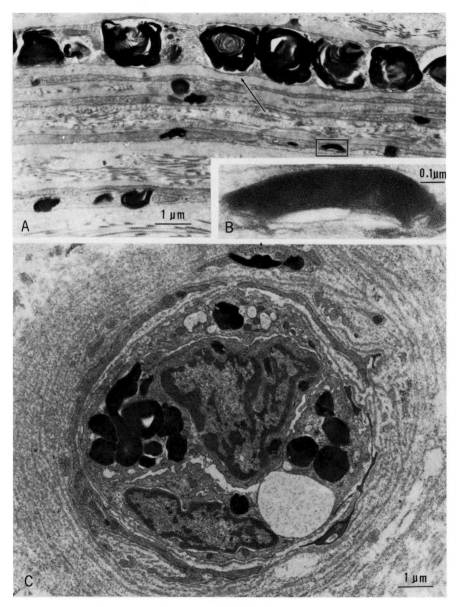

FIG. 4. Transverse sections from sural nerves from patient 2. **A:** Lamellated bodies in perineurial cells (*arrow*). **B:** Higher magnification of region in rectangle in **A. C:** Lamellated bodies in endothelial and perithelial cells of endoneurial capillary. (From ref. 17.)

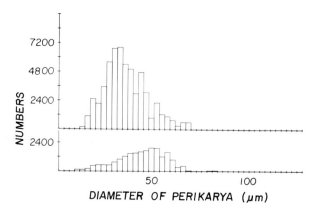

FIG. 5. Frequency distribution of diameters of perikarya of L-3 ganglion in patient 1 (*lower*) and in normal (*upper*) 43-year-old woman. (From ref. 17.)

The number of myelinated fibers per square millimeter and their diameter histograms were obtained using the techniques described earlier.

In the sural nerve, although the number of large myelinated fibers fell within the normal range, the number of small myelinated and of unmyelinated fibers was approximately one-half that of control nerves (Fig. 3). Large numbers of lamellated bodies, with different characteristics than Π granules, were found especially in endothelial and perineurial cells (Fig. 4).

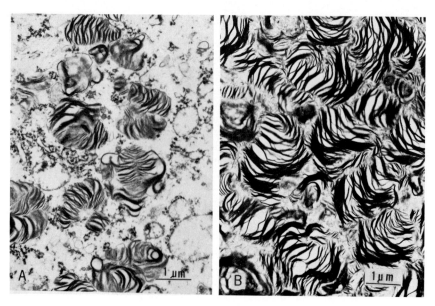

FIG. 6. Lamellated bodies in cytoplasm of perikarya in patient 1 are loosely packed among normal-looking **(A)** or tightly packed **(B)** cell organelles. (From ref. 17.)

Other electron microscopic abnormalities, especially of unmyelinated axis cylinders, were also seen (17).

The number of cytons in L-3 ganglion was approximately one-half of that of controls. There was a striking decrease from the normal of small-diameter cytons (Fig. 5). The number of myelinated fibers per square millimeter of fasciculus gracilis fell within the normal range.

Cytons of neurons containing an abnormal accumulation of lipids were found to contain a decreased amount of endoplasmic reticulum. In Fabry's disease, known to be due to an inborn error of lipid metabolism, we have shown that a preferential loss of small myelinated and unmyelinated fibers and of small cytons of spinal ganglia is present.

Thus these morphometric and pathologic studies have shown that in Fabry's disease the diseased cytons lose endoplasmic reticulum and accumulate abnormal amounts of lamellar lipid material (Fig. 6). There is a selective degeneration of small neurons, which is thought to account for the pain and absence of sweating characteristic of this disorder.

PATTERNS OF PATHOLOGY THAT MIGHT BE RECOGNIZED BY THREE-DIMENSIONAL STUDIES

Interstitial

INFLAMMATORY, DEMYELINATING

Foci of mononuclear cell infiltration, often in a pericapillary distribution and associated with demyelination, have been recognized in a variety of neurologic diseases. This pattern is found in experimental allergic encephalitis (EAE) and experimental allergic neuritis (EAN), in which immunologic mechanisms are known to be present.

INFILTRATIVE

Nerve fibers may be damaged by compressive lesions, either by pressure from the outside or from infiltration of cells or fluid into the endoneurial space. Although it is not yet known with certainty how amyloid damages nerve fibers, nodules may compress fibers as shown in Fig. 7. It is thought that various lymphomas, reticulosis, and myelomas damage nerve fibers by compression of nerve roots at foramina of exit and behind tight fascial sheaths.

VASCULAR

The pattern of nerve fiber degeneration from atherosclerosis is quite different from that of necrotizing angiopathy described earlier. Peripheral

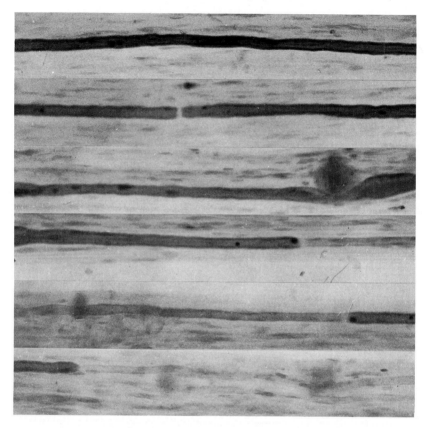

FIG. 7. Consecutive portions of myelinated fiber from sural nerve of case III.11, kinship 84–67. Note marked indentation of myelinated fiber (third row from top) by nodule of amyloid. In lowest two consecutive portions of this fiber, three clumps of amyloid are seen adjacent to thinly myelinated short internodes. [From Dyck, P. J., and Lambert, E. H. (1969): *Arch. Neurol.*, 20:490–507.]

vascular disease from atherosclerosis affects the distal nerves of the lower limbs along with other tissues.

Parenchymatous

The term "parenchymatous" implies a metabolic derangement within the neuron, the Schwann cell, or both. Perhaps in some diseases the entire neuron is affected (as is implied by the use of such terms as "anterior horn cell disease"), and in others only the terminal axons are affected (dying back). Particularly with the advent of the electron microscope, several patterns of axonal change have been described: dissolution of microtubules and neurofilaments within axons—as seen in wallerian degeneration and many axonal degenerations; proliferation of endoplasmic reticulum—as seen in tri-ortho-cresyl-phosphate (TOCP) toxicity; increased density of neurofilaments—as seen in acrylamide, cyanate, and other disorders; and increased glycogen—as seen in hypothyroidism (6).

DISEASES IN WHICH THREE-DIMENSIONAL STUDIES MIGHT BE USEFUL

Muscular Dystrophy

Early pathologic studies of patients dying with muscular dystrophy suggested that the pathologic changes were principally and predominantly in skeletal muscles. Predominantly from estimates of motor units, McComas et al. (15) have predicted that a neural abnormality may underlie the muscle weakness. In an evaluation of muscle nerve in myotonic dystrophy, Pollock and co-worker (18) were unable to show a morphologic abnormality. Because of the admixture of efferent and afferent fibers in muscle nerve, an abnormality may have gone undetected. To test the neural hypothesis of muscular dystrophy, it would be important to obtain reliable morphometric data on the number and size distribution of the: ventral horn alpha and gamma cytons, alpha and gamma axons of ventral roots, and myelinated fibers of defined muscle nerves in patients with dystrophy coming to postmortem examination.

Results of such an examination would have to be interpreted with caution. If an abnormality of morphology of alpha motor neurons could be demonstrated, this would not necessarily indicate that neural factors are primary in muscular dystrophy. A biochemical defect might affect both nerve and muscle, producing morphologic changes in each. Alternatively, morphologic changes in nerve might be secondary to the loss of the target tissue (muscle) from primary disease in muscle.

Neuropathy Associated with Uremia and Hemodialysis

Although a single pathogenetic mechanism may underlie the development of uremic peripheral neuropathy, the occurrence of different clinical neuropathies in uremia suggests that several mechanisms are involved. In what is probably the commonest variety (a symmetric sensorimotor neuropathy predominantly affecting the distal extremity of lower limbs), our studies suggested that the peripheral nerve cells may be affected by a parenchymatous axonal atrophy and degeneration (8). In the second variety, the onset and course, the characteristics of nerve conduction, and the EMG and spinal fluid findings resemble those of an acute or chronic inflammatory polyradiculoneuropathy, even though pathologic confirmation is not available. The third variety is that of mononeuropathy. Some of these neuropathies may be from compression, others may be related to the creation of access to the arterial system by means of cannulae or fistulas, and still others appear to be unrelated to the above.

Careful morphometric and pathologic studies along the length of the peripheral nervous system in patients dying with these syndromes should provide information on whether inflammatory-demyelinating (?immunologic), ischemic (from large- and small-artery disease), or infiltrative mechanisms are involved, *or* whether the pattern is that of parenchymatous involvement. If the latter is found, the search should be continued for toxins, deficiency states, or some other metabolic derangement.

Neuropathy Associated with Diabetes Mellitus

In diabetes mellitus, as in the uremic syndrome, there are a variety of clinical types of peripheral neuropathies (19). Of the cranial neuropathies associated with diabetes mellitus, the Cr III neuropathy with involvement of extraocular muscles but with sparing of pupillomotor fibers has been most completely studied and is known to be owing to central fascicular demyelination of the nerve approximately 1 cm behind the globe. Additionally, patients with diabetes mellitus develop a symmetric distal neuropathy. This tends to take two forms—an ataxic form (pseudo-tabes diabetica) and a hyperalgesic form. Femoral neuropathy (also sometimes called diabetic amyotrophy), which from the EMG characteristics is known to involve a greater distribution than could be explained by involvement of the femoral nerve, is probably a lumboradiculoplexus neuropathy.

A careful three-dimensional study along the length of appropriate parts of the peripheral nervous system, using control tissue, should provide at least an initial insight into the possible mechanism for the development of the neuropathy.

Brachial Plexus and Lower Lumbar and Sacral Plexus Neuropathy

Three-dimensional studies along the length of nerve roots (through the plexus) and nerve trunks during the height of these disorders would probably provide an insight into the mechanism of their development.

CONCLUSION

Research into the cause and treatment of the peripheral neuropathies should be directed broadly at understanding the cell biology of the peripheral nervous system and specifically at elucidating the mechanisms underlying the development of nerve cell degeneration in various diseases associated with neuropathy and with the development of symptomatology. Careful three-dimensional study of portions of the peripheral nervous system has provided an understanding of: (a) the nature of the Cr III neuropathy associated with diabetes mellitus, (b) the relationship between occluded small arteries and regions of nerve fiber degeneration in angiopathic neuropathy (a model of an interstitial neuropathy), and (c) the mechanism of painfulness and of the fact and possible mechanism of the degeneration of small neurons in Fabry's disease (a model of a parenchymatous neuropathy). It is our opinion that three-dimensional morphometric and pathologic studies of the peripheral nervous system in such common disorders as muscular dystrophy and neuropathy associated with uremia and diabetes mellitus would provide useful initial insights into the mechanisms of their development.

ACKNOWLEDGMENTS

This investigation was supported in part by grants NSO 5811, NSO 7541, AM2-2200, and MDA 12, and by the Upton and Herrick Funds.

REFERENCES

1. Asbury, A. K., Aldredge, H., Herschberg, R., and Fisher, C. M. (1970): Oculomotor palsy in diabetes mellitus: a clinico-pathological study. *Brain*, 93:555.
2. Asbury, A. K., Victor, M., and Adams, R. D. (1962): Uremic polyneuropathy. *Trans. Am. Neurol. Assoc.*, 87:100.
3. Dejerine, J., and Sottas, J. (1893): Sur la nevrite: interstitielle, hypertrophique et progressive de l'enfance. *C. R. Soc. Biol. (Paris)*, 45:63.
4. Denny-Brown, D. (1951): Hereditary sensory radicular neuropathy. *J. Neurol. Neurosurg. Psychiatry*, 14:237.
5. Dreyfus, P. M., Hakim, S., and Adams, R. D. (1957): Diabetic ophthalmoplegia. *Arch. Neurol. Psychiatry*, 77:337.
6. Dyck, P. J. (1975): Pathologic alterations of the peripheral nervous system of man. In: *Peripheral Neuropathy*, edited by P. J. Dyck, P. K. Thomas, and E. H. Lambert, pp. 296–336. W. B. Saunders Co., Philadelphia.
7. Dyck, P. J., Conn, D. L., and Okazaki, H. (1972): Necrotizing angiopathic neuropathy: Three-dimensional morphology of fiber degeneration related to sites of occluded vessels. *Mayo Clin. Proc.*, 47:461–475.
8. Dyck, P. J. et al. (1971): Severe hypomyelination and marked abnormality of conduction in Dejerine-Sottas hypertrophic neuropathy: Myelin thickness and compound action potential of sural nerve in vitro. *Mayo Clin. Proc.*, 46:432–436.
9. Eichorst, H. (1887): Neuritis acuta progressiva. *Virchows Arch. [Pathol. Anat.]*, 69:265.
10. Gombault, A., and Mallet, R. (1889): Un cas de tabes ayant debute dans l'enfance: autopsie. *Arch. Med. Exp. Anat. Pathol.*, 1:385.
11. Gombault, M. (1880): Contribution a l'etude anatomique de la nevrite parenchymateuse subaigue et chronique: nevrite segmentaire peri-axile. *Arch. Neurol.(Paris)*, 1:11.
12. Gombault, M. (1886): Sur les lesions de la nevrite alcoolique. *C. R. Acad. Sci. [D] (Paris)*, 102:439.
13. Jughenn, H., Krucke, W., and Wadulla, H. (1949): Zur frage der familiaren syringomyelie: klinisch-anatomische untersuchungen uber "familiare neuro-vasculare dystrophie der extremitaten." *Arch. Psychiatr. Nervenkr.*, 182:153.
14. Leyden, E. (1880): Ueber poliomyelitis und neuritis. *Z. Klin. Med.*, 1:387.
15. McComas, A. J., Sica, R. E. D., and Currie, S. (1970): Muscular dystrophy: Evidence for a neural factor. *Lancet*, 226:1263–1264.

16. Offord, K., Ohta, M., Oenning, R. F., and Dyck, P. J. (1974): Method of morphometric evaluation of spinal and autonomic ganglia. *J. Neurol. Sci.,* 22:65–71.
17. Ohnishi, A., and Dyck, P. J. (1974): Preferential loss of small sensory neurons in Fabry's disease: Histological and morphometric evaluation of cutaneous nerves, spinal ganglia and posterior columns. *Arch. Neurol.,* 31:120.
18. Pollock, M., and Dyck, P. J. (1976): Peripheral nerve morphometry in myotonic dystrophy. *Arch. Neurol.,* 33:33.
19. Thomas, P. K., and Eliasson, S. G. (1975): Diabetic neuropathy. In: *Peripheral Neuropathy,* edited by P. J. Dyck, P. K. Thomas, and E. H. Lambert, pp. 956–981. W. B. Saunders Co., Philadelphia.

Advances in Neurology, Vol. 17, edited by
R. C. Griggs and R. T. Moxley, III. Raven Press,
New York © 1977.

Treatment of Amyotrophic Lateral Sclerosis

David Goldblatt

*Department of Neurology, University of Rochester School of Medicine and
Dentistry, 601 Elmwood Avenue, Rochester, New York 14642*

INTRODUCTION

In reviewing therapy for amyotrophic lateral sclerosis (ALS), I shall consider mainly those forms of treatment that have been introduced, or continue to be employed, in the years since 1967, when a major conference on motor neuron diseases took place under the chairmanship of Drs. Forbes H. Norris, Jr. and Leonard Kurland (61). The proceedings of the conference should be consulted for many valuable contributions on topics that will not be included within the limited scope of the present chapter.

Treatment of any disease may be directed at halting, improving, or curing the underlying disease process, or at alleviating specific symptoms. To select an empirical treatment for a disease, the physician should be guided to some degree by his suppositions about its cause. To give symptomatic treatment, the therapist should understand the pathogenesis of the symptoms he is treating. And to propose a truly rational treatment, the scientist must understand both the cause and the pathophysiological mechanisms of the disorder. Everyone will agree that rational therapy is our long-term goal, but in the present unsatisfactory state of our understanding, symptomatic therapy offers the most substantial benefit to the individual patient, and in ALS it may distinctly alleviate some of the misery of what Cooper (15) has recently called "one of the cruelest, most demeaning, most unbearable of the chronic neurologic disorders, or of any of the intractable diseases."

The historical development of a unifying concept of ALS in its various clinical forms has been traced before (29,36), and I will not reconsider it here. In the classic form, the symptoms and signs of ALS indicate dysfunction or loss of lower motor neurons and of their regulatory systems in the central nervous system, at brainstem and at spinal levels. Characteristically, there are no signs of disturbance in ocular motility or in sensation, and there is little or no impairment of mentation. The illness begins in adult life and becomes progressively more severe. Survival is measured in months to a few years, with some patients living for a decade or considerably longer, occasionally in a stabilized condition. The clinical variability of the disease was well defined in a study reported by the late Dr. Roland Mackay (49); more recently, some authors (10,57) have emphasized variability in the relentlessly progressive course of illness; in so doing, they have underscored the likelihood that a given patient will become increasingly disabled (7) until he succumbs to respiratory failure or infection, or dies suddenly, perhaps because of abnormal vagal mechanisms (55).

I exclude from consideration those disorders that to some extent may resemble idiopathic ALS, but in which a cause has been identified. The differential diagnosis of ALS (55) includes cervical spondylosis, neurosyphilis, syringomyelia and hematomyelia, myopathies, diabetic amyotrophy, perhaps some instances of organomercurial poisoning, and polyneuropathies, including especially bilateral ulnar compression neuropathy and the neuropathy (or motor neuron disease) produced by lead.

I shall first review some of the recent empirical treatments for ALS, each placed under the heading of the causative hypothesis that lends an aura of rationality to that treatment. Then I shall discuss some of the practical modes that have been developed for improving specific symptoms that accompany the advancing illness.

EMPIRICAL TREATMENT

Genetically Determined Aging as Cause

Recently, McComas et al. (50), writing in *Lancet,* have suggested that "motor-neurone disease [is an] accelerated form of normal ageing," determined genetically but possibly influenced by secondary factors such as athletics, upper motor neuron lesions, viruses (polio and perhaps others), malabsorption, neoplasms, toxins (endogenous and exogenous, such as lead), shock, hypoglycemia, and trauma. When some cells are lost, the survivors are used to excess and they become exhausted. One of the numerous examples of an "inciting cause" is to be found in the report of Alpers and Farmer (1), who described two patients in whom "there appeared to be a direct relation between the use of a pneumatic drill and the onset of symptoms." (They suggested a vasospastic mechanism.)

McComas does not refer to Sir William Gowers (38), who, in an earlier edition of the same journal, discussed the subject of accelerated aging in the same way: after describing "abiotrophy"—i.e., "degeneration or decay in consequence of a defect of vital endurance"—in earlier life, Gowers went on to describe such degeneration "at the other end of life. While general life shall seem full of vigour the nutrition of some neurons fails; they slowly die. The neurons which most frequently thus decay are the spinal motor neurons. . . . According to the position of the tracts which suffer first and most the effect is the symptoms of spinal progressive muscular atrophy or of labio-glossal paralysis. . . . These maladies often come on without any apparent cause simply because the term of life for those structures is reached and they decay in a true abiotrophy. When any exciting cause can be traced it is usually one which is alone inadequate. . . . The apparent cause does not lessen the significance of the facts which show these affections to be essentially senile abiotrophy." The postulate of hereditary predisposition to premature aging, or abiotrophy, might seem to be most applicable to familial forms of ALS, but it has been extended to the more common, sporadic cases as well.

A treatment conveniently discussed under the "aging" hypothesis involves the use of inosiplex (Isoprinosine®), a salt of an inosine-alcohol complex, first tested for its effect on polyribosomes. (More recently, the drug has been investigated for its potential usefulness in treating virus diseases, including subacute sclerosing panencephalitis.)

The choice of inosiplex for treating ALS came about in a way that is typical for a "hopeless" disease: a physician developed ALS. His twin brother worked in a medical school where a colleague was giving rats RNA-stimulatory compounds, including inosiplex, thought to be potentially useful in treating senile dementia. On the postulate that RNA stimulation might offset the neuronal degeneration in ALS, and before the compound inosiplex had been shown to have any clinical effectiveness for anything, the physician-patient obtained the drug through his brother and, in 1968, began a treatment regimen that eventually proved completely ineffective. Meanwhile, solely on the strength of that one uncontrolled clinical trial, the drug was given to a group of supposed ALS patients in Mexico, one of whom was alleged to have improved promptly. The encouraging news was reported in a broadcast from Los Angeles, and another treatment program was under way.

By the time that controlled studies had been completed (10,30,65) indicating the lack of effectiveness of the drug in ALS, the rationale for its use had become a dual one—reconstitution of polyribosomes, and "general antiviral activity." The antiviral action had not been an original postulate because of the lack of supportive laboratory data.

I give these details not because it was wrong to have tried a compound "off the shelf," but because before controlled trials of the drug could be carried out, "rumors of its effectiveness in two patients had appeared in the paramedical journals and in the lay press" (30). The unfortunate publicity surrounding the early, uncontrolled trials (certainly not the fault of the original physician-patient) led to the spending of additional thousands of dollars to investigate a useless treatment.

Environmental Factors as Cause

Guamanian ALS, despite its decline in the last decade (67), remains unusually prevalent in that island population and is currently thought to be related to some unidentified environmental factor, perhaps acting on genetically predisposed victims. No genetic pattern for the disorder has been established, although there is a familial aggregation of cases (68), and no cohort phenomenon has been observed. Patients differ from controls in that they eat more raw pork and beef (not fish, shellfish, or cycad nuts), and in that they are of a somewhat lower socioeconomic level, with less education and more contact with animals. There is no difference in the number who work in metal mines, or in respect to childhood diseases. No Guamanian patients report having had poliomyelitis, hepatitis, meningitis, or epilepsy (67).

In a recent epidemiologic survey in the United States (33), patients with ALS differed from age-matched controls in their greater consumption of milk and more frequent exposure to heavy metals. In our experience, the occupation of arc-welding has in several instances been associated with the development of the disease. Boothby et al. (8) have recently reemphasized the close resemblance to ALS of lead "neuritis," which they consider to be a motor neuron disease; but they agree that "it seems unlikely that lead intoxication accounts for a substantial number of patients with ALS, except in individuals with clear occupational exposure." Nothing useful has been forthcoming from attempts to treat idiopathic ALS with chelating agents when the patients have given the history of exposure to lead, mercury, or arsenic (21). The patients of Kantarjian (42) with an ALS-like syndrome consequent to known organomercurial poisoning also were unimproved after treatment.

Metabolic Failure as Cause

Several reports have suggested an abnormality of metabolism in ALS, most commonly a disturbance in glucose utilization. Collis and Engel (14) concluded that elevated oral glucose tolerance tests in ALS are a nonspecific result of loss of muscle mass. Studies of this type continue, including a recent investigation on Guam (43), again reporting a high incidence of glucose intolerance in ALS. Diabetics were three to four times as common, however, among patients with parkinsonism-dementia as among those with ALS.

A causative relationship of impaired glucose metabolism to ALS remains an unproved hypothesis. Astin et al. (2) found no significant difference in plasma glucose and insulin values between patients with ALS and matched controls with other neurological disorders during an oral glucose tolerance test, or between ALS patients and controls with regard to CSF and plasma insulin and glucose in the fasting state and 1 hr after a glucose load. None of the patients had a diabetic curve in the glucose tolerance test. Astin and colleagues have considered the possibilities that the anterior horn cells of patients with motor neuron disease are less than normally responsive to available insulin, or that their cerebrospinal fluid may contain an insulin antagonist.

Therapy directed by the hypothesis of metabolic failure as a possible cause of ALS has included the use of amitriptyline, which was reported by Brown and Mueller (51) to improve glucose utilization in ALS patients. These investigators speculated that metabolic improvement was an indirect effect of treating the patients' suppressed depression.

Extending their interest to the exocrine function of the pancreas, Quick and Greer (66) in 1967 reported that in five ALS patients "the disturbance in the exocrine system was pronounced." Support for the findings of Quick and Greer came from a study by Charchaflie et al. (13), who found that ALS patients had a deficient amylase response in the endogenous secretin-pancreozymin test, which depends on indirect, neuroendocrine mechanisms. Indirect salivary stimulation, using citric acid, was also deficient, but direct stimulation with pilocarpine was normal. The authors postulate that "pancreatic and parotid deficiencies" do not follow a primary disease of the exocrine glands but are more likely to be owing to "modifications of the neuroendocrine mechanisms that regulate their secretory activity."

The initial report by Quick and Greer (66) of a beneficial effect from treatment with pancreatic extract and vitamin E has not been substantiated by subsequent investigators in published reports (26) or, anecdotally, by the experience of individual clinicians, including the author.

Circulating Neurotoxin as Cause

Recent attempts (41,48) to identify a neurotoxic or myelinolytic effect of ALS serum, using tissue culture techniques, have failed to confirm an earlier positive report (78). The attenuated cobra venom therapy directed by Dr. Murray Sanders in Florida, which has been well publicized over the years, finds its hypothetical basis in the attempt to create resistance or immunity to an unknown toxin through repeated exposure to small amounts of neurotoxin. The work has not yet been evaluated by means of accepted double-blind techniques, although such a trial is now being carried on in another clinic. Norris (*personal communication*) has evaluated at least 50 patients before and after the snake venom treatment and has seen no benefit from it in any of them. He adds that he is presently following 13 patients with typical ALS who are showing functional improvement, which he considers to be coincidental to any empirical therapy they may be receiving.

Virus Infection as Cause

Several diseases of animals and man, previously classified as heredo-familial or degenerative, actually are caused by a transmissible agent. This startling discovery has prompted a renewed search for such an agent — either a previously unknown virus or a known virus behaving in an unusual manner—as a cause of ALS. Poliomyelitis and mumps viruses have been held in suspicion. An unexpectedly high incidence of preceding poliomyelitis in patients who develop ALS has been reported several times (12) and can be confirmed in my experience and in that of other members of our department (R. C. Griggs, *personal communication*). Mumps in adult life has been noted to occur frequently in ALS patients. These associations have been reviewed by Lehrich and his colleagues (45). Their data, as well as earlier studies, fail to provide any serological evidence that ALS patients differ from controls with regard to antibodies against poliovirus or mumps virus. By analogy with other slow or latent virus diseases of the central nervous system, ALS could well have such a cause without a serological clue to betray it. The recent observation that in an instance of altered host immunity, poliovirus vaccine has induced a chronic neurological disorder (23) helps to keep poliovirus under suspicion. Poliovirus cannot be demonstrated in tissues by fluorescent antibody techniques, even when it is known to be present in high titer (56, and A. B. Sabin, *personal communication*), and it has not been convincingly demonstrated within neurons by electron microscopy. These difficulties make establishing a link between poliovirus and ALS frustrating and uncertain. Oshiro et al. (63) have reviewed the problems besetting the search for any unknown virus in ALS.

Gibbs and Gajdusek (35) have recently reviewed the past 8 to 10 years of their own work, which has included numerous unsuccessful attempts to transmit ALS to primates, small animals, and tissue cultures. They remain unconvinced, also, by Russian reports that a transmissible agent causing motor neuron disease in primates is the etiological agent of motor neuron disease in man.

In a colony of wild mice, Gardner and Henderson (34) found an increased incidence of naturally occurring lymphoma and of a lower motor neuron disease with hind leg paralysis, "both caused by a raised level of endogenous type-C oncornavirus activity." Costa et al. (18) suggested that a similar association should be sought in man, because they had observed a rapidly advancing form of progressive muscular atrophy, bulbar and spinal, in the teen-aged sister of a young woman with granulocytic leukemia. Unable to confirm or deny the presence of type-C oncornaviruses in the tissue (poorly preserved for electron microscopy), they suggested that muscle be studied for C particles, known to appear there in affected mice.

Gardner and Henderson report also finding no familial excess of lymphoma or other malignancies in 31 patients with ALS as compared with 24 controls. They identified no neutralizing or complement-fixing antibodies against the type-C virus strain in the sera of 40 patients, including 5 Guamanian cases; and, by electron microscopy, no type-C virus particles in anterior horn cells or other sites in 8 patients (2 Guamanian). The findings failed to support an association between overt type-C virus activity and ALS.

In a study carried out by Cremer et al. (19), cell cultures established from tissues of nine patients with ALS and maintained for from several months to more than a year gave no indication of the presence of virus, as revealed by cell fusion and co-cultivation techniques, direct and indirect fluorescent antibody methods, and electron microscopic examination of tissues and of pelletted cells from tissue culture. Hemabsorption techniques were also used on tissue cultures. Serum antibody titers to 15 viruses, including polioviruses, in 34 ALS patients did not differ from those of matched controls.

Therapy directed at a virus-related cause of ALS has included trials of amantadine hydrochloride, a compound used for prophylaxis of Asian influenza (and, acting through presumably different mechanisms, as an adjuvant therapy for Parkinson's disease). Amantadine has proved to be useless in the treatment of ALS (W. K. Engel and T. Munsat, *personal communication*).

Immune Disorder as Cause

The possibility has been considered that a virus may act indirectly via immune mechanisms in ALS. Immune complexes have been identified in renal glomeruli of patients with the disorder (62).

An abnormal cellular inflammatory reaction has been reported in ALS, as studied by the "skin window" technique. The altered pattern of response, with failure of migration of macrophages into the inflammatory field, has been seen also in Hodgkin's disease, chronic leukemia, hypogammaglobulinemia, and disseminated cancer, as well as during treatment with ACTH and after anti-inflammatory X-ray therapy (76). The patients studied were not cachectic. To the authors, the abnormal response suggested "a latent disorder of the autonomic nervous system"; they did not discuss a possible alteration or failure of immune mechanisms.

I am not aware of any major trial of immunosuppressive drugs in therapy for ALS. Most clinical investigators have been reluctant to employ these toxic agents with so little to justify their use on theoretical grounds.

"Purely" Empirical Therapy

The use of guanidine hydrochloride $- C(NH_2)_3Cl -$ in ALS by Norris (57) was initially empirical, and he felt that his study provided "no information about a rationale for this treatment." In his opinion, "the lack of immediate benefit indicates that the mechanism is not neuromuscular facilitation, while some of the side effects indicate that guanidine affects the central nervous system, at least in sensitive individuals." In their more recent experience with the drug, Norris and co-workers (58) found that the number of patients with "stable disease" was greater at 6 months in a group treated with 25 mg/kg/day than in a group receiving 2 mg/kg/day, and that the mortality of the high-dose group was lower. "The number of stable cases lost significance by 10 months, and no patient improved." They observed increased paralysis in two Chinese men (60) given the drug and considered the episodes to be caused by "dose-related sensitivity to guanidine." The drug has been administered "for long periods without toxic effects in doses up to 40 mg/kg/day," but guanidine has also occasionally caused depression of the bone marrow when given in smaller doses (59). Norris (*personal communication*) has abandoned the use of guanidine in doses higher than 10 mg/kg/day because he considers the risk of increasing weakness or suppressing the bone marrow to be unacceptable. He continues to use the drug in the 10 mg/kg/day dosage.

Securinine (24), an alkaloid that has been compared with strychnine, has been recommended for its symptomatic effect in ALS (improving muscle strength, alleviating fatigue, and restoring sexual potency). It is administered as the nitrate in oral doses of up to 16 mg b.i.d., or subcutaneously up to 0.2 to 0.3 mg/kg daily. It has not been reported to produce a remission or to slow the progression of the disease. The comment of the physicians reporting their trial of securinine could be applied broadly to many similar attempts at drug treatment: "We were primarily trying to treat a patient, and we were not studying either the disease or the drug" (16,17).

SYMPTOMATIC TREATMENT

Symptomatic treatment of ALS concerns itself with details important to the well-being of the patient. Manifestations of disease that may require treatment are weakness of various limb muscles; disability in motor performance associated with release of reflexes [i.e., spasticity, upper motor neuron syndrome (UMNS) in Landau's (44) definition of the term]; pain induced by traction on muscles, ligaments, and the capsules of joints; necrosis caused by pressure on tissues overlying bony prominences (rare in ALS); difficulty in swallowing and in speaking; lack of control over bowels and bladder (also unusual); and release of emotional display, with sobbing and choking. Emotional problems are always present because of the progressive nature of the disease, and they include frustration and depression, denial of illness, and, occasionally, loss of intellectual capabilities.

Treatment of Weakness

Painless footdrop in a man over the age of 50 suggests the possibility of ALS. Even a slight amount of footdrop may result in tripping and falling, with a painful or disabling injury. For that reason, early bracing of the foot is recommended, with a cosmetic brace if the plantar flexors of the foot are spastic, or if there is knee weakness along with the footdrop. A plastic posterior clip-on brace has been used successfully for limited walking outside the home by patients with footdrop who have adequate extension of the knee (C. Schmidt, *personal communication*). As in most other neurological disorders, it will rarely be efficacious to provide the patient with a long leg brace to stabilize the knee. Quadriceps muscles are likely to become seriously weakened only late in the disease, by which time braces will soon lose their usefulness as aids to walking.

In the upper limb, similarly, the biceps is usually relatively spared, and the most useful brace is likely to be a cock-up splint for the wrist, bringing the hand into that position in which the fingers can exert maximal strength of grip. The occupational therapist or some other resourceful person can provide aids to the activities of daily life. These include a pen or pencil wrapped in foam rubber to provide a large surface that is easy to grasp, and large handles for eating utensils, which can be weighted if the tremor associated with weakness and reinnervation of muscle leads to lack of control of voluntary movement. Utensils for writing and eating can also be attached directly to the hand. A plate guard provides a baffle for food that aids in getting it onto the fork. More elaborate devices have, of course, been developed experimentally.

Exercise

Ideally, the patient will have the services of a nurse and a physiotherapist to help him maintain mobility and avoid contracture. Because of the clinical impression that previous heavy work (or exercise) may predispose to the development of ALS (9,33), physicians may be reluctant (55) to permit the patient with early disease to exercise heavily. Exercise may induce painful cramps or lead to a prolonged feeling of exhaustion in the patient. On the other hand, the propensity for collateral sprouting to occur in ALS (77), with reinnervation of denervated muscle fibers and the development of giant motor units (11), makes exercise seem an attractive mechanism for improving strength. Lenman (46) studied six patients with ALS and concluded that their weakness was unaffected by exercise, unless it had resulted from disuse. I favor the continued use of exercise, short of exhaustion, for whatever potential benefit it may have, but the question of the usefulness of training, as opposed to less well-regulated exercises, should be studied scientifically. Active and passive exercises for home use are described in the pamphlet "Strike Back at Stroke" (74), and methods of aiding the partially paralyzed patient in activities of daily living are described in a booklet "Up and Around" (75), both available from the Superintendent of Documents in Washington, D.C.

Treatment of Spasticity

The use of drugs for spasticity has been criticized by Landau (44) because they lack specific effectiveness, because they must necessarily interfere with purposeful movement, and because they exert a sedative action. Dantrolene sodium, which, Landau asserts, "must have an overall weakening action identical with that of curare" (47), has been employed in ALS, but a recent letter by Rivera and associates (69) reports that "in our experience, dantrolene is very poorly tolerated by these patients." Patients with progressive muscular atrophy and primary lateral sclerosis, as well as fully developed ALS, experienced generalized weakness, dysphagia, sialorrhea, or respiratory depression soon after starting the drug in low dosage (usually 75 mg/day). Many physicians, including me, have found that diazepam may also produce weakness in the patient with ALS, even when there is no noticeable improvement in spasticity. Baclofen (Lioresal®), chemically related to gamma-aminobutyric acid, administered intravenously has been reported to depress hyperactive stretch reflexes caused by either a spinal or a cerebral lesion, without reducing voluntary power (64); but when given by mouth, it does not "lead to the complete disappearance or pronounced depression of . . . spasticity." As pointed out by Duncan et al. (28), individual components of the "global syndrome" of spasticity are differentially affected by the drug: they found that when given by mouth, it "regularly alleviated" involuntary flexor or extensor spasms and acted to diminish pathologically increased resistance to passive movement of the legs, but it did not alter strength, gait, stretch reflexes, or clonus. Some investigators (F. H. Norris, Jr., *personal communication*), have found it more useful than diazepam in treating ALS, but I have also received a report of a disappointing result in a controlled trial in patients with primary lateral sclerosis.

Treatment of Dysarthria

In the dysarthric, dysphagic patients with progressive bulbar palsy on whom they reported more than half a century ago, Critchley and Kubik (20) found severe disease in the nucleus ambiguus and atrophy in all muscles of articulation and deglutition. However, they emphasized the concomitant loss of upper motor neuron control, so that a given muscle might show little atrophy but severe dysfunction.

Clinically, the dysarthria of the ALS patient begins with nasality or with loss of the ability to sing high, falsetto, or loud notes. Labial and lingual consonants (p, b; l, r) are affected early. Then dentals (d, t) are impaired as weakness of the tongue commences at its tip. Eventually, the patient becomes anarthric, although not aphonic, and rarely is there dyspnea because of paralytic adduction of the vocal cords. "The speech gestalt distinctive of ALS, then, consists of grossly defective articulation of both consonants and vowels, often rendering the speech unintelligible; laborious, extremely slow production of words in very short phrases; marked hypernasality, with severe harshness and strained-strangled squeezing out of low-pitched tones; and complete disruption of prosody, with monotony suppressing meaningfulness and intervals between words and phrases becoming excessive" (22).

Other results of weakness of the posterior tongue and the palate are impaired ability to hum, to sniff, and to blow the nose. Weakness of the lips and anterior tongue may result in inability to spit. The role of upper motor neuron disease is shown by loss of voluntary laughing and coughing, although, when they occur reflexly, these acts are preserved and even released.

When the speech of the ALS victim becomes utterly unintelligible, and when loss of verbal communication is coupled with essentially complete paralysis, the patient's life may become an imprisonment better portrayed by Edgar Allen Poe than by a neurologist. Above all other needs, the need for communication must be met until the end of the patient's life. Illustrative of this is my experience with a remarkable physician, Dr. Alan Brown of Ithaca, New York, who, while he was in the early stages of ALS, attended the Symposium on Motor Neuron Diseases in San Francisco (61). He then devoted his remaining life to personal research in ALS, submitting, for example, to repeated lumbar puncture in order to study interferon levels in his spinal fluid after various procedures designed to stimulate interferon production.

When I visited Dr. Brown in his home on what proved to be his last day of life, he was propped up in bed, immobile except for his eyes, and hard at work on a revision of his programmed text on small boat racing. By using a board lettered with the alphabet, and directing his gaze to a quadrant of the board from which his wife, Nancy, read the letters until he signalled that the correct one had been found, he was able to spell words. And by directing the movement of magnetized toy sailboats attached to another board, he was able to develop the situations that formed the basis for his book. His agile mind had been permitted an outlet of creativity through the patience of his family; he did not ask for more.

The role of the speech therapist in progressive bulbar or pseudobulbar palsy may be regarded lightly by the physician but given great value by the patient, who should be the one to decide the question. Darley and his collaborators (22) at the Mayo Clinic in their recent text on the dysarthrias emphasize that, in speech therapy, the patient must learn "to make maximum use of the remaining potential." The goal of "simply being heard and understood replaces the former [goal] of being quick and expressive in a highly personal way." They consider it important for the patient to start early to monitor his speech, learning "speech conservation" before it becomes impossible to speak well. The speech therapist will try to encourage the patient to do his best and reassure him that the efforts are worthwhile. To this I would add that the physician who refers a patient for speech therapy and then conveys to the patient or his family the attitude that "it can't do any harm" — or, worse, the idea that the speech therapist is no more than a well-paid babysitter — is doing the patient and the therapist both a disservice. Admittedly, not everyone will agree that in progressive disorders "speech therapy started early can help retard speech impairment" (31). If the doctor wants to administer a placebo, however, it should not be in the form of speech therapy.

When speech therapy is not enough (and sooner or later, in ALS, it will not be enough), other aids can be tried. Gonzalez and Aronson (37) employed a palatal lift in patients with neurological disorders, including four with ALS and "mixed spastic-flaccid paralysis of the velum." The lift is a prosthesis attached to the upper teeth or to a removable partial denture, which may be effective in overcoming palatopharyngeal incompetence. The device produces "marked to moderate reduction of hypernasality and nasal emission and increased intelligibility of speech" (37). Similar results have been obtained by injecting Teflon into the nasopharynx to produce a bulge that aids contact of the pharynx with the soft palate (5).

Injection of Teflon, a permanent material, into the vocal fold has also been used successfully to manage paralytic weakness of that structure. A similar result has been achieved with silicone (73), which lasts for a few months, or with glycerine, which is also less permanent. Despite recent admonitions concerning the need for a precise technique (71), the Teflon procedure remains useful and effective in skilled hands (C. D. Bluestone, *personal communication*).

Electronic amplifiers for the telephone and other amplifiers to be worn on the body are available from several sources. The places from which they may be obtained are listed in the book by Darley et al. (22).

For the patient unable to write but able to point, a communication board or book is indispensable. An example of a useful booklet is Lessing's "Silent Spokesman" (47), which includes pictures of common objects such as those needed for personal care. I have also employed a spot of light projected from a surgical headlamp as a pointer for a patient literally unable to lift a finger but still able to move his head slightly. Several types of boards, and the instructions for making them, are presently available (25,32,40,52), and electromechanical signalling devices have been described (40).

Treatment of Dysphagia

In the experience of Critchley (20), the early difficulty with swallowing affects hard solids as often as it does liquids. Later, liquids are more difficult to swallow. Soft, ground material is easiest to get down. Patients tend to throw the head back in order to get liquid past the tongue; they may do better by drinking from a straw. Maneuvering solids into the oropharynx may require much effort — flexing the chin on the chest, tilting the head back, or even pushing food with a finger. Patients may lose fluid through the lips and often get it into the air passages, but they do not commonly regurgitate through the nose, probably because wasting of lips and tongue prevents elevation of pressure inside the mouth sufficient to force fluid past the weakened velum against gravity (20).

Elaborate instructions are available for the retraining of children and adults with functional disorders of swallowing, but applying these to the patient with neurogenic weakness is not easy. The patient can, however, be taught to keep the head erect or the chin tilted somewhat forward during swallowing; to position the posterior tongue down and back by making the /k/ sound (not "kay" or "kuh"), keeping the mouth open while doing so, "freezing" in that position, and then quickly swallowing (3); and to say "gah" at the very end of the swallow.

Aspiration of liquid is a common difficulty. It is helpful to maintain the intake of semisolid foods with a high water content, such as gelatin, in order to reduce the amount of liquid that must be consumed. Recently, Teflon injection of the vocal cord has been employed for the prevention of chronic aspiration (70), as well as for restoration of voice. A competent glottis is required both to build subglottic pressure preparatory to coughing and also to prevent reaspiration when foreign material has been expelled. Clinically, glottic competence can be evaluated by testing not only the patient's ability to cough but also his ability to sustain a note, to hold his breath, and to laugh.

The cricopharyngeus is a striated muscle, separate from the inferior constrictor of the pharynx, that has recently received much attention for its role in deglutition. The passage of food from the hypopharynx into the esophagus may be seriously disrupted in many neurogenic disorders, and malfunction of the cricopharyngeus has been a suspected cause. There is much debate about the nature of the obstructive action of the muscle. Some refer to its being in "spasm"; others prefer the term "achalasia." Doty (27) notes that, although the pharyngoesophageal junction is closed at rest, and "it might . . . seem reasonable to suppose that closure of the rostral esophageal orifice is maintained by constant activity of the inferior constrictor, . . . this would be metabolically inefficient, and no electromyographic evidence of such tonically maintained contraction has ever been found either in anesthetized or decerebrate cat, dog, and macaque; or in unanesthetized rabbit, dog, or man." The sphincteric quality of the junction in man may be owing in part to a rich venous plexus in the region and the tightly investing cricopharyngeus muscle. The junction "must be normally closed only by passive elasticity of surrounding tissues. . . . Active closure is readily induced by a variety of reflexes serving to contract the cricopharyngeus, and . . . during swallowing the orifice is opened passively by hyoid and laryngeal movements while all contraction of cricopharyngeus is initially forestalled by the swallowing center exerting a powerful inhibition on cricopharyngeal motoneurons."

Abnormally maintained closure of the sphincter is not, however, clearly or at least exclusively an "upper motor neuron sign," as it has been observed in bulbar poliomyelitis (6), in polymyositis associated with gastric carcinoma (R. C. Griggs, *personal communication*), and in oculopharyngeal muscular dystrophy (54). In all of these instances, excision or division of the muscle resulted in improved swallowing.

The operation of "cricopharyngeal sphincterotomy" or "myotomy" has proved highly efficacious (53,54) not only for the relief of dysphagia but also for the control of aspiration, which is an inevitable consequence when an appreciable amount of food or fluid remains trapped in the hypopharynx after the supposed completion of the swallow and the resumption of breathing. This aspirated fluid may be removed by coughing or by clearing the throat, or it may not be removed effectively and may lead to aspiration pneumonia, a common cause of death in ALS.

The patient, therefore, who has dysphagia and a tendency toward aspiration should have cineradiographic studies and, if a suitable candidate, should undergo sphincterotomy. From his own experience, Mills (53) concludes that "where a person with motor-neurone disease is reduced to taking a semisolid diet very slowly and with each mouthful there is some degree of spillover, a sphincterotomy might be contemplated. Although it is far better if the patient can feed himself, the operation is worthwhile even though a nurse or relation has to do the feeding. The best results are obtained in those cases where there is a moderate degree of tongue movement. If the tongue can be protruded as far as the lower lip, there is enough propulsion to initiate deglutition. If the patients have good hand and finger movement, it is still possible to improve their lives even though the tongue is paralyzed. In these circumstances, the food is pushed to the back of the tongue, the patient being in a semirecumbent position, allowing the bolus to slide down the pharynx."

The patient who aspirates solid food and suffers obstruction of the respiratory passage, so that he is suddenly in distress and aphonic, may be helped to expel the bolus by employing the abdominal "hug of life," or Heimlich maneuver, presently under evaluation by the National Research Council: the victim, standing, is bent forward over a chair or the rescuer's arms, so that his head is lower than his chest. The rescuer, standing behind the victim and encircling him with his arms, hands interlocked, presses forcefully upward on the upper abdomen, forcing the diaphragm upward, expelling residual air in the chest cavity, and dislodging the obstructing foreign body.

Lesser degrees of obstruction, accompanied by stridor (and therefore continued passage of air), produced by aspiration of saliva or food, must be dealt with as calmly as possible. Supplemental oxygen may help. Oropharyngeal suction is also important: a suction machine should be placed in the home before it is needed in an emergency, and family members should be instructed in its use.

Feeding via a nasogastric tube is often unpleasant for the patient and may cause irritation or ulceration of the mucosa, the nasal passage, or the pharynx. The tube must be changed competently to avoid entering the airway. The alternative method of alimentation for the patient no longer able to take food by mouth has commonly been gastrostomy, which may serve very well (72). (The patient can still place food in the mouth to obtain its taste, if he desires, but sometimes with a risk of aspirating.) Cervical esophagostomy (39) is preferred by some surgeons, in order to avoid the risk of peritonitis as associated with gastrostomy (C. D. Bluestone, *personal communication*). The tube passes into the piriform recess, through the esophagus, and into the stomach. It is changed every 3 or 4 weeks and can remain in place for at least a year (39).

Parenteral administration of fluids can be used during a temporary exacerbation of illness, for example, during a bout of pneumonia, but it cannot be recommended just for the sake of keeping the patient alive. Intravenous hyperalimentation is fraught with the danger of fungal infection and is too unnatural to be employed in the ambulatory patient, too heroic for the bedridden patient. In all of the methods of alimentation that bypass the mouth, the wishes of the patient should be respected: a patient for whom life has literally lost its savor cannot be compelled to accept any of them.

Psychological Support

Most physicians who deal with patients who have a chronic, progressive disease come to believe that it is better to tell the patient his diagnosis, and not have him learn it, inadvertently or by their intent, from family, friends, or personnel involved in his care. When that does happen, the terror of the disclosure is greater than when the information comes from the doctor. I believe that no characterization such as "a degeneration of motor nerve cells" should be given to the disease unless the doctor also tells the patient the names used by the medical community and by the public.

The only additional advice (difficult to follow!) in which I will indulge myself is to recommend that treatments already known to be without value (e.g., injections of vitamin B_{12}) not be used at all.

In Beckett's play, *Endgame* (4), the protagonist, Hamm, is an invalid, living out his days in a postapocalyptic world from which most of the requirements of ordinary life have disappeared. When, for example, he asks for bicycle wheels in order to construct a wheelchair, his manservant replies, "There are no more bicycle wheels."

One recurrent question, however, he asks in a different way: "Is it time for my painkiller?" The answer is always the same—a straightforward, "No." But the question has not been the one that Hamm fears to ask. When, finally, his poignant request, "Is it time for my painkiller?" is answered, "Yes," and he exclaims, "Ah! At last! Give it to me! Quick!" there comes his servant's shattering response: "There's no more painkiller."

It is wrong to encourage our patients in false hopes or to create unrealistic expectations. It is necessary to answer the question they do not dare to ask. With cautious, realistic support, they must be given reason to believe that, at every stage of illness, *something* can still be done to make existence a little more bearable. That approach is far better than trying one "curative" after another, in effect making the patient wait for the potent painkiller, and allowing him to discover at last that there is no painkiller—none at all.

REFERENCES

1. Alpers, B. J., and Farmer, R. A. (1949): Role of repeated trauma by pneumatic drill in production of amyotrophic lateral sclerosis. *Arch. Neurol. Psychiatry,* 62:178–182.
2. Astin, K. J., Wilde, C. E., and Davies-Jones, A. B. (1975): Glucose metabolism and insulin response in the plasma and CSF in motor neurone disease. *J. Neurol. Sci.,* 25:205–210.
3. Barrett, R. H., and Hanson, M. L. (1974): *Oral Myofunctional Disorders.* C. V. Mosby Co., St. Louis.
4. Beckett, S. (1950): *Endgame.* Grove Press, New York.
5. Bluestone, C. D., Musgrave, R. H., McWilliams, B. J., and Crozier, P. A. (1968): Teflon injection pharyngoplasty. *Cleft Palate J.,* 5:19–22.
6. Bofenkamp, B. (1958): *Arch. Otolaryngol.,* 68:165. Cited in Mills (ref. 53).
7. Boman, K., and Muerman, T. (1967): Prognosis of amyotrophic lateral sclerosis. *Acta Neurol. Scand.,* 43:489–498.
8. Boothby, J. A., deJesus, P. V., and Rowland, L. P. (1974): Reversible forms of motor neuron disease. Lead "neuritis." *Arch. Neurol.,* 31:18–23.
9. Breland, A. E., and Currier, R. D. (1967): Multiple sclerosis and amyotrophic lateral sclerosis in Mississippi. *Neurology (Minneap.),* 17:1011–1016.
10. Brody, J. A., Chen, K.-M., Yase, Y., Holden, E. M., and Morris, C. E. (1974): Inosiplex and amyotrophic lateral sclerosis. *Arch. Neurol.,* 30:322–323.
11. Brown, W. F. (1973): Functional compensation of human motor units in health and disease. *J. Neurol. Sci.,* 20:199–209.
12. Campbell, A. M. G., Williams, E. R., and Pearce, J. (1969): Late motor neuron degeneration following poliomyelitis. *Neurology (Minneap.),* 19:1101–1106.
13. Charchaflie, R. J., Bustos Fernandez, L., Perec, C. J., Gonzalez, E., and Marzi, A. (1974): Functional studies of the parotid and pancreas glands in amyotrophic lateral sclerosis. *J. Neurol. Neurosurg. Psychiatry,* 37:863–867.
14. Collis, W. J., and Engel, W. K. (1968): Glucose metabolism in five neuromuscular disorders. *Neurology (Minneap.),* 18:915–923.
15. Cooper, I. S. (1976): *Living with Chronic Neurologic Disease—a Handbook for Patient and Family.* W. W. Norton Co., New York.
16. Copperman, R., Copperman, G., and der Marderosian, A. (1973): Securinine—a central nervous stimulant is used in treatment of amytrophic (sic) lateral sclerosis. *Pa. Med.,* 76:36–41.
17. Copperman, R., Copperman, G., and der Marderosian, A. (1974): Letter. *J.A.M.A.,* 228:288.
18. Costa, J. C., Rabson, A. S., Tralka, T. S., Engel, W. K., Canellos, G. P., and Bratenahl, C. G. (1974): Letter: leukaemia and lower-motor-neurone disease. *Lancet,* 2:107–108.
19. Cremer, N. E., Oshiro, L. S., Norris, F. H., Jr., and Lennette, E. H. (1973): Cultures of tissues from patients with amyotrophic lateral sclerosis. *Arch. Neurol.,* 29:331–333.
20. Critchley, M., and Kubik, C. S. (1925): The mechanisms of speech and deglutition in progressive bulbar palsy. *Brain,* 48:492–534.
21. Currier, R. D., and Haerer, A. F. (1968): Amyotrophic lateral sclerosis and metallic toxins. *Arch. Environ. Health,* 17:712–719.
22. Darley, F. L., Aronson, A. E., and Brown, J. R. (1975): *Motor Speech Disorders.* W. B. Saunders Co., Philadelphia.
23. Davis, L. E., Bodian, D., D'Souza, B. J., Butler, I. J., and Price, D. L. (1977): Chronic

progressive poliomyelitis. Presented at Am. Assoc. Neuropathol., May 30, 1975. *J. Neuropathol. Exp. Neurol.* (*in press*). Cited by D. Bodian (1976) in *Johns Hopkins Med. J.,* 138:130–136.

24. Dimond, E. G. (1971): Medical education and care in People's Republic of China. *J.A.M.A.,* 218:1552–1557.
25. Dixon, C., and Curry, B. (1965): Some thoughts on the communication board. *Cerebral Palsy J.,* 26:12–15.
26. Dorman, J. D., Engel, W. K., and Fried, D. M. (1969): Therapeutic trial in amyotrophic lateral sclerosis: lack of benefit with pancreatic extract and DL-alpha tocopherol in 12 patients. *J.A.M.A.,* 209:257–258.
27. Doty, R. W. (1959): Neural organization of deglutition. In: *Handbook of Physiology,* edited by John Field, pp. 1861–1902. American Physiological Society, Washington, D.C.
28. Duncan, G. W., Shahani, B. T., and Young, R. R. (1976): An evaluation of baclofen treatment for certain symptoms in patients with spinal cord lesions: a double-blind cross-over study. *Neurology (Minneap.),* 26:441–446.
29. Eaton, L. J. (1957): Symposium on amyotrophic lateral sclerosis: introduction. *Mayo Clin. Proc.,* 32:425–426.
30. Fareed, G. C., and Tyler, H. R. (1971): The use of isoprinosine in patients with amyotrophic lateral sclerosis. *Neurology (Minneap.),* 21:937–940.
31. Farmakides, M. N., and Boone, D. R. (1960): Speech problems of patients with multiple sclerosis. *J. Speech Hear. Disord.,* 25:385–390. Cited in Darley et al. (ref. 22).
32. Feallock, B. (1958): Communication for the non-verbal individual. *Am. J. Occup. Ther.,* 12:60–63, 83.
33. Felmus, M. T., Patten, B. M., and Swanke, L. (1976): Antecedent events in amyotrophic lateral sclerosis. *Neurology (Minneap.),* 26:167–172.
34. Gardner, M. B., and Henderson, B. E. (1974): Letter: Lower-motor-neuron disease in mice and amyotrophic lateral sclerosis in man. *Lancet,* 2:952.
35. Gibbs, C. J., and Gajdusek, D. C. (1972): Amyotrophic lateral sclerosis, Parkinson's disease and the amyotrophic lateral sclerosis-Parkinsonism-dementia complex in Guam: a review and summary of attempts to demonstrate infection as the aetiology. *J. Clin. Pathol.* [*Suppl. 25*], 6:132–140.
36. Goldblatt, D. (1969): Motor neuron disease: historical introduction. In: *Symposium on Motor Neuron Diseases: Research on Amyotrophic Lateral Sclerosis and Related Disorders, San Francisco, 1967,* edited by F. H. Norris and L. T. Kurland. Grune & Stratton, New York.
37. Gonzalez, J. B., and Aronson, A. E. (1970): Palatal lift prosthesis for treatment of anatomic and neurologic palatopharyngeal insufficiency. *Cleft Palate J.,* 7:91–104.
38. Gowers, W. R. (1902): A lecture on abiotrophy. *Lancet,* 1:1003–1007.
39. Graham, W. P., and Royster, H. P. (1967): Simplified cervical esophagostomy for long term extraoral feeding. *Surg. Gynecol. Obstet.,* 125:127–128.
40. Hagen, C., Porter, W., and Brink, J. (1973): Nonverbal communication: an alternative mode of communication for the child with severe cerebral palsy. *J. Speech Hear. Disord.,* 38:448–455.
41. Horwich, M. S., Engel, W. K., and Chauvin, P. B. (1974): Amyotrophic lateral sclerosis sera applied to cultured motor neurons. *Arch. Neurol.,* 30:332–333.
42. Kantarjian, A. D. (1961): A syndrome clinically resembling amyotrophic lateral sclerosis following chronic mercurialism. *Neurology (Minneap.),* 11:639–644.
43. Koerner, Donald R. (1976): Abnormal carbohydrate metabolism in amyotrophic lateral sclerosis and Parkinsonism-dementia on Guam. *Diabetes,* 25:1055–1065.
44. Landau, W. M. (1974): (Editorial: Spasticity: the fable of the neurological demon and the Emperor's new therapy. *Arch. Neurol.,* 31:217–219.
45. Lehrich, J. R., Oger, J., and Arnason, B. G. W. (1974): Neutralizing antibodies to poliovirus and mumps virus in amyotrophic lateral sclerosis. *J. Neurol. Sci.,* 23:537–540.
46. Lenman, J. A. R. (1959): Clinical and experimental study of the effects of exercise on motor weakness in neurological disease. *J. Neurol. Neurosurg. Psychiatry,* 22:182–194.
47. Lessing, W. W. (1956): *Silent Spokesman: an Aid to the Speechless.* Hospital Topics (30 W. Washington St.), Chicago.
48. Liveson, J., Frey, H., and Bornstein, M. B. (1975): The effect of serum from ALS patients on organotypic nerve and muscle tissue cultures. *Acta Neuropathol. (Berl.),* 32:127–131.

49. Mackay, R. P. (1963): Course and prognosis in amyotrophic lateral sclerosis. *Arch. Neurol.,* 8:117–127.
50. McComas, A. J., Upton, A. R. M., and Sica, R. E. P. (1973): Motoneurone disease and ageing. *Lancet,* 2:1477–1480.
51. Medical News: "Lou Gehrig disease" – drug may arrest or slow ALS. *J.A.M.A.,* 207:249–250, (1969).
52. Miller, J., and Carpenter, C. (1964): Electronics for communication. *Am. J. Occup. Ther.,* 18:20–23.
53. Mills, C. P. (1973): Dysphagia in pharyngeal paralysis treated by cricopharyngeal sphincterotomy. *Lancet, 1:455–457.*
54. Montgomery, W. W., and Lynch, J. P. (1971): Oculopharyngeal muscular dystrophy treated by inferior constrictor myotomy. *Trans. Am. Acad. Ophthalmol. Otolaryngol.,* 75:986–993.
55. Mulder, D. W. (1957): The clinical syndrome of amyotrophic lateral sclerosis. *Mayo Clin. Proc.,* 32:427–436.
56. Nathanson, N., and Goldblatt, D. (1964): Spinal ganglion involvement in experimental poliomyelitis. *Neurology (Minneap.),* 14:1132–1148.
57. Norris, F. H., Jr. (1971): Prognosis in amyotrophic lateral sclerosis. *Trans. Am. Neurol. Assoc.,* 96:290–291.
58. Norris, F. H., Jr., Calanchini, P. R., Fallat, R. H., Panchari, S., and Jerwett, B. (1974): The administration of guanidine in amyotrophic lateral sclerosis. *Neurology (Minneap.),* 24:721–728.
59. Norris, F. H., Jr., Eaton, J. M., and Mielke, C. H. (1974): Depression of bone marrow by guanidine. *Arch. Neurol.,* 30:184–185.
60. Norris, F. H., Jr., Fallat, R. J., and Calanchini, P. R. (1974): Increased paralysis induced by guanidine in motor neuron disease. *Neurology (Minneap.),* 24:135–137.
61. Norris, F. H., Jr., and Kurland, L. T. (Eds.) (1969): *Symposium on Motor Neuron Diseases: Research on Amyotrophic Lateral Sclerosis and Related Disorders, San Francisco, 1967.* Grune & Stratton, New York.
62. Oldstone, M. B. A., Wilson, C. B., Dalessio, D., Norris, F. H., Jr., and Nelson, E. (1973): Immunoglobulin deposits in amyotrophic lateral sclerosis. *Trans. Am. Neurol. Assoc.,* 98:181–182.
63. Oshiro, Lyndon S., Cremer, N. E., Norris, F. H., Jr., and Lennette, E. H. (1976): Virus-like particles in muscle from a patient with amyotrophic lateral sclerosis. *Neurology (Minneap.),* 26:57–60.
64. Pedersen, E., Arlien-Søborg, P., and Mai, J. (1974): The mode of action of the GABA derivative baclofen in human spasticity. *Acta Neurol. Scand.,* 50:665–680.
65. Percy, A. K., Davis, L. E., Johnston, D. M., and Drachman, D. B. (1971): Failure of Isoprinosine in amyotrophic lateral sclerosis. *N. Engl. J. Med.,* 285:689.
66. Quick, D. T., and Greer, M. (1967): Pancreatic dysfunction in patients with amyotrophic lateral sclerosis. *Neurology (Minneap.),* 17:112–116.
67. Reed, D. M., and Brody, J. A. (1975): Amyotrophic lateral sclerosis and parkinsonism-dementia on Guam, 1945–1972. I. Descriptive epidemiology. *Am. J. Epidemiol.,* 101:287–301.
68. Reed, D. M., Torres, J. M., and Brody, J. A. (1975): Amyotrophic lateral sclerosis and parkinsonism-dementia on Guam, 1945–1972. II. Familial and genetic studies. *Am. J. Epidemiol.,* 101:302–310.
69. Rivera, V. M., Breitbach, W. B., and Swanke, L. (1975): Dantrolene in amyotrophic lateral sclerosis. *J.A.M.A.,* 233:863–864.
70. Rontal, E., Rontal, M., Morse, G., and Brown, E. M. (1976): Vocal cord injection in the treatment of acute and chronic aspiration. *Laryngoscope,* 86:625–634.
71. Rubin, H. J. (1965): Intracordal injection of silicone in selected dysphonias. *Arch. Otolaryngol.,* 81:604–607.
72. Schwartz, S. I., Lillehei, R. C., Shires, G. T., Spencer, F. C., and Storer, E. H. (1974): *Principles of Surgery, 2nd Ed.* McGraw-Hill, New York.
73. Smith, R. O., Sands, C. J., Goldberg, N. M., Massen, R. V., and Gay, J. R. (1967): Injection of silicone lateral to a vocal cord in a patient with progressive bulbar palsy. *Neurology (Minneap.),* 17:1217–1218.

74. "Strike Back at Stroke" (1958): D.H.E.W. Publication No. 596, U.S. Government Printing Office, Washington, D.C.
75. "Up and Around": Public Health Publication No. 1120, revised August, 1964.
76. Urbánek, K., and Jansa, P. (1974): Amyotrophic lateral sclerosis: abnormal cellular inflammatory response. *Arch. Neurol.,* 30:186–187.
77. Wohlfart, G. (1957): Collateral regeneration from residual motor nerve fibers in amyotrophic lateral sclerosis. *Neurology (Minneap.),* 7:124–134.
78. Wolfgram, F., and Myers, L. (1973): Amyotrophic lateral sclerosis: effect of serum on anterior horn cells in tissue culture. *Science,* 179:579–580.

Advances in Neurology, Vol. 17, edited by
R. C. Griggs and R. T. Moxley, III. Raven Press,
New York © 1977.

Clinical Electromyography:
Definition, Application, and Innovation

Michael P. McQuillen

*Department of Neurology, The Medical College of Wisconsin, 8700 West
Wisconsin Avenue, Milwaukee, Wisconsin 53226*

INTRODUCTION

Since their introduction into clinical medicine almost 50 years ago (1),
the techniques of electromyography (EMG) have added immeasurably to
the recognition, understanding, and direction of therapy for neuromuscular
disease in man. This review attempts a definition of some of these techniques
that are useful *in vivo;* a discussion of their application, limitations, and
value in disorders of the motor unit; and a precis of some of the innovative
developments of recent years. It is by no means a compendium of a field that
has already nurtured five international congresses, one from which several
standard texts are extant (12,18,27,46). Specifically not covered are the
topics of reflexology and kinesiology (3), in which adaptations of EMG
technique have added greatly to the understanding of movement control
and central nervous system disease productive of weakness and disordered
muscle tone.

NERVE CONDUCTION

Since the classic paper of Hodes, Larrabee, and German (23), a vast
body of data has been accumulated on the results of nerve stimulation
in man. The basic technique for the determination of *motor nerve conduction
velocity* involves the application of an electrical stimulus derived from an
isolation transformer to a peripheral nerve at more than one point in its
course through a limb, and the recording of the resultant muscle action
potential (MAP) from surface electrodes placed over the belly and tendon
of a muscle supplied by that nerve (Fig. 1). In the study of motor nerve, it
is necessary to stimulate a nerve at a minimum of two points in order to
derive a valid nerve conduction time between the points of stimulation, from
which nerve conduction velocity can be estimated. That this is so can be
seen from considering that the stimulus is applied to nerve (which generally
conducts at a rate approximating 40 to 60 meters/sec), while the response

STIMULUS
SITE

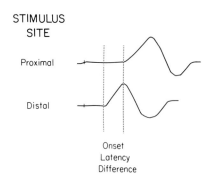

Proximal

Distal

Onset
Latency
Difference

FIG. 1. Schematic of technique for the measurement of motor nerve conduction velocity.

is recorded from muscle (the conduction velocity of which approximates 4 to 6 meters/sec): one cannot tell when nerve conduction time ends and muscle conduction time begins. Also involved are other times of different orders of magnitude, including the time required for the stimulus to elicit a response in nerve; slower conduction in fine nerve terminals compared to the main nerve trunk; and neuromuscular transmission.

Several kinds of information are derived from this method, including MAP size, distal latency, and conduction velocity.

MAP Size

MAP size is taken as a measure of the number of motor units, each with its given number of muscle fibers, responding to nerve stimulation. Ordinarily, size is expressed in millivolts of amplitude (either of the negative phase of the MAP, or of its peak-to-peak amplitude)—the easiest parameter of the MAP to measure. Normal variance in MAP size is considerable. New techniques, which look at MAP area as automatically derived (38), show the same or greater variance. McComas et al. (29) have reckoned that one can determine average motor unit size by threshold nerve stimulation and thereby estimate motor unit number by division of average size into the MAP evoked by maximal nerve stimulation. By using this approach, McComas and co-workers (30) and others (2) have suggested a decrease in the number of motor units—i.e., a neuropathic change—in many illnesses previously thought to be of myopathic origin. Aside from the discomfort of a new hypothesis, others have taken issue with some of the technical factors involved (42) or have been unable to duplicate his findings (43). Basically, MAP size will decrease whenever there is a functional or anatomical decrease in muscle, of whatever cause. Decrease in MAP size may reflect failure of impulse propagation in nerve—a phenomenon more commonly observed with proximal nerve stimulation than with stimulation distally, especially in some neuropathies that affect myelin segmentally.

Distal Latency

Distal latency is the time from a distal stimulus to the onset of the muscle response. Since this time comprises part of the time from a more proximal stimulus to the onset of the muscle response (proximal latency), it can be subtracted from proximal latency to derive the conduction time between the two stimulus points, and using this time conduction velocity *per se* is calculated. Such a latency difference technique eliminates the problem of events with different time frames (*vide supra*). One would think, from this analysis, that latency would be directly proportional to distance. With long distances such as are involved in the genesis of a "late" wave that can be recorded in small hand or foot muscles (the "F" wave[1]), this appears to be true; and one can analyze motor nerve root disease by this technique (9). However, distal latencies bear little relation to distal distances (32), and they are abnormal only with reference to upper limits established in studies of normal individuals of varying age. Since distal latency is a measure of function in the portion of nerve furthermost removed from the nerve cell body—the part of a nerve most susceptible to disease—an increase in distal latency is a useful and often the sole abnormality signaling the presence of a neuropathy. Focal increase in distal latency is the hallmark of some entrapment neuropathies (25), but is not an obligatory finding, even in that setting.

Conduction Velocity

Conduction velocity, considering motor nerve fibers, is the derivative of the distance between stimulus points and their latency differences, and is expressed in meters per second. The range of normal values is quite large; and serial studies in normal subjects (32) and even in some disease states (24) show such fluctuation that the usefulness of motor nerve conduction velocities has serious limitations (35), especially in the study of a single individual. In other disease states such as idiopathic polyneuritis (31), some of the hereditary neuropathies (13), and other peripheral nerve disorders primarily involving myelin, motor nerve conduction velocities are of great use, with slowing in velocity appearing so regularly as to be obligatory for a diagnosis.

Considering these limitations, and because many peripheral neuropathies are purely or largely sensory in clinical character, other techniques of study of peripheral nerve function have been developed. Since Dawson (11) ob-

---

[1] The "F" wave is felt to result from an impulse that travels antidromically up the motor axon to the anterior horn cell, around the Renshaw circuit, and orthodromically back out the axon again (28). Thus, in its travels the impulse traverses the motor nerve root in and out. It follows logically that the latency to onset of the "F" wave can be delayed by selective disease in the motor nerve root.

served that one could record a nerve action potential *in vivo* from stimulation of sensory nerve, Buchthal and Rosenfalck (7) have shown that a compound *sensory nerve action potential* (SNAP) can be derived using averaging techniques. Changes in the amplitude and/or velocity of various components of the SNAP parallel changes in the anatomical composition of nerve (8). These changes may predict the pathological character of the neuropathy and thus permit a focus on cause in a category of disease remarkable for its multiplicity of causes (14). Techniques for the study of *nerve excitability* generally are too cumbersome for clinical usefulness (17); but Heckmann (22) has proposed a simple modification of the standard strength-duration concept for judging excitability, which may have real value in the analysis of neuropathies with normal nerve conduction velocities (51).

NEUROMUSCULAR TRANSMISSION

Harvey and Masland (21) introduced the concept that, with repetitive supramaximal stimulation of motor nerve and recording of sequential MAPs, one could express changes in MAP size as a percentage of initial size and thereby define the character of a block in neuromuscular transmission (Fig. 2). To be certain that the MAP changes result from a defect in transmission rather than in nerve or in muscle, sometimes it is necessary to record simultaneously from nerve, and to stimulate and record from muscle directly: if the changes are observed only in muscle with nerve stimulation, then the defect must be in transmission (33). At times, the simultaneous recording of isometric muscle tension adds useful information (45). These techniques have had their greatest application in myasthenia gravis, in which an extremely specific kind of block may be observed. This block involves an "early dip" fall off and repair of MAP size, and often a late fall off as well, with an immediate post-tetanic increase (facilitation) in MAP size and a later post-tetanic decline (exhaustion) (20). Many illnesses affecting other levels of the motor unit, and indeed even normal fatigue, are associated with a late fall off in MAP size, especially at fast (e.g., 20 impulses/sec or greater) rates of repetitive stimulation. The techniques are useful in the study of uncommon defects in neuromuscular transmission

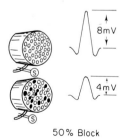

8mV

4mV

50% Block

FIG. 2. Schematic of technique for analysis of neuromuscular transmission (from R. J. Johns, M.D., with permission). MAP response to a supramaximal stimulus at the start of (*top*) and during (*bottom*) a train of repetitive nerve stimulation, showing a 50% decline in MAP amplitude.

(26) such as the myasthenic syndrome sometimes associated with small cell carcinoma of the bronchus (33) or botulism (34). Since the techniques will not identify every patient with myasthenia gravis (39), methods to impose a regional curarization have been introduced, which may uncover latent myasthenia (5).

NEEDLE ELECTROMYOGRAPHY

The clinical physiology of muscle can be analyzed by recording the electrical activity of muscle directly, using needle recording techniques. Two types of needles are in general clinical use: a concentric electrode (or needle-within-a-needle), and a monopolar electrode (with which a surface or subcutaneous electrode is used as reference). The two needles give different information, especially during voluntary activation of muscle (*vide infra*). When doing a needle EMG study, one must pay attention to the activity observed.

At Rest

In normal muscle, except for a few random potentials that appear with insertion or after needle movement and last less than 15 to 30 sec, electrical silence is observed at rest. "Sick" muscle fibers discharge spontaneously as brief, simple wave forms (fibrillations), or with a simple monophasic event (positive sharp waves). Fibrillations must be distinguished from the activity observed in the zone of innervation of a muscle ("end-plate noise"), which is thought to represent the electrical consequence of spontaneous release of neurotransmitter, recorded extracellularly (19). "End-plate noise" is more often observed in small muscles, wherein the statistical chance of penetrating the motor point is greater. Fibrillations and positive sharp waves are more common when there is denervation, but they may be seen when there is active degeneration of muscle from any cause—e.g., polymyositis (37). They may be observed in the paravertebral muscles in the presence of nerve root disease: when fibrillations and positive sharp waves are seen there in profusion at multiple levels, some investigators have drawn a strong correlation with the presence of cancer, although others have not found this correlation to be so specific (50). Whole motor units may discharge spontaneously (fasciculations) at rest—by themselves especially in some myopathies [e.g., thyrotoxic myopathy (40)]. Unique repetitive discharges are sometimes observed. When these increase and later decrease in amplitude and frequency, the term "myotonia" is used, and the phenomenon is specific for the various myotonic disorders of muscle—a useful feature distinguishing them from the contracture associated with some rare disorders of energy metabolism of muscle, as well as from the even rarer states of persistent muscle contraction (36). Repetitive discharges of constant amplitude and frequency, which turn on and off crisply, form a "pseudomyotonic" pattern that may be observed in many active disease states, especially neuropathies.

With Effort

Traditionally, there are two ways of analyzing motor unit discharge that occurs during voluntary effort. With the concentric electrode, attention is paid primarily to motor unit shape and duration. Less heed is given to motor unit amplitude, since multielectrode recording has demonstrated what anyone who has ever listened to a radio knows intuitively: the further away you go from the source of a wave form, the softer (i.e., smaller in amplitude) it is, whereas its pitch (i.e., duration) is affected only slightly (Fig. 3). The duration of a motor unit is directly related to its size. Normal parameters for various muscles at differing ages have been established (6). Deviations from normal imply disease that may be neuropathic or myopathic in origin. Usually such deviations are associated with an increase in the percentage of polyphasic motor units observed as well. Deviations are defined as mean values, derived from the analysis of 20 or more separate nonpolyphasic potentials. Longer, larger motor units suggest an increase in motor unit size, which can be seen only in a neuropathy, when there has been reinnervation or simultaneous firing of adjacent anterior horn cells; and brief, small motor units suggest a reduction in motor unit size that commonly occurs with the spotty fiber atrophy of a myopathy. King Engel (16) has criticized the concept of a "myopathic" EMG, citing many mechanisms — neuropathic, congenital, or fiber type–specific — that could reduce motor unit size and (hence) action potential duration. Nevertheless, the concept has excellent utilitarian value, as demonstrated by correlation with other descriptors of neuromuscular disease (4). The other way of looking at the

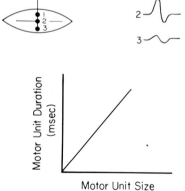

FIG. 3. Theoretical basis for analysis of muscle action potential parameters with concentric needle recording techniques. See text for details.

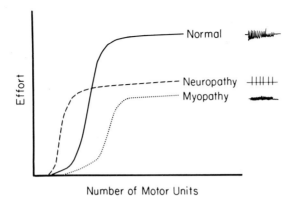

FIG. 4. Schematic representation of method for analysis of motor unit disease with monopolar needle recording techniques.

electrical behavior of muscle with effort—a technique applied when using monopolar electrodes—is to correlate recruitment of motor units with increasing force of contraction (Fig. 4). When neuropathic disease is present, whole motor units may be lost and recruitment is less per unit effort so that at maximal effort a pattern of single motor units is seen. In the setting of myopathy, increased recruitment occurs at each level of effort. Electronic averaging devices have been developed to quantitate recruitment in terms of numbers of units or summated electrical activity per quantity of effort (41). When all of these techniques are compared in the same patient by the same electromyographer, the concentric needle, mean duration estimate method appears to be the most reliable (10).

To these standard methods of analysis has been added a new technique using a small-diameter (0.5 mm) electrode with multiple leading off surfaces that are quite small (25 μm) with respect to the average diameter of a muscle fiber (50 μm) (15). Using one or another of the recording surfaces of such an electrode with reference to a subcutaneous or surface electrode, and with slight voluntary activation of a muscle or submaximal stimulation of the nerve to that muscle, one can record an action potential that is identical with consecutive discharges, usually one that is a smooth, biphasic spike often followed by terminal phases of small amplitude and long duration. Considerable data have been published to support the concept that this spike is derived from a single muscle fiber; the technique, therefore, is referred to as single-fiber electromyography (SFEMG). With SFEMG one can measure propagation velocity of single muscle fibers (47) and study the microphysiology of the motor unit (48). One phenomenon that has received particular attention is the variability of the time interval between two action potentials generated by two adjacent muscle fibers belonging to the same unit ("jitter") (49). Although a variability in the time course of impulse propagation in terminal nerve twigs to each muscle fiber, or in the muscle fibers themselves, can increase jitter, the most marked increases in jitter are observed in disorders of neuromuscular transmission (44). Because such disorders ultimately arise from pathophysiology affecting individual neuromuscular junctions, SFEMG is a welcome refinement for the study of diseases of neuromuscular transmission.

SUMMARY

Clinical EMG techniques, useful in the study of patients with neuromuscular disease, are defined. These include measurement of motor and sensory nerve conduction velocities; analysis of the size, shape, and latency of response of muscle and nerve action potentials after nerve stimulation; estimates of nerve excitability; study of the response to repetitive nerve stimulation as a measure of neuromuscular transmission; and observation of the electrical activity of muscle with needle recording electrodes (monopolar, bipolar, and multielectrodes). From a consideration of the application, limitations, and value of these various techniques, it can be concluded logically that to assure the highest probability of reliable information in regard to an individual patient, the choice of technique(s) and the part(s) to be studied should be intimately tied to a clinical analysis of that patient's problem. EMG as a fishing expedition is rarely fruitful; EMG as an exercise in clinical physiology is often exciting.

ACKNOWLEDGMENT

The secretarial assistance of Mrs. Howard Maney is most gratefully acknowledged.

REFERENCES

1. Adrian, E. D., and Bronk, D. W. (1929): The discharge of impulses in motor nerve fibres. II. The frequency of discharge in reflex and voluntary contraction. *J. Physiol.*, 67:119–151.
2. Ballantyne, J. P., and Hansen, S. (1974): A new method for the estimation of the number of motor units in a muscle. I. Control subjects and patients with myasthenia gravis. *J. Neurol. Neurosurg. Psychiatry*, 37:907–915.
3. Basmajian, J. V. (1967): *Muscles Alive. Their Functions Revealed by Electromyography.* Williams & Wilkins Co., Baltimore.
4. Black, J. T., Bhatt, G. P., DeJesus, P. V., Schotland, D. L., and Rowland, L. P. (1974): Diagnostic accuracy of clinical data, quantitative electromyography and histochemistry in neuromuscular disease. A study of 105 cases. *J. Neurol. Sci.*, 21:59–70.
5. Brown, J. C., Charlton, J. E., and White, D. J. K. (1975): A regional technique for the study of sensitivity to curare in human muscle. *J. Neurol. Neurosurg. Psychiatry*, 38:18–26.
6. Buchthal, F. (1957): *An Introduction to Electromyography.* Glydendahl, Copenhagen.
7. Buchthal, F., and Rosenfalck, A. (1966): Evoked action potential and conduction velocity in human sensory nerves. *Brain Res.*, 3:1–122.
8. Buchthal, F., and Rosenfalck, A. (1971): Sensory potentials in polyneuropathy. *Brain*, 94:241–262.
9. Conrad, B., and Aschoff, J. C. (1975): The diagnostic value of the F-wave latency. *Fifth International Congress of Electromyography*, abstracts of communications.

10. Daube, J. P. (1975): Comparison of methods of quantitating electromyography. *Fifth International Congress of Electromyography*, abstracts of communications.
11. Dawson, G. D. (1956): The relative excitability and conduction velocity of sensory and motor nerve fibres in man. *J. Physiol.*, 131:436–451.
12. Desmedt, J. E. (Ed.) (1973): *New Developments in Electromyography and Clinical Neurophysiology*. Karger, Basel.
13. Dyck, P. J., and Lambert, E. H. (1968): Lower motor and primary sensory neuron diseases with peroneal muscular atrophy. *Arch. Neurol.*, 18:603–625.
14. Dyck, P. J., Thomas, P. K., and Lambert, E. H. (Eds.) (1975): *Peripheral Neuropathy*. W. B. Saunders Co., Philadelphia.
15. Eckstedt, J., Äggqvist, D., and Stålberg, E. (1969): The construction of needle multi-electrodes for single fibre electromyography. *Electroencephalogr. Clin. Neurophysiol.*, 27: 540–543.
16. Engel, W. K. (1975): Brief, small, abundant motor-unit action potentials. A further critique of electromyographic interpretation. *Neurology (Minneap.)*, 25:173–176.
17. Gilliatt, R. W., and Willison, R. G. (1963): The refractory and supernormal periods of human median nerve. *J. Neurol. Neurosurg. Psychiatry*, 26:136–147.
18. Goodgold, J., and Eberstein, A. (1972): *Electrodiagnosis of Neuromuscular Diseases*. Williams & Wilkins Co., Baltimore.
19. Grob, D. (1971): Spontaneous end-plate activity in normal subjects and in patients with myasthenia gravis. *Ann. N.Y. Acad. Sci.*, 183:248–269.
20. Grob, D., Johns, R. J., and Harvey, A. M. (1956): Studies in neuromuscular function. *Johns Hopkins Med. J.*, 99:125–238.
21. Harvey, A. M., and Masland, R. L. (1941): A method for the study of neuromuscular transmission in human subjects. *Johns Hopkins Med. J.*, 68:81–93.
22. Heckmann, J. R. (1972): Excitability curve: A new technique for assessing human peripheral nerve excitability in vivo. *Neurology (Minneap.)*, 22:224–230.
23. Hodes, R., Larrabee, M. C., and German, W. (1948): The human electromyogram in response to nerve stimulation and the conduction velocity of motor axons. *Arch. Neurol. Psychiatry*, 60:340–365.
24. Kominami, N., Tyler, H. R., Hampers, C. L., and Merrill, J. P. (1971): Variations in motor nerve conduction velocity in normal and uremic patients. *Arch. Intern. Med.*, 128:235–239.
25. Kopell, H. D., and Thompson, W. A. L. (1963): *Entrapment Neuropathies*. Williams & Wilkins Co., Baltimore.
26. Lambert, E. H. (1966): Defects of neuromuscular transmission in syndromes other than myasthenia gravis. *Ann. N.Y. Acad. Sci.*, 135:367–384.
27. Licht, S. (Ed.) (1971): *Electrodiagnosis and Electromyography*. Waverly Press, Baltimore.
28. Mayer, R. F., and Feldman, R. G. (1967): Observation on the nature of the F wave in man. *Neurology (Minneap.)*, 17:147–156.
29. McComas, A. J., Fawcett, P. R. W., Campbell, M. J., and Sica, R. E. P. (1971): Electrophysiological estimation of the number of motor units within a human muscle. *J. Neurol. Neurosurg. Psychiatry*, 34:121–131.
30. McComas, A. J., Sica, R. E. P., and Campbell, M. J. (1971): "Sick" motoneurones. A unifying concept of muscle disease. *Lancet*, 1:321–325.
31. McQuillen, M. P. (1971): Idiopathic polyneuritis: serial studies of nerve and immune functions. *J. Neurol. Neurosurg. Psychiatry*, 34:607–615.
32. McQuillen, M. P., and Gorin, F. J. (1969): Serial ulnar nerve conduction velocity measurements in normal subjects. *J. Neurol. Neurosurg. Psychiatry*, 32:144–148.
33. McQuillen, M. P., and Johns, R. J. (1967): The nature of the defect in the Eaton-Lambert syndrome. *Neurology (Minneap.)*, 17:527–536.
34. McQuillen, M. P., and Josifek, L. A. (1972): An unusual neuromuscular defect in a case of possible botulism. *Arch. Neurol.*, 26:320–325.
35. McQuillen, M. P., Procopis, P. G., and Luke, R. G. (1973): Nerve excitability in chronic renal disease. *Trans. Am. Soc. Artif. Intern. Organs*, 19:337–339.
36. McQuillen, M. P., Tucker, K., and Pellegrino, E. D. (1967): Syndrome of subacute generalized muscular stiffness and spasm. *Arch. Neurol.*, 16:165–174.
37. Mechler, F. (1974): Changing electromyographic findings during the chronic course of polymyositis. *J. Neurol. Sci.*, 23:237–242.

38. Montgomery, E., and McQuillen, M. P. (1973): Grouped muscle action potential area. *Arch. Phys. Med. Rehabil.*, 54:243–248.
39. Özdemir, C., and Young, R. R. (1971): Electrical testing in myasthenia gravis. *Ann. N.Y. Acad. Sci.*, 183:287–302.
40. Ramsay, I. D. (1965): Electromyography in thyrotoxicosis. *Q. J. Med.*, 34:255–267.
41. Rose, A. L., and Willison, R. G. (1967): Quantitative electromyography using automatic analysis. Studies in healthy subjects and patients with primary muscle disease. *J. Neurol. Neurosurg. Psychiatry*, 30:403–410.
42. Rosselle, N., and Stevens, A. (1973): Unexpected incidence of neurogenic atrophy of the extensor digitorum brevis muscle in young normal subjects. In: *New Developments in Electromyography and Clinical Neurophysiology*, edited by J. E. Desmedt. Karger, Basel.
43. Scarpalezos, S., and Panayiotopoulos, C. P. (1973): Duchenne muscular dystrophy: reservation to the neurogenic hypothesis. *Lancet*, 2:458.
44. Schwartz, M. S., and Stålberg, E. (1975): Single fibre electromyographic studies in myasthenia gravis with repetitive nerve stimulation. *J. Neurol. Neurosurg. Psychiatry*, 38:678–682.
45. Slomić, A., Rosenfalck, A., and Buchthal, F. (1968): Electrical and mechanical responses of normal and myasthenic muscle. *Brain Res.*, 10:1–78.
46. Smorto, M. P., and Basmajian, J. V. (1972): *Clinical Electroneurography*. Williams & Wilkins Co., Baltimore.
47. Stålberg, E. (1966): Propagation velocity of human muscle fibres in situ. *Acta Physiol. Scand.* [*Suppl. 287*], 70:1–112.
48. Stålberg, E., and Ekstedt, J. (1973): Single fibre EMG and microphysiology of the motor unit in normal and diseased human muscle. In: *New Developments in Electromyography and Clinical Neurophysiology*, edited by J. E. Desmedt. Karger, Basel.
49. Stålberg, E., and Thiele, B. (1972): Transmission block in terminal nerve twigs. A single fibre electromyographic finding in man. *J. Neurol. Neurosurg. Psychiatry*, 35:52–59.
50. Watson, R., and Waylonis, G. W. (1975): Paraspinal electromyographic abnormalities as a predictor of occult metastatic carcinoma. *Arch. Phys. Med. Rehabil.*, 56:216–218.
51. Wright, E. A., and McQuillen, M. P. (1973): Excitability of peripheral nerve in patients with normal motor nerve conduction velocities. *J. Neurol. Neurosurg. Psychiatry*, 23:78–83.

Advances in Neurology, Vol. 17, edited by
R. C. Griggs and R. T. Moxley, III. Raven Press,
New York © 1977.

Understanding the Floppy Baby

Gary J. Myers

*University of Rochester School of Medicine and Dentistry, 601 Elmwood Avenue,
Rochester, New York 14620*

Abnormalities of muscle tone are often observed in newborns, and hypotonia is the most frequent change. It is especially important for the clinician to understand hypotonia since it may be an early and striking indication of neuromuscular disease or dysfunction of the central nervous system. To interpret hypotonia in the newborn properly, the clinician must understand maturation of mechanisms controlling muscle tone. This control develops in an orderly manner during gestation and is incomplete even in the term newborn. Premature infants have prominent hypotonia, which steadily improves as they mature. In these instances hypotonia is a normal finding.

In infancy a variety of pathological conditions also alter whatever muscle tone is present. These changes have important prognostic significance at this age. Muscle tone is part of the Apgar rating, a widely used clinical scale to evaluate newborns in the first few minutes after birth. Hypotonia in the newborn is an indication for active intervention. It is not clear why hypotonia is associated so closely with such a diversity of disease states in the newborn.

Careful observation of the presence and pattern of infantile hypotonia can be very useful to the clinician. However, the normal pattern must be understood before pathological variations can be appreciated. This chapter reviews the normal development of muscle tone and then proceeds to the clinical evaluation of the floppy infant. Since the mechanisms underlying normal tone are essential background for understanding the floppy baby, the basis for normal muscle tone is briefly considered.

MUSCLE TONE

Muscle tone is the resistance of a muscle to passive elongation or stretch. At least two factors contribute to this resistance. The first is the viscoelasticity inherent in the muscle, its tendon, surrounding connective tissues, and the fibrous tissues around the joint it influences. This provides some tone even when the muscle is completely at rest.

The second factor is the neural activity that controls muscle contraction and relaxation. Muscle contraction reflects the activity of alpha motor neurons. Their activity can be changed voluntarily or by reflex mechanisms. The reflex changes are mediated by muscle spindles, and their development can be correlated with muscle tone changes in infancy.

MUSCLE SPINDLES

Muscle spindles, the primary sensory receptors monitoring changes in skeletal muscle, are nearly as rich in nerve fibers and endings as the receptors of special senses such as the eye and ear (20). Muscle spindles are present in all muscles and are most numerous in muscles that perform delicate movements (5). There are fewer muscle spindles in the axial musculature (head, neck, and trunk) than in muscles that bear weight and are under postural stress (8).

The muscle spindle consists of a fibrous capsule surrounding from 4 to 10 muscle fibers. Figure 1 illustrates a typical muscle spindle and its major components. Muscle fibers within the spindle are termed intrafusals and differ in several ways from the extrafusal fibers.

There are two types of afferent fibers that leave the muscle spindle. A single primary afferent (Ia fiber) arises from the midportion of both types of intrafusal fibers, and up to five secondary afferents (II fibers) also arise from both types. Secondary endings arise from the distal striated portions of the intrafusal fibers, mostly nuclear chain fibers. Both fiber types respond to

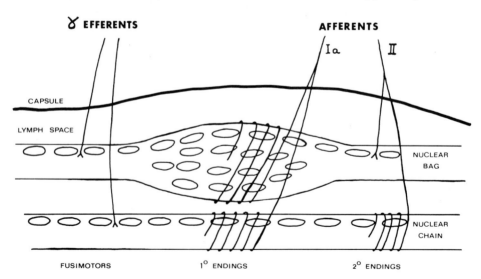

FIG. 1. Diagrammatic view of a muscle spindle to illustrate the two muscle fiber types and their neural supply. Afferents arise from the muscle fiber equators (Ia, 1° endings) or from the distal portions (II, 2° endings). Efferents or fusimotors supply the striated portions of the fibers. The intrafusal fibers are of two types, nuclear bag and nuclear chain. Each spindle has a capsule and a lymph space between the capsule and fibers. (Modified from ref. 20.)

TABLE 1. *Innervation of the cat soleus muscle*

Afferent fibers		Efferent fibers[a]
50 Ia (1° endings) ⎱ 50 II (2° endings) ⎰ 40 Ib (GTOs)[b]	50 spindles	150 alpha motor (25,000 extrafusal fibers) 100 gamma motor (300 intrafusal fibers in 50 spindles)

[a] Note that 40% of efferent fibers are for control of muscle spindles and not for contraction of extrafusal muscle.
[b] GTO, Golgi tendon organ.
Modified from ref. 20.

changes in muscle spindle length, but the primary endings are more sensitive to the rate at which the length is changing.

Each muscle spindle also receives several efferent (fusimotor) fibers from gamma motor neurons. These account for approximately 40% of all efferent fibers going to muscles. The relative proportion of efferent fibers to spindles has been compared to the alpha-efferent fibers to the extrafusal muscle. Table 1 shows this relationship in the cat soleus muscle, in which the ratio of gamma efferents to spindles is 2:1, whereas that for alpha efferents to extrafusal fibers is 1:166 (20). The majority of efferent fibers to muscle are involved in the regulation of muscle spindles.

DEVELOPMENT OF MUSCLE SPINDLES

Histologically muscle spindles can first be recognized in the human embryo at 11 weeks gestation (9). Initially they appear as a spiral nerve surrounding several myoblasts. By 12 weeks gestation the spindle capsule has also formed. At 14 weeks the lymphatic space has developed, and myelination of large nerves to the spindle is first seen. At 15 weeks the motor end plates are visible, and by 16 weeks the subneural apparatus is present (4). By 24 to 31 weeks mature-appearing spindles can be seen (9,10). Table 2 outlines this development. These observations pertain to the biceps

TABLE 2. *Development of muscle spindle formation in the human fetus*

Anatomical structure	Gestational age (weeks) when first seen
Annulospiral endings around myoblasts	11
Capsule	12
Lymphatic space	14
Myelination of large nerves to muscle spindles	14
Myoneural junctions	15
Subneural apparatus of end plate	16
Some muscle spindles appear mature	24

Data based on observations in the biceps brachii muscle (9).

brachii muscle, and spindle development in other sites may vary slightly. Appendicular muscle fibers generally mature after axial musculature (23), and in cats the muscle fiber differentiation begins in the forelegs earlier than in the hindlegs (22).

Although spindle development seems complete by 31 weeks, there is evidence to suggest that mature structure and function are not achieved until much later. In the human fetus the neuromuscular end plates all appear similar, but in the adult there are a variety of different types (4). The human subneural apparatus, which first appears at 16 weeks, may not reach its final form until after a year of age (4). In rats the spindle development continues for a month after birth (33), and in kittens and rabbits the spindle function differs from that in the adult until several weeks after birth (29).

The development of tone and coordinated movement can be correlated with spindle development. Infants at 36 weeks gestation begin to develop flexion postures in all extremities, and at this time their nerve conduction velocity is approximately 20 m/sec (28). This conduction rate in the cat is the critical level for muscle spindle activity. At about the same age the Moro reflex becomes complete and the infant's tone approaches that of the term baby (26).

GOLGI TENDON ORGANS

In addition to muscle spindles, the tendons contain receptors. These are termed Golgi tendon organs, and their fibers are the Ib afferents. They are stimulated by tension resulting from either active or passive stretch of the muscle. They require more stretch than spindles to be activated, and they are thought to prevent overcontraction of the muscles, partly by activating antagonists. In most muscles there are nearly equal numbers of spindles and Golgi tendon organs.

STRETCH REFLEXES

Neural control of muscle tone depends on the muscle stretch reflex. The stretch reflex consists of two distinct types termed tonic (static) and phasic (transient). Both depend on the spinal reflex arc. The stimulus receptor for both reflexes is the muscle spindle or Golgi tendon organ. Afferent fibers from these receptors travel via dorsal roots to the spinal cord gray matter where connections are made with efferent fibers. Figure 2 illustrates this relationship. The efferent impulses then travel to intrafusal and extrafusal fibers.

The phasic stretch reflex represents the most direct pathway from receptor to spinal cord to muscle. This is the pathway tested clinically by the deep tendon reflex. Although the pathway is simple, it can be modified by neural influences from as far away as the cortex. Figure 3 outlines cortical

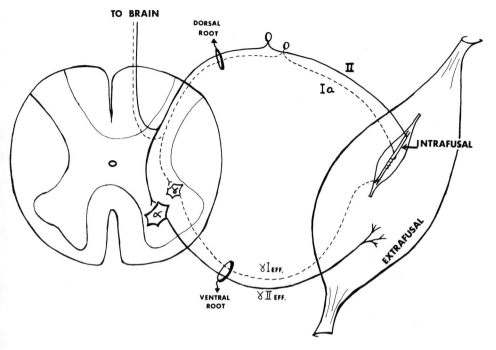

FIG. 2. Simplified diagram of the peripheral reflex arcs involved in stretch reflexes. The motor neurons actually receive multiple afferent inputs. α, alpha motoneuron; γ, gamma motoneuron; γI eff., type I efferent; γII eff., type II efferent; Ia, type Ia afferent; II, type II afferent.

areas known to modify this reflex. The cerebellum and reticular formation are particularly influential in this regulation (15). The knee jerk can first be demonstrated by electromyography at 25 weeks (28), but it is not clinically apparent until near term when the response is more coordinated.

The tonic stretch reflex maintains the muscle in a state of partial contraction and is the primary mechanism behind resting tone. It is this reflex that maintains static posture. During gestation tonic spindle discharges increase as myelination of nerves progresses (28). The degree of myelination also affects the amplitude of the action potential and consequently synaptic transmission at the myoneural junction. Immaturity of tonic reflex activity may be one factor in the hypotonia of prematures and newborns.

GENERAL CLINICAL ASPECTS OF HYPOTONIA

The first fetal movement occurs at approximately 8 weeks of gestation with turning of the head, and this is soon followed by spinal movements (16). Despite the lack of neural myelination and the immaturity of the myoneural junction, even these early movements appear to result from

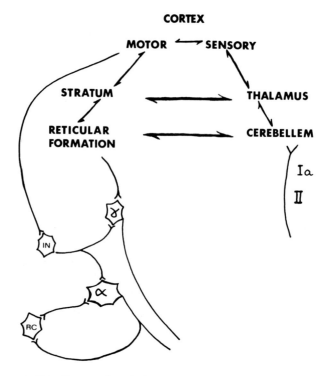

FIG. 3. Diagrammatic pathways of central nervous system areas that can influence stretch reflexes. These can be Renshaw cells (RC) which modify alpha motoneuron (α) activity, or structures within the brain. γ, gamma motoneuron; Ia, type Ia afferent fiber; II, type II afferent fiber; IN interneuron; stratum, corpus striatum (caudate, putamen).

nervous system activity. Clinically recognizable muscle tone is not seen until approximately 26 weeks gestation, nearly 4 months after the first movement.

The clinical evaluation of muscle tone is hampered by the lack of objective tests. The evaluation is thus subjective, and the clinician compares the tone in a given patient to his experience with muscle tone in other circumstances. This is fairly reliable when dealing with marked deviations from normal, but it is increasingly difficult when the patient's tone approaches normal or he is uncooperative. Despite the generally involuntary nature of the control of muscle tone, any adult can consciously alter his muscle tone. A patient faking hypotonia can temporarily mislead most physicians (3). This conscious control may also be one element of self-hypnosis. Changes in muscle tone can occur with mood (5) and can accompany rapid eye movement sleep.

The neural component of tone is so dynamic that it can vary from moment to moment. The act of passively moving an extremity may alter its muscle tone by stimulating stretch reflexes. This sometimes leads to a difference between muscle tone evaluated by passive stretch as opposed to palpation. For instance, after capsular hemiplegias the involved muscles may be flaccid on palpation and hypertonic when manipulated.

The speed with which the passive movement is carried out can also influence the tone (14), as can the patient's ability to cooperate in relaxing the muscles so that resting tone can be evaluated. Despite these complicating factors, it is possible to determine clinically the general state of a patient's muscle tone. Experienced clinicians often become very astute at assessing it.

Weakness must be separated from hypotonia. Strength may be normal in cerebellar disease although muscle tone is markedly diminished (34). In patients who can cooperate, this distinction can be made easily. However, in infancy it is more difficult, and observation of movements made either spontaneously or after stimulation must be used. The infant's strength is then inferred from his functional ability. In this age group a clear distinction between strength and tone cannot be made.

The distribution of hypotonia in an infant is essential to determine in any clinical evaluation. Its pattern is helpful in determining the site of the lesion, its etiology, and the prognosis. An interruption of the peripheral reflex arc either in its afferent or efferent limb leads mainly to distal hypotonia. In contrast, lesions within the central nervous system in infancy usually produce hypotonia that involves axial (trunk and limb girdle) musculature more than appendicular (limb). Metabolic changes or defects in neuromuscular transmission usually produce hypotonia affecting all muscles.

In infancy axial hypotonia associated with normal muscle tone in the limbs is a particularly helpful sign. When this pattern is combined with brisk or easily elicited deep tendon reflexes, the clinician should strongly suspect a lesion within the central nervous system. This may be the only clue to the underlying etiology, and laboratory tests may fail to confirm positively the site of the lesion. Until language begins at approximately 1 year of age, the evaluation of cortical function may be quite difficult, and hypotonia itself can delay motor development, regardless of its etiology.

Hypotonia in a single limb during the newborn period is usually the result of a plexus lesion. These are most common in the brachial plexus and vary widely in severity. Some regress within days whereas others are permanent deficits. Nerve injuries of all types can lead to hypotonia in the muscles which that nerve supplies, and injuries to the brachial or lumbar plexus can affect the tone in an entire extremity. Damage to sensory roots or afferent nerves produces hypotonia (21) similar to that seen with ventral root or motor nerve lesions. Any interruption of the peripheral reflex arc interferes with the sensitive neural mechanisms controlling tone and leads to hypotonia.

Hypotonia affecting all muscle groups is usually a secondary phenomenon related to metabolic problems or interference with neuromuscular transmission. A diffuse depression of nervous system function resulting from hypoxia, hypoglycemia, or oversedation is the most common neonatal cause. Impairment of neuromuscular transmission is less common but can be seen with hypermagnesemia, myasthenia gravis, or after administration of aminoglycoside antibiotics.

TESTING HYPOTONIA IN NEWBORNS AND INFANTS

The steady development of tone during gestation makes it a useful criterion for assessing an infant's maturity. Several investigators have studied the development of tone after the birth of premature infants (2,12,27). Since the extrauterine development of the nervous system is similar to that occurring in the uterus (28), it is reasonable to assume that the development of muscle tone progresses similarly. In premature infants special criteria have been developed to evaluate tone because of its generally reduced level. This gestational hypotonia results from both reduced neural control and laxity of tissues. The difficulties in distinguishing hypotonia from weakness should be kept in mind.

Resting postures are important to observe since infants develop flexion first of the legs and later of the arms as they mature. The term infant with normal tone lies with all extremities partially flexed. To confirm that the observed postures are not simply positioning artifacts, the clinician should

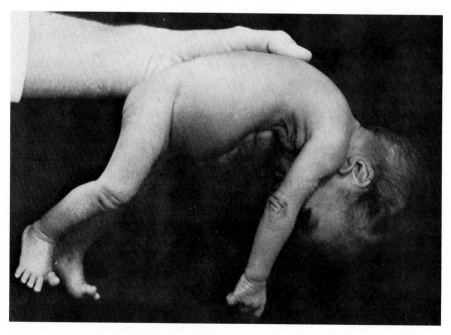

FIG. 4. Ventral suspension. Note truncal curvature, head droop, and extension of limbs. A premature infant of 30 weeks gestation.

test recoil in the limb by first flexing the limb for 5 sec and then holding it extended for 5 sec before releasing it. The important observation is the amount of flexion following this maneuver. Both upper or both lower extremities are usually tested simultaneously.

Muscle tone in the truncal musculature is tested by ventral suspension and the infant's ability to control head movements. Ventral suspension consists of placing the infant across the palm of the examiner's hand and observing the infant's head, trunk, and limb postures (Fig. 4). The hypotonic or weak infant lies like a piece of cloth, but with increasing tone or strength the trunk is partially or fully extended, the limbs flexed, and the head elevated. The term infant in ventral suspension lies with the back straight, head up, and limbs strongly flexed.

Neck flexors are examined by pulling the supine infant to the sitting position while holding both hands (Fig. 5). The ability to control the head is observed. Healthy infants at term have partial control. This same maneuver is also helpful in testing limb muscles. Infants with normal tone and strength pull against the examiner. This leads to arm flexion and is termed the traction response. Hypotonic infants fail to flex the arms, either at elbows or shoulders, as they are pulled upright.

Tone of muscles around the limb girdles can be tested several ways.

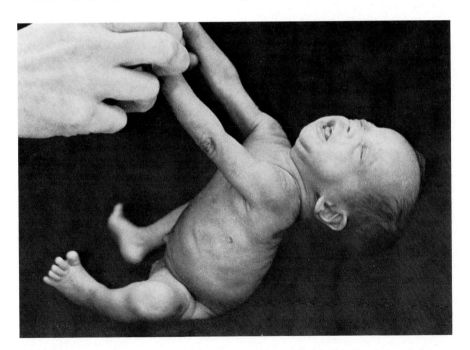

FIG. 5. Traction response to test muscle tone in arms, shoulder girdle, and neck flexors. Note poor head control and absence of flexion at elbows and shoulders. A premature infant of 30 weeks gestation.

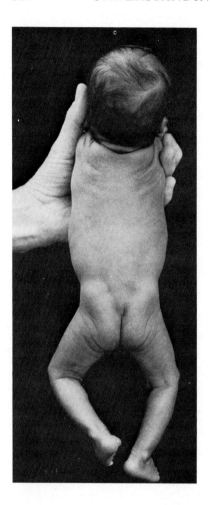

FIG. 6. Shoulder girdle hypotonia being tested by lifting infant with pressure under the axillae. Notice how the scapulae ride up, the arms fail to adduct well, and the legs are only partly flexed. A premature infant of 30 weeks gestation.

Suspension of the infant by lifting with the examiner's hands in each axilla (Fig. 6) tests the infant's ability to fix the shoulder girdle. Normal infants adduct their arms and fix their scapulae so that they can be readily lifted. However, the hypotonic infant fails to do this and the examiner finds himself holding the thorax tightly as the shoulder girdle and arms rise upward and the baby begins slipping through his hands. In more immature infants the scarf sign is helpful. This is elicited by pulling the arm across the midline (Fig. 7) toward the opposite shoulder. With hypotonia the elbow crosses the midline and the arm can be placed like a scarf across the baby's neck. As muscle tone increases this becomes impossible. A similar test, the heel to ear, can be used for the pelvic girdle (Fig. 8). With the infant lying supine and the pelvis flat, the baby's foot is moved toward the head. The knee is left free and may lie lateral to the abdomen. In premature infants less than

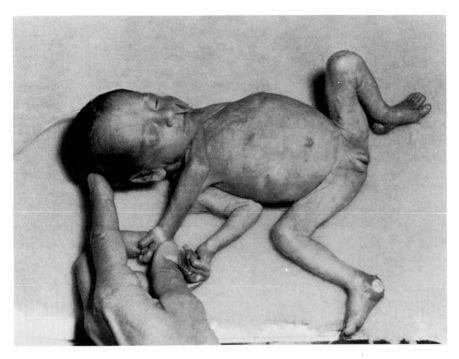

FIG. 7. Scarf sign. Notice how the arm can be pulled across the midline and the elbow reaches the opposite axilla. A premature infant of 27 weeks gestation.

30 weeks gestation, the heel can be readily touched to the ipsilateral ear. This becomes increasingly difficult as the infant matures.

In addition to these specific tests, reflex activity is also impaired in the presence of hypotonia. The Moro reflex is a good example, but stepping, placing, trunk incurvation, rooting, and other reflexes are similarly impaired. The Moro reflex first appears at 28 weeks gestation. At this age it is rapidly exhausted and not well coordinated. As neural integration improves and muscle tone becomes more organized, components such as adduction of the arms, extension of the legs, and opening of the hands are added. In the presence of severe hypotonia all components of the Moro reflex are virtually absent. Asymmetries of the Moro are seen with injuries to a nerve plexus, such as a brachial palsy.

These gestational changes in specific tests are outlined in Fig. 9, and the normal variability of muscle tone is compared further in Table 3. Evaluation of muscle tone in babies requires an understanding of these changes since normal findings in a premature infant vary with the gestational age, and all of these findings would be considered abnormal in a term or older infant. During the first few months of life, muscle tone and strength can be evaluated with many of the same tests. Ventral suspension, head lag, postures,

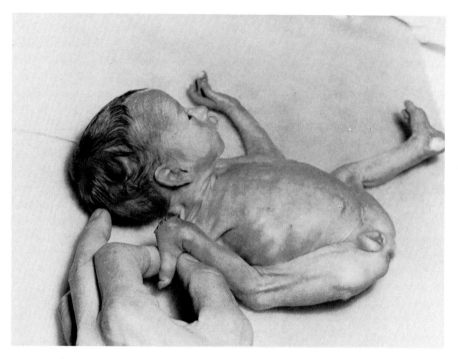

FIG. 8. Heel to ear sign. Notice how the heel can be brought to the ear while the pelvis is flat. A premature infant of 27 weeks gestation.

shoulder suspension, and the traction response are especially helpful. In older children observation of sitting postures can also be useful since fixation of the spine is required.

The difference between proximal and distal hypotonia is especially important in older children. The use of distal musculature requires that proximal structures such as the spine and shoulder girdle be fixed adequately. Failure to do so seriously impairs the ability to use the hands, arms, and legs. This can lead to delayed motor development involving the limbs even when they are normal. Why such differences between axial and appendicular muscles occur is not clear, but differences in their origin, development, and spindle distribution (Table 4) may be important.

Other clinical features may also help in localizing the site of hypotonia. Fasciculations in the muscles are seen in anterior horn cell disease. These are easiest to observe in the tongue where there is no subcutaneous tissue overlying the muscle. In newborns this finding must be used cautiously since it may be normal.

Changes in deep tendon reflexes often reflect the site of the neurologic lesion. Depressed or absent reflexes are seen with interruption of the peripheral reflex arc, whereas exaggerated ones are present with damage or dys-

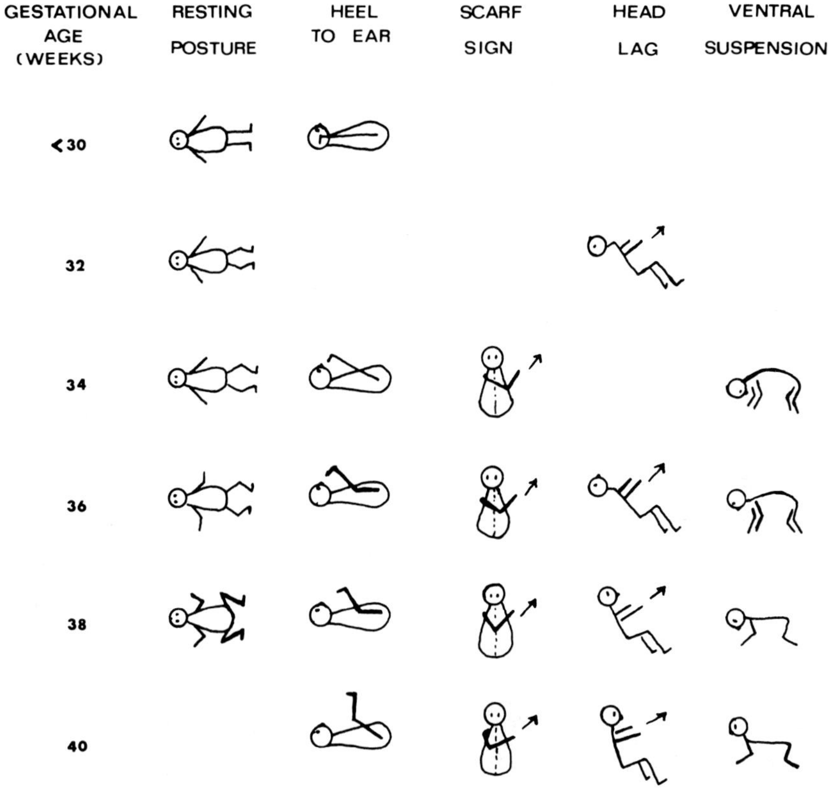

GESTATIONAL AGE (WEEKS)	RESTING POSTURE	HEEL TO EAR	SCARF SIGN	HEAD LAG	VENTRAL SUSPENSION
< 30					
32					
34					
36					
38					
40					

FIG. 9. Diagrammatic outline of the specific tests for hypotonia that are most useful in newborns. The gestational ages when they first appear are indicated, but there is some individual variation. (Modified from ref. 12.)

function of the brain or spinal cord. The combination of brisk deep tendon reflexes and axial hypotonia is quite characteristic of a central lesion. The presence of even mild microcephaly helps to confirm this. When deep tendon reflexes are difficult to obtain and the child is old enough to cooperate, it is worthwhile to use the Jendrassik maneuver. This activates the muscle spindle afferents and enhances these reflexes (32). The maneuver is performed by having the child hook his hands together and pull laterally while the examiner tests the reflexes.

LABORATORY EVALUATION

Laboratory evaluation may also be helpful in pinpointing the source of hypotonia. Although there are no direct tests of hypotonia itself, many components of the system controlling muscle tone can be tested. Muscle biopsy, electromyography, and nerve conduction are especially helpful in evaluating the peripheral reflex arc, and negative studies can indicate that

Table 3. Normal maturation of the major clinical tests influenced by muscle tone in the newborn[a]

Test	Weeks gestation												
	26	28	30	31	32	33	34	35	36	37	38	39	40
Tone													
Heel to ear	No resistance		→	Slight resistance			→ Difficult		→ Almost impossible	→	→	→ Impossible	
Scarf		No resistance						→ Minimal resistance	→ Fair resistance		→ Difficult		
Neck													
Extension	Absent		→ Slight		→								
Flexion		Absent					→ Fair Minimal		→ Good		→ Fair		
Postures													
Resting	Hypotonic		→ Legs flexed			→ Some arm flexion			→ Total flexion				
Recoil	None		→ Legs slight				→ None arms Good legs			→ Slow arms		→ Good arms	
Trunk extension (ventral suspension)				Absent				→ Slight		→ Good			
Reflexes													
Moro	Barely apparent	→ Complete exhaustible		→		Complete without arm adduction					→ Complete		
Grasp		→ Feeble	Fair	→	Solid with arms Good								
Root	Minimal	→ Good with reinforcement		→							→ Can lift infant		

[a] Arrows indicate the approximate time when the test matures to the next developmental level. Modified from Dubowitz (11).

TABLE 4. *Differences in axial and appendicular muscles that may contribute to clinical patterns of hypotonia*

	Trunk	Limb
Origin	Myotomes	Lateral plate mesoderm
Spindles	Relatively few	Many
Development	Early	Later

this portion of the system is intact. A decrease in the motor or sensory nerve conduction velocity can indicate a peripheral neuropathy. In infants, however, nerve conduction is slower than in adults (31), and values need to be compared to age-related standards. The electromyogram is particularly helpful in detecting fibrillations. In limb muscles these are abnormal at any age and indicate anterior horn cell dysfunction.

The muscle biopsy can also help and may indicate either a myopathy or a neuropathy. Muscle spindles are present in some biopsies, and several studies have tried to relate these to disease states (6,30). So far this has not proven clinically useful, but no studies have been reported in newborns. In the rat, denervation of muscle spindles postnatally results in no significant anatomic changes, even after many months. However, prenatal denervation of developing muscle spindles leads to atrophy of the intrafusal fibers (33). It is not known if this occurs in man.

Evidence that lesions of the central nervous system account for hypotonia is often more difficult to obtain. There can be serious problems with cortical, subcortical, basal ganglia, cerebellar, and other central structures without concomitant changes in the electroencephalogram, skull films, brain scan, or cerebrospinal fluid. The diagnosis then rests on clinical evidence and must be inferred after negative or nondiagnostic laboratory evaluations. Table 5 presents a simplified clinical and laboratory approach to evaluation of the level of involvement producing hypotonia.

DIFFERENTIAL DIAGNOSIS OF HYPOTONIA

The classification of floppy infants can be approached in various ways (11,19,34). Zellweger et al. (34) have divided the hypotonias into those caused by chemical and endocrine abnormalities and those resulting from neuromuscular dysfunction. Jebsen (19) classifies them as metabolic, motor unit, or central nervous system diseases. Rabe (25) classifies only those within the neuromuscular system and has separated them accordingly to site of the lesion. From the neurologic standpoint this orderly arrangement provides a good basis for clinical thinking about the hypotonic infant. Dubowitz (11) has approached the problem by separating hypotonia with normal strength from that with weakness. This system seems logical, but

TABLE 5. *A diagnostic approach to hypotonia.*

Level of lesion	Clinical		Laboratory		
	Babinski	DTRs[a]	Muscle biopsy	EMG	Nerve conduction
Cortical or subcortical	N or ↑	N or ↓	N	N	N
Cerebellar	N or ↑	N or ↑	N	N	N
Spinal cord	N or absent	N or absent	N	N	N
Peripheral reflex arc					
Receptor (muscle spindles)			?N	N	N
Afferent			N	N	Sensory abn
Anterior horn cell			Grouped atrophy	Fibrillations	N
Efferent			Grouped atrophy	Fibrillations	Motor abn
Neuromuscular junction			N	Facilitation	N
Muscle			Variable	Abn	N

These are the most useful clinical and laboratory criteria in evaluations and the changes usually seen with lesions at each level.
a DTR, deep tendon reflex; N, normal; abn, abnormal; ↑, increased; ↓, decreased.

clinically the distinction can not always be made. Indeed, the younger the infant the more difficult it becomes.

Some metabolic problems are difficult to classify since they can impair muscular tone in several ways. For example, hypoxia produces muscle spindle dysfunction (35) and also has serious central nervous system effects. Other metabolic changes may have similar widespread effects on neural control.

In a number of hypotonic infants no cause of the defect can be found. Many of these infants show steady improvement in muscular tone and at some later time have normal neuromuscular function. Infants with perinatal asphyxia are often hypotonic, and their muscle tone improves over hours or days. The length of time to recovery seems roughly proportional to the severity of the hypoxic insult. An adequate history of the labor, delivery, and immediate postnatal period is essential to making this diagnosis.

Some hypotonic infants who develop normal muscle tone are diagnosed as having benign congenital hypotonia. This diagnosis can be made only in retrospect, and its frequency seem inversely related to the thoroughness of the diagnostic evaluation. Many infants diagnosed initially as having benign congenital hypotonia later fit into the Prader-Willi syndrome.

Table 6 presents a combined classification that emphasizes the distinction between metabolic problems with secondary hypotonia and neurological problems that primarily interfere with the control of muscular tone.

Among the various causes of hypotonia, those resulting from central nervous system dysfunction are most frequent. In various series this percentage ranges from 58 to 80% (Table 7) (13,19,24). These series do not include newborns or infants who are transiently hypotonic but reflect the etiology when hypotonia is persistent beyond the newborn period.

COMPLICATIONS ASSOCIATED WITH HYPOTONIA

The hypotonic infant presents several management problems. Feeding difficulties are usually the earliest problem and are especially prominent with diseases affecting facial and bulbar musculature, such as congenital myasthenia gravis or myotonic dystrophy. Infants with generalized hypotonia for other reasons are also difficult to feed. In either instance gavage feedings may be necessary, and care must be taken to prevent aspiration. In peripheral myopathies and anterior horn cell diseases, feeding is usually normal.

The decreased tone and consequently movement may lead to several related problems. An abnormal head shape can result from constantly lying in one position. The head is usually flattened occipitally with hair loss over the most prominent area. Contractures may develop, such as the jug handle arms seen in anterior horn cell disease. These are due to arm positioning when lying supine and resulting contractures of the muscles about the

TABLE 6. *Classification of the hypotonic infant*

I. Gestational (developmental)
II. Metabolic
   A. Nutritional (matnutrition, rickets, scurvy, celiac disease)
   B. Endocrine (hypothyroidism, Cushing's syndrome, hyperparathyroidism)
   C. Connective tissue (arachnodactyly, Ehlers-Danlos and Marfan's syndromes, osteo- genesis imperfecta)
   D. General (hypoglycemia, hypomagnesemia, hypercalcemia, hyper- or hypokalemia, hypophosphatemia, acidosis, hypoxia, hyperbilirubinemia, amino aciduria, de- hydration)
   E. Transplacental intoxication (bromine, magnesium, phenobarbital, sedatives, anesthetics)
III. Neuromuscular
   A. Central nervous system
      1. Cortical or subcortical damage
      2. Chromosomal abnormalities (trisomy 21, Turner's syndrome)
      3. Degenerative diseases (lipidoses, mucopolysaccharidosis)
      4. Cerebellar diseases (agenesis, inflammation, infarction)
      5. Prader-Willi syndrome
   B. Spinal cord
      1. Trauma (birth injury)
      2. Malformation (spina bifida)
      3. Anterior horn cell (Werdnig-Hoffmann's disease, myelopathic arthrogryposis, poliomyelitis)
   C. Spinal roots or peripheral nerves
      1. Trauma (plexus palsies, nerve injuries)
      2. Peripheral neuropathy (acute, chronic, polyneuritis)
   D. Myoneural junction
      1. Myasthenia gravis
      2. Antibiotics (kanamycin, colistin, neomycin)
   E. Muscle
      1. Congenital myopathy (Duchenne, rod, central core, myotubular, nemaline, myotonic dystrophy, glycogen storage)
      2. Polymyositis
IV. Environmental (congenital blindness, maternal deprivation)
V. Benign congenital

shoulders. Scoliosis may develop because of spinal column positioning. It can result from the infant's lying in one position, or, if the child is able to sit, from the pull of gravity.

Pulmonary problems are perhaps the most serious since the infant's reserve may be limited and any compromise can impair adequate gas

TABLE 7. *Primary site of pathology in several large series of hypotonic infants.*

Author	CNS	Peripheral reflex arc	Metabolic or benign
Jebsen et al. (19)	18 (58%)	13 (42%)	0
Paine (24)	96 (72%)	9 (6%)	28 (22%)
Eng (13)	265 (80%)	59 (15%)	7 (5%)

These series include mainly infants who were referred for hypotonia persisting beyond the newborn period.

exchange. A depressed cough reflex may be present, making clearance of secretions difficult and any respiratory infection potentially serious. Scoliosis may further compromise pulmonary reserve.

When spinal cord lesions, such as transections, are present, there may be poor autonomic regulation of cutaneous vessels and of sweating below the lesion. This compromises thermal control, especially in infants, and can result in potentially serious hyperthermia.

Retarded development often accompanies hypotonia, and it is important to differentiate its motor and intellectual aspects. Hypotonia due to CNS lesions is usually accompanied by cognitive impairment, whereas with spinal cord or peripheral reflex arc lesions this is not true. For example, most children with anterior horn cell disease are mentally normal unless hypoxia has occurred. The parent-infant interaction is another factor that can affect the infant's development. Parents are stimulated to provide more interaction when infants respond to their attentions. Even newborns can provide positive reinforcement to parents by eye contact, moving when stimulated, and quieting when comforted. The hypotonic infant, however, has a smaller repertoire of these responses, and this can result in his receiving a reduced amount of stimulation.

Problems such as cardiac failure can be a complication if there is primary (myopathies) or secondary (glycogen storage diseases) muscle involvement. However, most hypotonic infants have no cardiac problems.

TREATMENT

The correct diagnosis is essential before any rational treatment can be undertaken since therapy must be directed toward the basic cause. Unfortunately, in newborns there may not be adequate time to follow this dictum, and some treatment may be called for immediately — particularly if sepsis or hypoglycemia is suspected — for any delay could have serious consequences. If sepsis is suspected, appropriate cultures should be taken and antibiotic coverage should be started. Studies of blood sugar, calcium, magnesium, and electrolytes should also be performed. Hypoglycemia is very common and should always be of concern. Use of the Dextrostix for immediate estimation of blood sugar should supplement quantitative blood sugar determinations. If the Dextrostix is low or unavailable, it is safest to give the infant 0.5 cc/kg of 50% dextrose intravenously while awaiting the quantitative blood sugar value since prolonged hypoglycemia can lead to permanent neurological damage. Other metabolic problems can be approached with less urgency.

The treatment of hypotonia itself is difficult except when it is secondary to an underlying metabolic problem. In those instances treatment is directed toward correction of the metabolic derangement. In trisomy 21 (Down's syndrome), in which hypotonia is a prominent feature, treatment with 5-

hydroxytryptamine (5-HT) has been shown to improve tone (1). Some patients have received 5-HT for up to 2 years. While on treatment they achieved milestones more rapidly than untreated controls, but the long-range benefit of this treatment is unknown. One side effect appears to be infantile spasms (7).

In most hypotonic infants treatment is symptomatic. Feeding problems may necessitate special nipples, small and frequent feedings, gavage feedings, or occasionally placement of a gastrostomy tube. When hypotonia impairs pulmonary reserve or reduces the cough reflex, it is important to provide postural drainage, suctioning, and vigorous treatment of respiratory illnesses. Constipation and abdominal distention may further impair pulmonary reserve. Dietary control, stool softeners, or laxatives may be needed to prevent this. All infants need sensory stimulation, but especially those unable to explore their environment actively. This is most apparent in blind children: approximately one-third of those who are congenitally blind and without other neurological problems have hypotonia. These children need encouragement to sit, creep, stand, walk, and perform other motor activities, but as they learn these activities their muscle tone improves (17,18). Stimulation must be constantly encouraged because the hypotonic infant provides parents with fewer rewards for interaction than does the normal infant.

SUMMARY

Muscle tone develops in an orderly sequence through gestation and continues to change after birth. Hypotonia is frequently found in infants, and pathological degrees must be differentiated from normal variations. This distinction is possible if the clinician understands how muscle tone is regulated and modifies his examination to include some special clinical signs. A variety of pathological conditions can influence muscle tone, and hypotonia can be an early and valuable clue to recognizing neuromuscular, CNS, metabolic, and other disease states in this age group.

REFERENCES

1. Airaksinen, E. M. (1974): Tryptophan treatment of infants with Down's syndrome. *Ann. Clin. Res.,* 6:33–39.
2. Amiel-Tison, C. (1968): Neurological evaluation of the maturity of newborn infants. *Arch. Dis. Child.,* 43:89–93.
3. Basmajian, J. V. (1957): New views on muscular tone and relaxation. *Can. Med. Assoc. J.,* 77:203–205.
4. Beckett, E. B., and Bourne, G. H. (1972): Histochemistry of developing skeletal and cardiac muscle. In: *The Structure and Function of Muscle, 2nd Ed., Vol. I,* edited by G. H. Bourne, pp. 150–180. Academic Press, New York.
5. Brodal, A. (1969): *Neurological Anatomy in Relation to Clinical Medicine, 2nd Ed.,* pp. 117–150. Oxford University Press, New York.
6. Cazzato, G., and Walton, J. N. (1968): The pathology of the muscle spindle. *J. Neurol. Sci.,* 7:15–70.

7. Coleman, M. (1971): Infantile spasms associated with 5-hydroxytryptophan administration in patients with Down's syndrome. *Neurology (Minneap.)*, 21:911–919.
8. Crosby, E. C., Humphrey, T., and Lauer, E. W. (1962): *Correlative Anatomy of the Nervous System,* pp. 24–27. The Macmillan Co., New York.
9. Cuajunco, F. (1940): Development of the neuromuscular spindle in human fetuses. *Contrib. Embryol.,* 28(173):97–128.
10. Cuajunco, F. (1942): Development of the human motor end plate. *Contrib. Embryol.,* 30(195):129–152.
11. Dubowitz, V. (1969): The floppy infant. In: *Clinics in Developmental Medicine,* pp. 1–109. Spastics International Medical Publications, London.
12. Dubowitz, L. M. S., Dubowitz, V., and Goldberg, C. (1970): Clinical assessment of gestational age in the newborn infant. *J. Pediatr.,* 77:1–10.
13. Eng, G. D. (1975): Neuromuscular diseases. In: *Neonatology, Pathophysiology and Management of the Newborn,* edited by G. B. Avery, pp. 821–837. J. B. Lippincott Co., Philadelphia.
14. Gilman, S. (1969): The mechanism of cerebellar hypotonia. *Brain,* 92:621–638.
15. Granit, R., and Kaada, B. R. (1952): Influence of stimulation of central nervous structures on muscle spindles in cat. *Acta Physiol. Scand.,* 27:130–160.
16. Hamburger, V. (1975): Fetal behavior. In: *The Mammalian Fetus,* edited by E. S. E. Hafez, pp. 68–81. Charles C Thomas, Springfield, Ill.
17. Jan, J. E., and Scott, E. (1974): Hypotonia and delayed early motor development in congenitally blind children. *J. Pediatr.,* 84:929–930.
18. Jan, J. E., Robinson, G. C., Scott, E., and Kinnis, C. (1975): Hypotonia in the blind child. *Dev. Med. Child. Neurol.,* 17:35–40.
19. Jebsen, R. H., Johnson, E. W., Knobloch, H., and Grant, D. K. (1961): Differential diagnosis of infantile hypotonia. *Am. J. Dis. Child.,* 101:8–17.
20. Matthews, P. B. C. (1972): *Mammalian Muscle Receptors and Their Central Actions,* pp. 1–630. Williams & Wilkins Co., Baltimore.
21. Nathan, P. W., and Sears, T. A. (1960): Effects of posterior root section on the activity of some muscles in man. *J. Neurol. Neurosurg. Psychiatry,* 23:10–22.
22. Nystrom, B. (1968): Histochemistry of developing cat muscles. *Acta Neurol. Scand.,* 44:405–439.
23. Olkowski, Z. L., and Manocha, S. L. (1973): Muscle spindle. In: *The Structure and Function of Muscle, 2nd Ed., Vol. II,* edited by G. H. Bourne, pp. 365–482. Academic Press, New York.
24. Paine, R. S. (1963): The future of the 'floppy infant': a follow-up study of 133 patients. *Dev. Med. Child Neruol.,* 5:115–124.
25. Rabe, E. F. (1964): The hypotonic infant. *J. Pediatr.,* 64:422–440.
26. Robinson, R. J. (1966): Assessment of gestational age by neurological examination. *Arch. Dis. Child.,* 41:437–447.
27. Saint-Anne Dargassies, S. (1955): La maturation neurologique du premature. *Etudes Neonat.,* 4:71–122.
28. Schulte, F. J., Linke, I., Michaelis, R., and Nolte, R. (1969): Excitation, inhibition, and impulse conduction in spinal motoneurones of preterm, term, and small-for-dates newborn infants. In: *Brain and Early Behavior. Development in the Fetus and Infant,* edited by R. J. Robinson, pp. 87–114. Academic Press, New York.
29. Schweiler, G. H. (1968): Respiratory regulation during postnatal development in cats and rabbits and some of its morphological substrate. *Acta Physiol. Scand. [Suppl.],* 304:1–123.
30. Swash, M., and Fox, K. P. (1975): The pathology of the muscle spindle in myasthenia gravis. *J. Neurol. Sci.,* 26:39–47.
31. Thomas, J. E., and Lambert, E. H. (1960): Ulnar nerve conduction velocity and H-reflex in infants and children. *J. Appl. Physiol.,* 15:1–9.
32. Wiesendanger, M. (1972): *Pathophysiology of Muscle Tone,* pp. 24–25. Springer-Verlag, Berlin.
33. Zelena, J. (1957): The morphogenetic influence of innervation on the ontogenetic development of muscle-spindles. *J. Embryol. Exp. Morphol.,* 5:283–292.
34. Zellweger, H. U., Smith, J. W., and Cusminsky, M. (1962): Muscular hypotonia in infancy; diagnosis and differentiation. *Rev. Can. Biol.,* 21:599–612.
35. Zimmerman, G. W., and Grossie, J. (1969): Sensitivity and behavior of muscle spindles to systemic arterial hypoxia. *Proc. Soc. Exp. Biol. Med.,* 132:1114–1118.

Advances in Neurology, Vol. 17, edited by
R. C. Griggs and R. T. Moxley, III. Raven Press,
New York © 1977.

Respiratory Failure as a Complication of Neuromuscular Disease

William J. Hall

*Department of Medicine, University of Rochester School of Medicine and
Dentistry, Rochester, New York 14642*

INTRODUCTION

For many years there has been a logical sharing of interests between physicians caring for patients with neuromuscular diseases and physicians interested in respiratory care. In fact, one of the key factors in the emergence of respiratory medicine as a specialty was the specialized needs of patients with acute poliomyelitis (14). Many of the basic physiologic and clinical principles, as well as advances in instrumentation, were developed during that era. The purpose of this chapter is to review the physiologic principles of respiratory failure owing to neuromuscular disease irrespective of the specific entity, describe some current methods of clinical assessment, and outline the specialized care of these patients.

Physiologic Background

MUSCLES OF RESPIRATION

The diaphragm is the principal muscle of inspiration. Its efferent nerves are derived from the third through the sixth cervical segments and run in the phrenic nerve. The number of muscle fibers per motor unit, the innervation ratio, of the diaphragm is quite low relative to other large skeletal muscles, resulting in few proprioceptors. Classic stretch reflexes are correspondingly minimal in the diaphragm. There is, however, anatomic evidence of afferent innervation (2). The gross action of the diaphragm may be thought of as analogous to a piston moving downward, thereby enlarging the thoracic cage downward. Under conditions of quiet breathing, intercostal muscles function primarily to stabilize the chest wall during changes in intrathoracic pressure. However, in cases of bilateral diaphragmatic paralysis, the external intercostal muscles may become the primary inspiratory muscles and sustain ventilation without leading to respiratory failure. Under conditions of quiet breathing, *expiration* is completely passive. However, the importance of adequate muscular contraction during coughing will be discussed below.

RESPIRATORY MECHANICS

In recent years, respiratory physiologists have focused on those physical properties of the lung important in understanding the mechanism of expiratory flow limitation, which is seen commonly in asthma, emphysema, and chronic bronchitis. An adequate understanding of these physiologic principles is beyond the scope of this review (11). In brief, it is now well known that the expiratory flow limitation seen in these entities is owing almost entirely to intrinsic properties of the lung parenchyma and airways, and not to primary defects in muscular contraction. To understand the pathophysiology of respiratory failure secondary to neuromuscular disease, it is more important to concentrate on the events surrounding inspiration. Figure 1 demonstrates the relationships among atmospheric, pleural, and alveolar pressures during various phases of respiration. In the normal lung at the end of a normal breath (functional residual capacity), pleural pressures are slightly negative relative to atmospheric, reflecting the opposing forces of the semirigid chest wall tending to hold the thoracic cage open and the opposing inward pressures from the elastic recoil of the lung itself. During inspiration, contraction of the diaphragm enlarges the thoracic cage, resulting in increased negative pressure in the pleural cavity relative to atmosphere. Thus air is sucked into the airways. In contrast, in the patient with neuromuscular disease, there are two important differences compared to the normal situation. First, lack of muscular tone in the thoracic musculature leaves the recoil pressures of the lung relatively unopposed, resulting in smaller resting lung volume (functional residual capacity). This may lead to actual airway closure, atelectasis, and impairment of oxygenation (10). Secondly, inspiratory forces will be proportionately lower, and to maintain normal levels of ventilation, accessory muscles of respiration—including neck and abdominal muscles—must be used, resulting in increased oxygen cost of breathing or progressively inadequate alveolar ventilation.

As previously mentioned, under conditions of quiet breathing, expiration

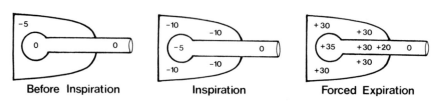

| Before Inspiration | Inspiration | Forced Expiration |

FIG. 1. Relationship among atmospheric, intrapleural, and intraalveolar pressures during various phases of respiration. Atmospheric pressure is represented as zero, and all other pressures are relative to atmospheric. See text for details.

is completely passive. However, the importance of muscular contraction during coughing, which may be thought of as a specialized form of forced expiration, is of particular interest in neuromuscular disease. A cough begins with a forced expiration against a closed glottis. The diaphragm, intercostals, and accessory muscles — including the muscles of the abdominal wall — are probably all contributory and necessary to generate the high intrathoracic pressure required for an effective cough. When the glottis is suddenly opened, the high-pressure gradient between the alveoli and the atmosphere results in extremely high linear velocity of air flow, often approaching 400 to 600 miles/hr (5). This high flow velocity effectively clears mucus and tracheobronchial secretions. Since the pressure gradient responsible for this flow is a direct function of muscle contraction, it is not surprising that one of the hallmarks of respiratory failure owing to neuromuscular disease will be retention of secretions secondary to a depressed cough mechanism.

EFFECTS ON GAS EXCHANGE

The mechanical alterations described above affect gas exchange in two important ways. First, the reduction in resting lung volume and retention of secretions result in alterations in the distribution of inspired air, particularly in the region of the lower lung fields. In general, in these areas, the amount of ventilation relative to regional perfusion of the pulmonary capillary surface is reduced, resulting in low ventilation to perfusion ratios. At times, if ventilation is severely reduced blood may be actually shunted from the right to left sides of the heart without benefit of oxygenation. The net result of these changes is progressive hypoxemia reflected in the arterial Po_2, even though the lungs may be completely structurally normal. Second, the reduction in ventilation associated with progressive muscular weakness impairs carbon dioxide excretion, resulting in elevations in arterial partial pressure of carbon dioxide (Pco_2). This in turn leads to further drop in arterial Po_2, and ultimately to respiratory acidosis.

In summation, impairment of the muscles of respiration affects primarily inspiratory flow rates, causes reductions in lung volumes, and results in impaired clearance of secretions because of a depressed cough. These changes result in hypoxemia and eventually hypercarbia.

CLINICAL ASSESSMENT OF NEUROMUSCULAR FUNCTION

Two aspects regarding the assessment of pulmonary function of these patients bear discussion: First, how to assess the mild or asymptomatic patient, and second, what guidelines to follow to recognize impending acute respiratory failure.

The Asymptomatic Patient

Even in the patient without manifest pulmonary symptomatology, we recommend some objective assessment of respiratory muscle function. This information is often of important prognostic significance as the natural history of the disease unfolds. Further, neuromuscular disease is often associated with mild degrees of dyspnea (6,12), and since it often occurs in the same age group as does chronic obstructive disease, it is important to differentiate this form of impairment from that of intrinsic lung disease. Several pulmonary function tests are of value in this regard. In clinical spirometry, the most commonly performed test, a patient performs a maximal inspiratory and expiratory breathing maneuver. The volume of air moved is plotted against time in seconds, and from this tracing various inspiratory and expiratory flow rates can be calculated. The normal pattern of inspiratory effort results in a rapid flow rate. There is normally some diminution in expiratory flow because of intrinsic compression of airways as previously described. The tracing obtained from the patient with chronic obstructive disease demonstrates a normal inspiratory flow rate with a markedly impaired expiratory limb. In contrast, the patient with neuromuscular disease shows a characteristic diminution in inspiratory flow rates. Thus almost at a glance one can distinguish obstructive lung disease from neuromuscular impairment, and this technique has wide applicability in the office setting. Another test obtainable with the spirometer, the maximal breathing capacity (9), is also impaired in neuromuscular disease, but it may also be abnormal in obstructive lung disease.

Recently, a more sensitive technique has been described (3). With the use of a simple hand-held device, patients generate a maximal inspiratory and expiratory effort, and the resultant pressures are recorded (Fig. 2). No actual flow of air results, and consequently these so-called maximal static respiratory pressures are a direct measure of respiratory muscle strength. In one recent study, maximal static respiratory pressures were abnormal in patients with neuromuscular disease even when spirometric abnormalities were absent (4). Moreover, since abnormalities of these pressures are not seen in various forms of intrinsic lung disease, they are of value in specifically defining neuromuscular impairment. These pressure measurements are reasonably reproducible in the same subject, and therefore serve as suitable means of serial evaluation of a patient, or of assessing results of various therapeutic interventions. Note that all of these tests are relatively simple to perform and use uncomplicated, readily available equipment, yet they provide highly specific objective data of respiratory muscle impairment.

The efficacy of various forms of respiratory therapy in mildly symptomatic neuromuscular disease is not clearly established. Some groups advocate a vigorous program of intermittent positive pressure breathing in children with Duchenne muscular dystrophy (1). A modest increase in

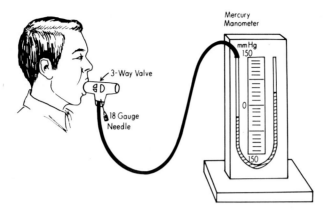

FIG. 2. Apparatus used to obtain maximal static inspiratory and expiratory pressures in assessment of neuromuscular disease.

lung volume over a 3-month period can be demonstrated (18), but it is not clear what effect these efforts have in altering overall prognosis.

Recognition of Impending Ventilatory Failure Secondary to Neuromuscular Disease

Although respiratory failure secondary to neuromuscular disease is less common today than during the poliomyelitis era, these problems continue to comprise from 5 to 10% of admissions to most respiratory intensive care units. In large measure, successful outcomes are related to accurate early assessment of impending respiratory failure, specifically early recognition of hypoxemia and hypercarbia.

The symptoms associated with hypoxia are entirely nonspecific. Confusion, restlessness, and a sensation of dyspnea are often all that are present even in life-threatening hypoxia. More severe hypoxia is often accompanied by a decreased sympathetic response, with bradycardia and hypotension. It should be emphasized that cyanosis is an extremely unreliable index of hypoxemia. Factors such as peripheral circulation, hemoglobin concentration, and degree of skin pigmentation all influence recognition of cyanosis. At best, it is an extremely late sign of hypoxemia, and serious end-organ damage can occur in its absence.

Similarly, impending CO_2 narcosis causes nonspecific symptoms, similar to those seen after administration of a general anesthetic. Headache, drowsiness, and eventual coma are seen. There is often evidence of peripheral vasodilatation and enhanced sympathetic discharge with hypertension and tachycardia.

Thus successful recognition of respiratory failure requires an appreciation of the nonspecificity of these signs and symptoms, and accordingly a high index of suspicion. For specific diagnosis, there is at present no substitute for arterial blood gas determinations.

MANAGEMENT OF ACUTE RESPIRATORY FAILURE

Successful outcome in these patients is related to two factors. First, the need for oxygen therapy, intubation, and mechanical ventilation must be assessed accurately. Second, careful attention to the specialized medical and nursing needs of these patients must be assured.

Since hypoxemia may be present without hypercarbia because of the physiologic mechanisms previously described, initial respiratory management can often be as simple as providing adequate supplemental oxygenation. Generally, arterial Po_2 levels should be kept at 60 mm Hg or higher, since at lower levels progressively increasing desaturation of hemoglobin occurs. This can very often be accomplished with use of simple face masks, and these measures should always be attempted before considering intubation in the treatment of uncomplicated hypoxemia. Although oxygen administration to patients with severe chronic obstructive pulmonary disease may be dangerous because of their dependency on hypoxic ventilatory drive, these considerations do not carry over to patients with neuromuscular disorders.

In contrast to hypoxemia, even slight elevations of arterial Pco_2 (normal less than 40 mm Hg) suggest severe ventilatory impairment and the potential need for intubation. Our usual indications for intubation are listed in Table 1.

Probably the most important clinical characteristic of neuromuscular respiratory failure is its often insidious onset. Medical and nursing personnel in respiratory intensive care settings are attuned to careful, sequential observation of arterial blood gases and ventilatory capacity in patients with intrinsic lung disease. Generally, respiratory failure is a progressive phenomenon in these patients. However, in neuromuscular disease, the natural history of respiratory failure may be quite explosive. It has been the experience in our hospital and elsewhere that such patients may be only slightly dyspneic, with no apparent need for specialized care, only to sustain a life-threatening respiratory arrest minutes later (13).

A full consideration of the care of the patient requiring ventilatory support has been reviewed elsewhere (16). Of special interest to the neurologist should be an appreciation of the rather excellent prognosis of these patients

TABLE 1. *Indications for intubation*

1. Protect airway
2. Mobilize secretions
3. Halt progressive hypoventilation
4. Prevent severe hypoxia

relative to other forms of respiratory failure. For instance, cumulative data over a 10-year span in the respiratory unit of the Massachusetts General Hospital (16) demonstrate an 80% survival rate in patients with neuro-muscular disease. In contrast, patients with respiratory failure secondary to emphysema demonstrated 50% survival, and those with neurosurgical-related illness, 60% survival. Similar data have been reported from Colorado (15). And although occasional reports appear of patients with neuromuscular disease requiring extraordinary time periods in intensive care units (19), recent prospective data show an average stay of only 13 days in an intensive care setting (13). The major management problems of these patients are as expected: nosocomial respiratory and urinary tract infection, decubiti ulcers, thrombophlebitis, pulmonary emboli, localized complications of tracheostomy, and generalized debilitation from malnutrition. Patients with neuromuscular disease in addition are prone to autonomic instability, especially manifest in wide swings in blood pressure and cardiac arrhythmias (13). Recent advances in our therapeutic approach hopefully will minimize these complications. These newer concepts include use of bedside fiberoptic bronchoscopy to assist clearance of secretions (17), low-dose heparin prophylaxis (8), and a more physiologic approach to parenteral hyper-alimentation (7).

In summary, assessment of respiratory failure in neuromuscular disease requires an understanding of the physiologic mechanisms involved. Im-portant pathophysiologic differences exist between this form of respiratory embarrassment and that resulting from intrinsic lung disease. Simple techniques, suitable for outpatient use, are readily available in most com-munities to provide early specific data. Although the therapy for acute respiratory failure may be associated with many potential complications, the overall prognosis of this form of respiratory failure is generally much better than that of respiratory failure owing to intrinsic lung disease.

REFERENCES

1. Adams, M. A., and Chandler, L. S. (1974): Effects of physical therapy program on vital capacity of patients with muscular dystrophy. *Phys. Ther.*, 54:494–496.
2. Agostini, E. (1964): Action of respiratory muscles. In: *Handbook of Physiology*, Section 3, edited by W. O. Fenn and H. Rahn. Waverly Press, Baltimore.
3. Black, L. F., and Hyatt, R. E. (1969): Maximal respiratory pressures: normal values and relationship to age and sex. *Am. Rev. Respir. Dis.*, 99:696–702.
4. Black, L. F., and Hyatt, R. E. (1971): Maximal static respiratory pressures in generalized neuromuscular disease. *Am. Rev. Respir. Dis.*, 103:641–650.
5. Comroe, J. H. (1965): *Physiology of Respiration.* Year Book Medical Publishers, Chicago.
6. Gillam, P. M. S., Heaf, P. J. D., Kaufman, L., and Lucas, B. G. B. (1964): Respiration in dystrophia myotonia. *Thorax*, 19:112–120.
7. Jeejeebhoy, K. N., Anderson, G. H., Nakhooda, A. F., Greenberg, G. R., Sanderson, I., and Marliss, E. B. (1976): Metabolic studies in total parenteral nutrition with lipid in man. *J. Clin. Invest.*, 57:125–136.
8. Kaakar, V. V. (1975): Efficacy of low dose heparin prophylaxis. *Curr. Ther. Res.*, 18:6–19.

9. Keltz, H. (1965): The effect of respiratory muscle dysfunction on pulmonary function: studies in patients with neuromuscular disease. *Am. Rev. Respir. Dis.,* 99:934.

10. Kilburn, K. H., Eagan, J. T., and Heyman, A. (1959): Cardiopulmonary insufficiency associated with myotonic dystrophy. *Am. J. Med.,* 26:269.

11. Mead, J., Turner, J. M., Macklem, P. T., and Little, J. B. (1967): Significance of the relationship between lung recoil and maximal expiratory flow. *J. Appl. Physiol.,* 23:646–662.

12. Miller, R. D., Mulder, D. W., Fowler, W. S., and Olsen, A. M. (1957): Exertional dyspnea: a primary complaint in unusual cases of progressive muscular atrophy and amyotrophic lateral sclerosis. *Ann. Intern. Med.,* 46: 119–125.

13. O'Donohue, W. J., Baker, J. P., Bell, G. M., Muren, O., Parker, C. L., and Patterson, J. L. (1976): Respiratory failure in neuromuscular disease. *J.A.M.A.,* 235:733–735.

14. Paul, J. R. (1971): *A History of Poliomyelitis.* Yale University Press, New Haven.

15. Petty, T. L., Laksminarayan, S., Sahn, S. A., Zwillich, C. W., and Nett, L. M. (1975): Intensive respiratory care unit—review of ten years' experience. *J.A.M.A.,* 233:34–37.

16. Pontoppidan, H., Geffin, B., and Lowenstein, E. (1972): *Acute Respiratory Failure in the Adult.* Little, Brown and Co., Boston.

17. Sackner, M. A., Wanner, A., and Landa, J. (1972): Applications of bronchoscopy. *Chest,* 62:70s–78s.

18. Siegel, I. M. (1975): Pulmonary problems in Duchenne muscular dystrophy. Diagnosis, prophylaxis, and treatment. *Phys. Ther.,* 55:160–162.

19. Whitehouse, A. C., and Petty, T. L. (1969): Recovery in Landry Guillain-Barre syndrome after prolonged respiratory support. *Lancet,* 1:1029–1030.

Advances in Neurology, Vol. 17, edited by
R. C. Griggs and R. T. Moxley, III. Raven Press,
New York © 1977.

Cardiac Manifestations of the Neuromuscular Disorders

Jules Cohen

Cardiology Unit, Department of Medicine, University of Rochester School of Medicine and Dentistry, 601 Elmwood Avenue, Rochester, New York 14642

INTRODUCTION

The interest of cardiologists in the neuromuscular disorders has several derivations. First, a broad understanding of disorders of muscle may provide clues to the pathogenesis of the unexplained cardiomyopathies. Little is known of the basic fault in the cardiomyopathies except when they are a part of some systemic disease process. Pathologic findings of cardiac hypertrophy and inflammatory or destructive myocardial lesions are not sufficiently specific to suggest possible etiologies. Even when there has been associated skeletal muscle disease, the availability of such tissue for study has not usually resulted in significant advances in our understanding. The unexplained primary heart muscle disorders, then, continue to represent a challenge to investigators, and some clues may yet come from the study of patients with specific neuromuscular diseases.

Second, cardiac dysfunction may be the presenting feature of certain of the neuromuscular disorders. In these situations, the characteristic shrewdness of the cardiologist is taxed to provide an explanation for symptoms and signs when their cause is uncertain. Furthermore, in several of the neuromuscular disorders, cardiac disability may dominate the natural history of the patients' illnesses.

Finally, as is the case with the cardiomyopathies generally, the treatment of cardiac dysfunction in the neuromuscular diseases can usually be no more than supportive, and such patients can be difficult and frustrating to manage.

Thus cardiologists respond to these challenges — of trying to understand the basic nature of the disorders, and of diagnosis and treatment — with continued interest. A host of publications dealing with cardiovascular manifestations of the neuromuscular disorders has appeared in the past 20 years, and the purpose of this chapter is not to recapitulate all of these published data. Rather, I will try to offer an approach to recognition and management of cardiac problems in the neuromuscular disorders based on altered physiology and on the manner in which such patients exhibit cardiac disability. Finally, several representative cases will be briefly presented.

SPECIFIC NEUROMUSCULAR DISORDERS ASSOCIATED WITH CARDIAC INVOLVEMENT

Friedreich's Ataxia

Although not afflicted with a disorder primary to *muscle,* patients with Friedreich's ataxia have been known, from the time of the earliest descriptions of the disease, to manifest disturbances in cardiac structure and function (5,12,15,17,31,33,39). In fact, it has been reported that over 90% of patients at some time in the course of their illness exhibit cardiac abnormalities. These include disorders of cardiac rhythm and abnormalities of ventricular function. Atrial and ventricular ectopic beats are common, as is paroxysmal supraventricular tachycardia. Ventricular hypertrophy and congestive failure both occur, and heart failure not uncommonly accounts for death. No correlation has been observed between the severity of the heart disease and the degree of neurologic disability. In fact, in some patients heart disease precedes manifest neurologic symptoms.

Of particular interest have been recent reports of hypertrophic obstructive cardiomyopathy (HOCM) complicating Friedreich's syndrome (2,4, 9,11,32,42,46). In patients with classic HOCM (14), massive hypertrophy, particularly of the ventricular septum, may be associated with pressure gradients across the outflow tracts of the ventricles reflecting intracavitary obstruction. In addition, disproportionately elevated ventricular filling pressures reflect reduced ventricular distensibility. Such hemodynamic findings have now been described in patients with Friedreich's syndrome, and in some cases the right ventricular and left ventricular angiograms recorded also demonstrate features suggestive of HOCM (47).

This possible association of Friedreich's syndrome and HOCM is fascinating since some features of this particular cardiomyopathy have long suggested that excessive sympathetic neural discharge might play a role in pathogenesis (34), and it has been reported that long-term administration of low-dose catecholamines can reproduce the disorder in experimental animals (3). If the neural abnormality characteristic of Friedreich's disease could in some way influence or be associated with excessive cardiac sympathetic drive, this fascinating association might have a reasonable pathophysiologic basis. But all of this is highly speculative, and there are important differences between the tissue pathology in HOCM and that found in the hearts of patients with Friedreich's, so that these disorders may well be wholly separate entities.

It has also been reported that the small intramural coronary arteries in Friedreich's syndrome exhibit intimal thickening and often occlusion (23). How this abnormality may relate to the cardiomyopathy is not at all clear. The arrhythmia and muscle dysfunction reported could be accounted for on an ischemic basis. HOCM is less easily explained, although this type of eccentric hypertrophy has occasionally been reported as a complication of ischemic heart disease. However, such lesions of the coronary arteries have not been uniformly found (18), so that their role in the cardiomyopathy of Friedreich's remains an open question.

The clinical history in Friedreich's syndrome may include awareness of ectopic beats or periodic rapid heart action, or a high-grade conduction disturbance may result in frank Stokes-Adams seizures. In patients with cardiac failure, the symptoms are those of pulmonary or systemic fluid retention. Angina pectoris is distinctly unusual. The physical examination reflects these functional disturbances and may reveal cardiac enlargement, biventricular hypertrophy, third or fourth heart sounds, or combinations thereof. Characteristically, a left sternal border systolic ejection murmur is present and may be of the sort heard in patients with hypertrophic cardiomyopathy, with or without obstruction to ventricular outflow. The precise character of these murmurs, however, has not been carefully studied — nor has their response to physiologic and pharmacologic interventions — so that it is not clear if they precisely mimic the murmurs present in patients with HOCM.

The EKG abnormalities are very nonspecific and include ST-T–wave changes, ectopic beats, conduction abnormalities ranging from bundle branch block to complete atrioventricular (AV) dissociation, and evidence of ventricular hypertrophy.

Nonspecific cardiac enlargement may be present on chest roentgenogram, accompanied by signs of pulmonary congestion.

Limited hemodynamic data are available. Reduced cardiac stroke output and raised filling pressure are found when ventricular dysfunction occurs. Outflow gradients have been found when obstructive disease has been present. As noted earlier, ventriculograms demonstrate evidence of hypertrophy, which may be of the eccentric type and suggestive of the radiographic appearances in HOCM.

Therapy is wholly symptomatic and includes stabilization of rhythm, including pacemaker implantation when indicated, and the usual measures for control of congestive cardiac failure.

The pathological features are nonspecific (20) and include myocardial fibrosis, cellular infiltration, and cardiac hypertrophy, sometimes with disproportionate septal enlargement.

MUSCULAR DYSTROPHIES

Cardiac involvement has been reported in all forms of the muscular dystrophies (Table 1), but it is more common in progressive muscular dystrophy of the Duchenne type (36,51,52) and in myotonic dystrophy (7,10,26). In both disorders cardiac failure and conduction disturbances contribute to disability, but in myotonic dystrophy AV block of varying degree is a particularly prominent feature (16,27,38).

TABLE 1. *Neuromyopathic disorders associated with cardiomyopathy*

Disorder	Pathogenesis of cardiomyopathy	Cardiac abnormality	Clinical features
Friedreich's disease	Unknown	Cardiac hypertrophy Muscle degeneration, fibrosis, and cellular infiltration Disproportionate septal hypertrophy	Cardiac rhythm disturbances Cardiac failure Hypertrophic obstructive features in some patients

The muscular dystrophies
1. Progressive muscular dystrophy
  a. Duchenne type
  b. Limb-girdle type
  c. Fascioscapulo-humeral type
 	
2. Other nonmyotonic dystrophies
  a. Late-onset distal myopathy
  b. Oculocranio-somatic dystrophy
3. Myotonic dystrophy
	Unknown	Cardiac dilatation and hypertrophy
		Interstitial myocardial fibrosis
		Cellular infiltration
			1a. Rhythm disturbances
			b. Congestive heart failure
			c. Cardiac involvement may be no more frequent than in general population
			
			2a. Rhythm disturbances or heart failure
			b. Conduction abnormalities may be present
			3. Conduction disturbances prominent in myotonic dystrophy

Alcoholic cardiomyopathy	Uncertain ? direct toxic effect of alcohol	Muscle fiber destruction Myocardial fibrosis Cellular infiltration	Cardiac enlargement/hypertrophy, heart failure Rhythm disturbances, especially supraventricular tachy-arrhythmias Pericardial effusion
Miscellaneous disorders			
1. Inflammatory myopathy	1a. Viral processes b. Immune disorder(s)	1. Cellular infiltration, muscle destruction, fibrosis	1. Tachyarrhythmia, conduction disturbances; congestive heart failure rare
2. Periodic paralyses (hypokalemic hyperkalemic)	2. K^+ imbalance presumed	2. –	2. Arrhythmia
3. Refsum's syndrome	3. Accumulation of phytanic acid	3. Nonspecific muscle damage and fibrosis	3. Arrhythmia, ventricular dysfunction
4. Mulibrey nanism	4. Unknown	4. Nonspecific muscle damage; pericardial fibrosis and calcification	4. Arrhythmia, pericardial constriction

Clinical heart disease in Erb's limb-girdle dystrophy and in fascioscapulo-humeral dystrophy (Landouzy-Dejerine) is much less common. In fact, Tyler and Stephens (49) believe that in the latter, clinical signs of heart disease are no more common than in the general population, although EKG changes may occur more often.

In myotonic dystrophy, clinical heart disease may precede muscle disease and confound diagnosis. Cardiovascular symptoms and signs when they do occur are entirely nonspecific, reflecting cardiac muscle dysfunction and cardiac rhythm disturbances. As in the case of Friedreich's syndrome, overt severe congestive heart failure may occur, and in such patients the presentation is that of congestive cardiomyopathy (14). Symptoms related to ectopic rhythm disturbances may be present, and preexcitation also has been described (1). High-grade AV block may develop and be associated with Stokes-Adams attacks and require artificial pacing. We do not know how to predict which patients with lower-grade AV block will advance to high-grade block, and who may therefore be at risk of sudden death. Studies of the conduction system in patients with myotonic dystrophy — using His bundle recording techniques — have been reported from this and other institutions (16,24) but have provided little information that allows a confident prediction of prognosis. Blocks both proximal and distal to the main His bundle have been described. What does seem important is that the use of procainamide for treatment of myotonia may aggravate AV block in those patients with preexisting conduction delay (16).

Although cardiac symptoms and signs are nonspecific in the muscular dystrophies, Duchenne's dystrophy is associated with distinctive electro-cardiographic changes (37). Loss of electrically active muscle and regional fibrosis in the posterobasal portion of the left ventricle produce abnormal Q waves in the inferior and lateral precordial leads and prominent anterior forces in the right precordial leads. The basis for this unique distribution of the cardiac disease is unknown.

Cardiomyopathy in patients with the muscular dystrophies, then, may be related to the presence of dystrophic muscle, to loss of fibers with scar formation, or to both. Disorders of rhythm are less readily explained. Abnormalities of small coronary arteries supplying pacemaker tissue and the conduction system have been reported in Duchenne's (21), but they have not always been found when rhythm disturbances have been present.

Hemodynamic and angiographic studies in these patients are few. In patients with Duchenne's dystrophy, a relatively localized wall motion abnormality, consistent with posterobasal scarring (*vide supra*) has been reported (50). Otherwise the findings are nonspecific and simply reflect generalized ventricular dysfunction.

Therapy for cardiac involvement in the muscular dystrophies is again symptomatic, but careful attention to the possible presence of conduction abnormalities is essential — especially in myotonic dystrophy — since the incidence of sudden cardiac death is not insignificant.

Alcoholic Cardiomyopathy

As is true for skeletal myopathy, cardiologists generally agree that over-indulgence in spirits may lead to so-called alcoholic cardiomyopathy. Exactly what constitutes overindulgence in respect to this disorder is unknown, nor has "clinical" alcoholic heart disease been reproduced experimentally. It has been puzzling, given the amount of alcohol consumed in the world, that the problem does not occur with very high frequency among heavy drinkers. For these reasons questions have been raised as to the specific role of alcohol in the pathogenesis of the disorder, but there is now considerable circumstantial evidence confirming that excessive alcohol intake can lead to cardiac enlargement, rhythm disturbances, and cardiac failure. Regan et al. (41), for example, have shown abnormalities in ventricular function in alcoholics without clinically evident heart disease. We (43) have reported that cardiac hypertrophy and cardiac muscle disease also can be found in alcoholics dying of other causes and in whom no heart disease was apparent during life. Although not entirely clear-cut, there is also evidence that structural or functional (40) myocardial abnormalities can be produced in experimental animals by long-term alcohol administration. Skeletal muscle abnormalities have been produced experimentally in man (45). Coupling all of this evidence with the extensive clinical experience of otherwise unexplained cardiomyopathy among heavy drinkers, it seems clear that there is an important relationship between alcohol and heart muscle damage and dysfunction.

Precisely how alcohol does its damage is not known. It is unlikely to be the result of the metabolism of alcohol by the heart since alcohol dehydrogenase activity is so low in heart muscle. Acetaldehyde has been incriminated as a possible culprit (22,44), and direct unknown toxic effects also have been suggested as playing a role in pathogenesis.

Clinically, alcoholic heart disease is most often characterized by unexplained cardiac enlargement with or without heart failure. The cardiomyopathy is usually of the congestive type, although we have seen several patients in whom restrictive features were important, or dominant (43), presumably because of extensive myocardial fibrosis. Pericardial effusion seems to occur out of proportion to other manifestations of heart failure (25), and in patients studied post-mortem, nonspecific unexplained pericardial inflammation has been found (43). We have been impressed by the high incidence of supraventricular rhythm disturbances, including atrial fibrillation, flutter, and paroxysmal atrial tachycardia, and otherwise unexplained sinus tachycardia. These tachyarrhythmias seem to occur more frequently among patients with alcoholic cardiomyopathy than in patients with other forms of primary heart muscle disease. It is tempting to suggest that the catecholamine-releasing properties of acetaldehyde (22) may be playing a role in the genesis of these rhythm disturbances, but occasionally we find that they persist as a problem long after (with documentation) the patient has stopped drinking.

Bundle branch block also has been seen, but higher grades of AV block have not been a problem in these patients, and in this respect they differ from patients with Duchenne's and myotonic dystrophy.

I have included alocholic cardiomyopathy in this chapter because alcohol can produce, independently, skeletal myopathy and because we have found a high incidence of nonspecific skeletal muscle disease in patients with alcoholic heart disease (R. C. Griggs and J. Cohen, *to be published*). In some there have been associated changes in muscle strength and in the EMG, but such cases have not been common. We still do not know if there is a specific and constant association of skeletal myopathy in patients with alcoholic cardiomyopathy, but we believe that skeletal muscle disease should be sought in all patients with cardiomyopathy and perhaps, particularly, in those with alcoholic heart disease.

MISCELLANEOUS DISORDERS ASSOCIATED WITH CARDIAC INVOLVEMENT

Inflammatory Myopathy

Nonspecific myositis accompanying a variety of viral illnesses can be accompanied by carditis. Screening studies have demonstrated nonspecific EKG changes in a large number of patients with a variety of viral syndromes. It has therefore been speculated that an occasional unexplained sudden death in an otherwise healthy person who has a viral illness may be the result of an arrhythmia related to myocarditis. Occasionally, too, viral myocarditis is complicated by severe and sometimes rapidly progressive cardiac dysfunction. But such cases are the exception, and usually carditis occurring as a part of a generalized viral illness is probably of little clinical importance and goes unnoticed.

Cardiac involvement also may occur in polymyositis, but few detailed studies of such patients are available. Conduction abnormalities (30) and otherwise unexplained supraventricular tachycardia have been described but have not been carefully studied. Anginal syndrome and overt cardiac failure have not been specifically associated with polymyositis. Most commonly, pathologic evidence of cardiac involvement can be found but without heart disease having been clinically apparent.

Periodic Paralysis

Both hypokalemic and hyperkalemic varieties of periodic paralysis have been described in which cardiac arrhythmias have been prominent. Ectopic beats and tachyarrhythmia, occasionally leading to syncope, have been described (28,29), but ventricular dysfunction does not seem to have been reported.

Refsum's Syndrome (Heredopathia Atactica Polyneuritiformis)

Another rare neuromuscular disorder in which cardiomyopathy has been reported is Refsum's syndrome (6). Inherited through autosomal recessive transmission, this syndrome includes the following signs: cerebellar ataxia, polyneuropathy, atypical retinitis pigmentosa, anosmia, altered pupillary reflexes, nerve deafness, skin and skeletal abnormalities, and cardiomyopathy.

The syndrome appears to be the result of accumulation of phytanic acid — a branched-chain fatty acid of dietary origin — in affected tissues, including both skeletal and cardiac muscle.

The cardiac disease is nonspecific. Some degree of cardiac involvement is common, and both ventricular dysfunction and rhythm disturbances have been reported (19).

Since manipulation of diet may provide some benefit (8), recognition of the disorder as a specific entity is important.

Mulibrey Nanism

Mulibrey nanism, a rare, inherited (probably autosomal recessive) disorder involving several systems and afflicting infants, children, and young adults, was reported originally in 1970 (35). Growth retardation, muscle hypotonia, distinctive pigmentary deposits in the optic fundi, enlarged cerebral ventricles, and hepatomegaly are reported to be characteristic. In addition, a high proportion of patients demonstrate cardiac disease. Pericardial constriction of clinically significant degree importantly influences the clinical course. Several patients have succumbed as a result; others have required pericardiectomy. In addition, cardiac rhythm disturbances have been noted including ectopic impulse formation, preexcitation, and degrees of AV block (48).

The cardiac abnormality — in addition to the pericardial fibrosis and calcification — is nonspecific: vacuolar degeneration of muscle fibers and myocardial fibrosis have been found.

Myasthenia Gravis

Although it has been suggested that there may be heart muscle involvement in myasthenics, the evidence for this is not convincing, except perhaps when myasthenia is associated with thymoma and polymyositis. Gibson (13) has carefully reviewed the data bearing on possible cardiac involvement in myasthenia and has reached a similar conclusion.

ILLUSTRATIVE CASES

Friedreich's Ataxia

A 25-year-old white man died of congestive cardiac failure 18 years after Friedreich's ataxia had been diagnosed originally and 8 years after cardiac symptoms had first appeared.

Development of ataxia at age 7 led to his initial evaluation and diagnosis. He became progressively more disabled and then was confined to a wheelchair at age 17, in 1965. Shortly thereafter he noticed effort dyspnea and palpitations and was admitted to a hospital for treatment of atrial fibrillation with rapid ventricular response. Cardiac enlargement was present at that time and he was digitalized.

His cardiac status was stable for the next several years but the neuromuscular disability progressed. On reevaluation in 1972 he was found to have evidence of mild cardiac failure and EKG signs of first-degree AV block and right ventricular hypertrophy (Fig. 1).

One year later, he came to the emergency department with overt biventric-

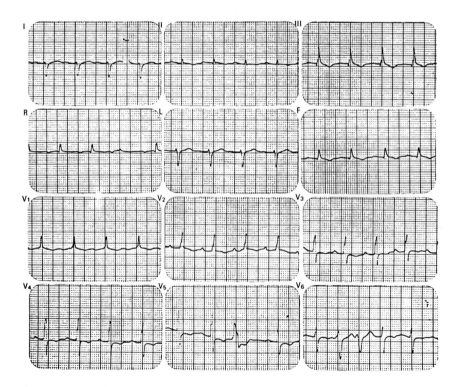

FIG. 1. Electrocardiogram of patient with Friedreich's syndrome showing right ventricular hypertrophy, supraventricular and ventricular premature beats, and nonspecific ST-T abnormalities.

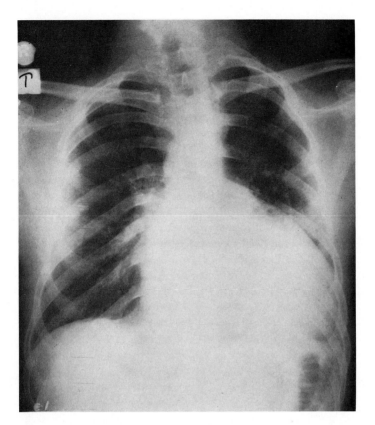

FIG. 2. Plain chest roentgenogram of patient with Friedreich's syndrome, showing generalized cardiac enlargement and evidence of congestive heart failure.

ular failure (Fig. 2). He was managed with digitalis, diuretics, and sodium restriction. Over the next 6 to 8 months congestive cardiac failure was a recurring problem, and its management was complicated by the patient's depression, which had developed in response to his progressive deterioration, and by his refusal to take medicines. In addition, bouts of paroxysmal supraventricular tachycardia began to occur and on several occasions were thought to be related to digitalis toxicity. More likely they were simply a manifestation of the underlying cardiomyopathy.

In mid-1973 an episode of hemiparesis occurred which was thought to be embolic; he recovered from this without residual deficit.

During the last months of the patient's life, his basic neurologic disability progressed so that it was difficult to tell how many of his symptoms were owing to the Friedreich's and attendant impaired chest function and how many were owing to heart disease. But in late 1973 cardiac failure clearly progressed. He had increasing shortness of breath and weakness, and unequivocal signs of biventricular failure on physical examination. He was admitted for the last time in November 1973, and on admission he was hypotensive, cyanotic, obtunded, and exhibited periodic breathing. He died 48 hr later.

At postmortem his heart weighed 570 g; all four chambers were dilated. There was an organizing mural thrombus in the left ventricle, and on microscopic study severe, diffuse, interstitial myocardial fibrosis was found (Fig. 3).

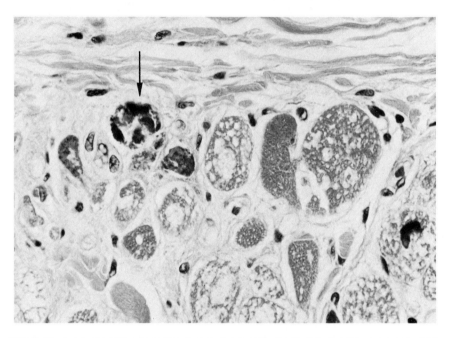

FIG. 3. Photomicrograph of cardiac muscle from patient with Friedreich's syndrome. Note extensive myocardial fibrosis, fiber damage, pleomorphism of fibers, and one almost wholly calcified fiber (*arrow*).

The tragic case of this young man illustrates the frustrations of trying to manage the relentless cardiac failure of primary heart muscle disease. It also illustrates the diagnostic confusion that can occur when intrinsic cardiac disease results in rhythm disturbances resembling those produced by digitalis or other drug intoxication, and when pulmonary disability owing to neuromyopathic disease resembles pulmonary dysfunction primarily of cardiac origin. Further, he suffered systemic embolization, a not uncommon complication of the mural thrombosis that often accompanies cardiomyopathy. Finally, this case clearly illustrates the frustration one encounters when even at postmortem study the pathologic findings are so nonspecific as to yield no helpful clue to the fundamental nature of the clinical disorder.

Myotonic Dystrophy

A 44-year-old black man was initially seen at age 38 in 1970 with a 4-year history of progressive myotonic weakness. Examination at that time revealed characteristic features of myotonic dystrophy, including muscle weakness, typical grip and percussion myotonia, characteristic facial features, high arched palate, nasal speech, temporal wasting, and testicular atrophy with impotence. No cardiac abnormality was found, and the EKG was normal. Diphenylhydantoin therapy was begun, but the drug provided little relief and was soon discontinued.

Because of persisting and progressive symptoms, a trial of quinine therapy was initiated. An EKG done after several months of treatment exhibited (for the first time) first-degree AV block but was otherwise normal. A chest X-ray at this time was within normal limits, but the heart looked bulky.

Muscular complaints continued, and because of the first-degree block quinine was stopped. The first-degree AV block disappeared. The patient was admitted for His bundle studies, and prolongation of both A-H and H-V conduction were found. A trial of first procainamide and then diphenylhydantoin produced some symptomatic relief, but a striking reduction in the PR interval from 0.24 to 0.18 sec was observed with the latter drug, so the patient was maintained on this therapy.

In late 1973, atrial flutter developed and digoxin was instituted. However, heart rates as low as 40/min occurred because of high-grade AV block (up to 7 to 9:1 conduction of the flutter), even with a very small dose of digoxin. Gentle carotid massage produced 3 sec of asystole, and because of the clear conduction disturbance and sensitivity to digitalis the drug was stopped.

The patient has subsequently remained in atrial flutter, with ventricular rates in the 80 to 100 range, without digitalis. There have never been any symptoms or signs of congestive cardiac failure, although his heart size is slightly increased.

This case illustrates the prominence of conduction abnormalities in patients with myotonic dystrophy and the real hazard of treatment with drugs that depress AV conduction.

Polymyositis

A 50-year-old white school nurse was originally seen at age 45. Several months of fatigue, muscle weakness, arthralgias, excessive sweating, mild effort dyspnea, and persistent tachycardia had followed a flu-like illness. Her history was otherwise completely unremarkable. On examination, she was overweight, with an office blood pressure of 180/108. Resting heart rate was 120/min. Her heart size was normal but both third and fourth heart sounds were audible. Her musculoskeletal examination was totally unremarkable and muscle strength was normal. First-degree AV block (PR

1970   **1974**   **1976**

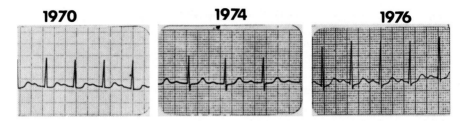

FIG. 4. Sequential EKG records (V$_5$ lead) from patient with polymyositis. Note that in 1976 first-degree AV block present in 1970 and 1974 is gone but resting tachycardia persists.

interval 0.22 sec) and ST-T abnormalities were present on her EKG (Fig. 4). Cardiothoracic ratio on her chest X-ray was 14/25 cm. The erythrocyte sedimentation rate was 40 mm/hr.

Because of persisting symptoms, she was admitted to the hospital for study. Although no musculoskeletal abnormalities were found on examination, the clinical picture, abnormal EKG, and an inconstantly elevated serum creatinine phosphokinase (CPK) level prompted skeletal muscle biopsy. The findings were those of polymyositis with variation in fiber size, central migration of nuclei, and foci of inflammatory cell infiltration (Fig. 5). A

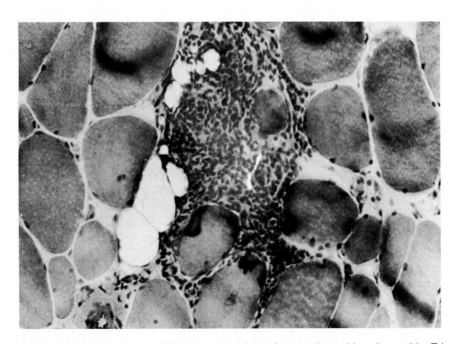

FIG. 5. Photomicrograph of skeletal muscle biopsy from patient with polymyositis. Trichrome stain. Variation in fiber size, centrally displaced nuclei, and a focus of inflammatory cell infiltration are demonstrated.

trial of prednisone improved her symptoms but resulted in depression and manifestations of Cushing's syndrome, so the drug had to be temporarily discontinued. Her symptoms of muscle weakness then recurred, typical nonspecific pericarditis with a three-component friction rub developed, an episode of atrial fibrillation occurred, and she was admitted to the hospital for reevaluation. Her muscle strength, on testing, was normal, but her EMG revealed changes compatible with a myopathic process. Antiskeletal, smooth, and cardiac muscle antibodies were absent from her serum (courtesy Dr. E. A. Schenk). A skin biopsy demonstrated minimal perivascular inflammatory reaction. Mild cardiomegaly was found on chest X-ray, and the PR interval was again slightly prolonged (0.21 sec).

Prednisone therapy was reinstituted, and her symptoms improved again.

Presently (March 1976) she is free of symptoms of overt cardiac failure, but she continues to have mild shortness of breath with effort. She has only mild muscle weakness and mild ease of fatigue. She is taking prednisone 40 mg every other day and daily diuretics. She has cushingoid features. Her blood pressure is significantly elevated (218/118), and her heart rate is still 115/min. There is no evidence of cardiac failure; a fourth heart sound is present but no S3. No pericardial rub can be heard. Her muscle strength is good. The EKG (Fig. 4) still shows tachycardia and ST-T abnormalities, but the PR interval is now normal and her serum CPK is within normal limits.

This patient illustrates the point that patients with neuromuscular disease may come initially to the cardiologist, often with a confusing clinical picture. Her case also is a happy example of the beneficial effects of steroids in the management of inflammatory myopathy. Symptoms, altered serum enzyme levels, and the abnormal EKG have all responded, if incompletely, to institution of prenisone therapy.

ACKNOWLEDGMENTS

Dr. Robert C. Griggs and Dr. Eric A. Schenk generously provided photomicrographs for inclusion in this chapter.

Mrs. Deborah Sheedy's excellent secretarial assistance in the preparation of the manuscript is gratefully acknowledged.

This work was supported in part by funds from the U.S.P.H.S., National Heart and Lung Institute, Postgraduate Training Grant No. HL05500.

REFERENCES

1. Agarwal, R. K., Misra, D. N., and Verma, R. K. (1973): Wolff-Parkinson-White syndrome with paroxysmal atrial fibrillation in pseudohypertrophic muscular dystrophy (Duchenne type). *Indian Heart J.*, 25:346–348.
2. Barrillon, A., Bensaid, J., Coirault, R., Scebat, L., Maurice, P., and Gerbaux, A. (1973): Myocardiopathie obstructive et maladie de Friedreich. *Arch. Mal. Coeur*, 66:1525–1535.

3. Blaufuss, A. H., Laks, M. M., Garner, D., Ishimoto, B. M., and Criley, J. M. (1975): Production of ventricular hypertrophy simulating "idiopathic hypertrophic subaortic stenosis" (IHSS) by subhypertensive infusion of norepinephrine (NE) in the conscious dog. *Clin. Res.,* 23:77A.

4. Boehm, T. M., Dickerson, R. B., and Glasser, S. P. (1970): Hypertrophic subaortic stenosis occurring in a patient with Friedreich's ataxia. *Am. J. Med. Sci.,* 260:279–284.

5. Boyer, S. H., IV, Chisholm, A. W., and McKusick, V. A. (1962): Cardiac aspects of Friedreich's ataxia. *Circulation,* 25:493–505.

6. Campbell, A. M. G., and Williams, E. R. (1967): Natural history of Refsum's syndrome in a Gloucestershire family. *Br. Med. J.,* 3:777–789.

7. Cannon, P. J. (1962): The heart and lungs in myotonic muscular dystrophy. *Am. J. Med.,* 32:765–775.

8. Eldjarn, L., Try, K., Stokke, O., Munthe-Kars, A. W., Refsum, S., Steinberg, D., Avigan, J., and Mize, C. (1966): Dietary effects on serum phytanic acid levels and on clinical manifestations in heredopathia atactica polyneuritiformis. *Lancet,* 1:691–693.

9. Elias, G., Fouron, J. C., and Davignon, A. (1972): Muscular subaortic stenosis and Friedreich's ataxia. *Union Med. Can.,* 101:474.

10. Fisch, C., and Evans, P. (1954): The heart in dystrophia myotonica. *N. Engl. J. Med.,* 251:527–529.

11. Gach, J. C., Andriange, M., and Franck, G. (1971): Hypertrophic obstructive cardiomyopathy and Friedreich's ataxia. Report of a case and review of literature. *Am. J. Cardiol.,* 27:436–441.

12. Gauthier, E. J. (1964): Cardiac disease in Friedreich's ataxia. *Ann. Intern. Med.,* 60:892–897.

13. Gibson, T. C. (1975): The heart in myasthenia gravis. *Am. Heart J.,* 90:389–396.

14. Goodwin, J. F. (1970): Congestive and hypertrophic cardiomyopathies. *Lancet,* 1:731–739.

15. Graham, G. R. (1964): Friedreich's disease. In: Cardiomyopathies. *A Ciba Foundation Symposium,* edited by G. E. W. Wolstenholme, and M. O'Connor, pp. 358–370. J and A Churchill Ltd., London.

16. Griggs, R. C., Davis, R. J., Anderson, D. C., and Dove, J. T. (1975): Cardiac conduction in myotonic dystrophy. *Am. J. Med.,* 59:37–42.

17. Heck, A. F. (1963): Heart disease in Friedreich's ataxia. *Neurology (Minneap.),* 13:587–600.

18. Hewver, R. (1969): The heart in Friedreich's ataxia. *Br. Heart J.,* 31:5–14.

19. Hudson, R. E. B. (1970): Refsum's syndrome. In: *Cardiovascular Pathology, Vol. 3,* edited by R. E. B. Hudson. Williams & Wilkins Co., Baltimore.

20. Ivemark, B., and Thoren, C. (1964): The pathology of the heart in Friedreich's ataxia. *Acta Med. Scand.,* 175:227–237.

21. James, T. N. (1962): Observations on the cardiovascular involvement, including the cardiac conduction system in progressive muscular dystrophy. *Am. Heart J.,* 63:48–56.

22. James, T. N., and Bear, E. S. (1967): Effects of ethanol and acetaldehyde on the heart. *Am. Heart J.,* 74:243–255.

23. James, T. N., and Fisch, C. (1963): Observations on the cardiovascular involvement in Friedreich's ataxia. *Am. Heart J.,* 66:164–170.

24. Josephson, M. E., Caracta, A. R., Gallagher, J. J., and Damato, A. N. (1973): Site of conduction disturbances in a family with myotonic dystrophy. *Am. J. Cardiol.,* 32:114–118.

25. Kerr, A., Jr. (1967): Myocardopathy, alcohol and pericardial effusion. *Arch. Intern. Med.,* 119:617–619.

26. Kilburn, K. H., Eyan, J. T., and Heyman, A. (1959): Cardiopulmonary insufficiency associated with myotonic dystrophy. *Am. J. Med.,* 26:929–935.

27. Kennel, A. J., Titus, J. L., and Meredith, J. (1974): Pathologic findings in the atrioventricular conduction system in myotonic dystrophy. *Mayo Clin. Proc.,* 49:838–842.

28. Levitt, L. P., Rose, L. I., and Dawson, D. M. (1972): Hypokalemic periodic paralysis with arrhythmia. *N. Engl. J. Med.,* 286:253–254.

29. Lisak, R. P., Lebeau, J., Tucker, S., and Rowland, L. P. (1972): Hyperkalemic periodic paralysis and cardiac arrhythmia. *Neurology (Minneap.),* 22:810–817.

30. Lynch, P. G. (1971): Cardiac involvement in chronic polymyositis. *Br. Heart J.,* 33:416–419.

31. Manning, G. W. (1950): Cardiac manifestations in Friedreich's ataxia. *Am. Heart J.,* 39: 799–816.
32. Moore, A. A. D., and Lambert, E. C. (1968): Cardiomyopathy associated with muscular and neuromuscular disease. In: *Pediatric Cardiology,* edited by H. Watson. C. V. Mosby, St. Louis.
33. Nadas, A. S., Alimurung, M. M., and Sieracki, L. A. (1951): Cardiac manifestations of Friedreich's ataxia. *N. Engl. J. Med.,* 244:239–244.
34. Oakley, C. M. (1974): Clinical recognition of the cardiomyopathies. *Circ. Res.,* 35 (Suppl. 2):152–167.
35. Perheentupa, J., Autio, S., Leisti, S., et al. (1973): Mulibrey nanism, an autosomal recessive syndrome with pericardial constriction. *Lancet,* 2:351–355.
36. Perloff, J. K., DeLeon, A. C., and O'Doherty, D. (1966): The cardiomyopathy of progressive muscular dystrophy. *Circulation,* 33:625–648.
37. Perloff, J. K., Roberts, W. C., DeLeon, A. C., and O'Doherty, D. (1967): The distinctive electrocardiogram of Duchenne's progressive muscular dystrophy. *Am. J. Med.,* 42:179–188.
38. Petkovich, N. J., Dunn, M., and Reed, W. (1964): Myotonia dystrophica with A-V dissociation and Stokes-Adams attacks. A case report and review of the literature. *Am. Heart J.,* 68:391–396.
39. Pitt, G. N. (1886): On a case of Friedreich's disease. Its clinical history and postmortem appearances. *Guys Hosp. Rep.,* 44:369–394.
40. Regan, T. J., Khan, M. I., Ettinger, P. O., Haider, B., Lyons, M. M., and Oldewurtel, H. A. (1974): Myocardial function and lipid metabolism in the chronic alcoholic animal. *J. Clin. Invest.,* 54:740–752.
41. Regan, T. J., Levinson, G. E., Oldewurtel, H. A., Frank, M. J., Weisse, A. B., and Moschos, C. B. (1969): Ventricular function in noncardiacs with alcoholic fatty liver: role of ethanol in the production of cardiomyopathy. *J. Clin. Invest.,* 48:397–407.
42. Ruschhaupt, D. G., Thilenius, O. G., and Cassels, D. E. (1972): Friedreich's ataxia associated with idiopathic hypertrophic subaortic stenosis. *Am. Heart J.,* 84:95–102.
43. Schenk, E. A., and Cohen, J. (1970): The heart in chronic alcoholism. *Pathol. Microbiol.,* 35:96–104.
44. Schreiber, S. S., Briden, K., Oratz, M., and Rothschild, M. A. (1972): Ethanol, acetaldehyde and myocardial protein synthesis. *J. Clin. Invest.,* 51:2820–2826.
45. Song, S. K., and Rubin, E. (1972): Ethanol produces muscle damage in normal volunteers. *Science,* 175:327–328.
46. Soulié, P., Vernant, P., and Gaudeau, S. (1966): Le coeur dans la maladie Friedreich: ètude hémodynamique droite et gauche. *G. Ital Cardiol.,* 7:369–386.
47. Thoren, C. (1964): Cardiomyopathy in Friedreich's ataxia. *Acta Paediatr. Scand. [Suppl. 153],* 53.
48. Tuuteri, L., Perheentupa, J., and Rapola, J. (1974): The cardiopathy of Mulibrey nanism, a new inherited syndrome. *Chest,* 65:628–631.
49. Tyler, F. H., and Stephens, F. E. (1950): Studies in disorders of muscle II. Clinical manifestations and inheritance of fascioscapulohumeral dystrophy in a large family. *Ann. Intern. Med.,* 32:640–660.
50. Ueda, K., Okada, R., Matsuo, H., Harumi, K., Yasuda, H., Tsuyuki, H., and Ueda, H. (1970): Myocardial involvement in benign Duchenne type of progressive muscular dystrophy. *Jpn. Heart J.,* 11:26–35.
51. Weisenfeld, C., and Messinger, W. J. (1952): Cardiac involvement in progressive muscular dystrophy. *Am. Heart J.,* 43:170–187.
52. Welsh, J. D., Lynn, T. N., and Haase, G. R. (1963): Cardiac findings in 73 patients with muscular dystrophy. *Arch. Intern. Med.,* 112:199–206.

Advances in Neurology, Vol. 17, edited by
R. C. Griggs and R. T. Moxley, III. Raven Press,
New York © 1977.

Orthopedic Correction of Musculoskeletal Deformity in Muscular Dystrophy

Irwin M. Siegel

*Department of Orthopaedic Surgery and Muscle Disease Clinic, Strauss Surgical
Group Associates, L.A. Weiss Memorial Hospital; and Department of
Orthopaedic Surgery, Abraham Lincoln School of Medicine, and Muscle
Disease Clinic, University of Illinois, Chicago, Illinois 60612*

INTRODUCTION

To paraphrase Steindler, surgery is but one moment in the total treatment of the child with muscular dystrophy. However, in few conditions is the timing of the moment as important a consideration as in the elective surgery of this disease.

As concerns ambulation, lower extremity contractures increase until the unstable base of support secondary to equinovarus and the pelvic imbalance produced by hip flexion contracture prohibit walking (Fig. 1). Surgery cannot be delayed beyond this point because, with rare exception, once a patient becomes wheelchair-bound, he will not walk again.

For this reason it is essential to recognize the signs of early difficulty in walking and to correct deformities impeding balance so that ambulation can be prolonged. At the same time, surgical procedures designed to do this must not require prolonged bedrest or entail excessive pain, as such measures would defeat themselves by restraining the patient in bed.

The muscles developing ambulation-limiting contractures in the lower extremities are (Fig. 2): (1) hip flexors, (2) tensor fasciae latae, and (3) triceps surae.

As quadriceps weakness progresses and contracture increases in these muscle groups, the base of support decreases and, in trying to balance, the child walks with a wide gait, characterized by equinus, heel varus, knee flexion, and hip flexion and abduction (8) (Fig. 3).

Increased lumbar lordosis is noted early as an attempt to compensate for pelvic imbalance secondary to weakened hip extension accompanied by hip flexion contracture. Abdominal and low back extensor weakness contribute to the grotesque and effortful gait, and loss of strength in the shoulder depressors makes torso balance awkward (11). Parascapular weakening draws the shoulders forward, increasing the need for lumbar lordosis to achieve torso balance (Fig. 4).

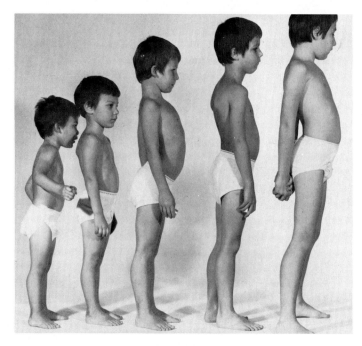

FIG. 1. Five brothers, all with Duchenne muscular dystrophy. Note increase in lordosis, hip abduction, and equinus as the disease progresses.

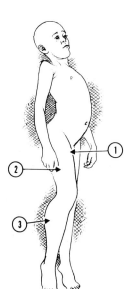

FIG. 2. Muscle groups that develop ambulation-limiting contractures. 1, Hip flexors; 2, tensor fasciae; 3, triceps surae.

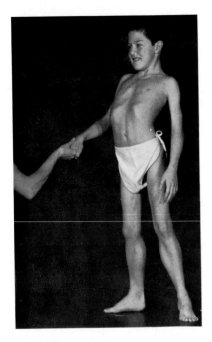

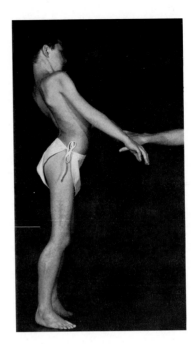

FIG. 3.   **FIG. 4.**

The aims of leg surgery are (a) to release lower-extremity contractures sufficiently to bring the body into adequate standing and walking equilibrium, and (b) to strengthen the lower limbs so that lightweight braces can be applied for support.

Generally speaking, bracing and the surgery necessary to place the lower limbs in braces are advised when, because of a combination of both weakness and contracture, balance becomes precarious and the patient begins to find walking increasingly difficult. This is usually heralded by more frequent loss of balance and falling. As a rule of thumb, functional abilities to rise from the floor, climb stairs, and walk are lost at approximate intervals of 1 year in the order stated (18).

Muscle strength assessment by functional testing and serial measurement of joint contracture aids in determining when surgery is necessary. With few exceptions, with equinovarus deformity present and a combined knee and hip antigravity extension lag greater than 90°, the line of gravity can no longer be maintained. Walking ends at this point (14) (Fig. 5). In this regard, the patient can tolerate knee extension lag better than extension lag of the hip because with fixed-ankle equinus the knee can be locked into stable extension, whereas the hip cannot. The combined extension lag measurement is, of course, without significance unless enough equinovarus to decrease lower extremity stability is present.

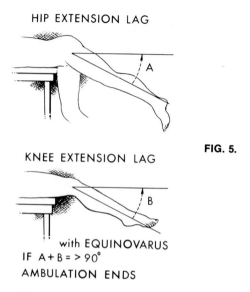

HIP EXTENSION LAG

KNEE EXTENSION LAG

FIG. 5.

with EQUINOVARUS
IF A + B = > 90°
AMBULATION ENDS

SURGICAL TECHNIQUE—LOWER EXTREMITY
CONTRACTURE RELEASE

Subcutaneous release of tendon contractures permits early mobilization, thus obviating the danger of prolonged inactivity. To preclude the need for a long scrub under anesthesia in a patient whose respiratory exchange is usually compromised, 24-hr skin preparation is desirable. A fracture table facilitates postoperative cast application, a double-holed lap sheet completes draping, and an adequate array of tenotomes decreases the possibility of infection, assuring that no knife need be used more than once in any wound.

The danger of damage to important neurovascular structures such as the femoral artery in the groin or the common peroneal nerve at the knee can be avoided by marking these sites with methylene blue.

Suxamethonium anesthesia should not be used (2). Some muscular dystrophics are also sensitive to halothane, an anesthetic that has caused cardiac toxicity and malignant hyperthermia (3), which may be related to low potassium storage. Additionally, myotonics have an increased sensitivity to thiopentone. These agents should be administered with caution, if at all, to patients with muscle disease undergoing surgery, however brief. Barbiturates depress respiration, and even standard doses of succinylcholine have deleterious effects. The anesthesiologist should carefully attend cardiac monitoring, provide adequate ventilation, and avoid potassium overload and gastric dilatation.

Subcutaneous tenotomy of hip flexors (including sartorius and straight head of rectus femoris) is accomplished by introducing the tenotome at the anterio-superior iliac spine and sweeping it distally and posteriorly. The knife is kept close to bone, and, if this is done while fully flexing the contralateral hip, flexion contracture can usually be decreased by at least 50%. Remaining contracture exists in the deeper hip flexors (e.g., iliopsoas) as well as in the anterior hip capsule.

Through the same stab wound, the tenotome severs the origin of the tensor fasciae latae at the lateral aspect of the anterior portion of the iliac crest. Bipolar tenotomy of the tensor is completed by subcutaneous release of the iliotibial band just proximal to the lateral aspect of the knee joint. Prognosis for correction is better if this structure is taut and narrow rather than thick and ill defined. Section of the lateral intermuscular septum is assured by completing this incision to the bone. Separation of approximately 1 inch in the palpable ends of the transsected iliotibial band, accompanied by correction of tensor fasciae contracture, is thus accomplished. Finally, percutaneous tenotomy of the heel cord is performed at its insertion into the calcaneus. It is important to tenotomize the Achilles tendon without a tourniquet as a hematoma forms quickly in this area and skin does not fall into the space created by separation of the cut ends of the tendon. Dressings or a cast applied with a tourniquet in use encourages such prolapse and can prevent the localization of the hematoma necessary for healing. The entire percutaneous procedure takes less than 5 min (Fig. 6).

If heel cord tenotomies are included in the surgery, toe-to-groin plaster casts are applied with the ankles at neutral and the knees in 5° of flexion. To assure plantigrade position in the casts, the plantar surfaces are flattened on a board during application. In those patients in whom heel cord lengthening is not performed (because it is unnecessary or was done previously), braces are fitted postoperatively.

When casts are applied they are worn for 3 weeks, and lower extremity braces are then fitted. These braces feature double uprights, drop-ring locks, spring-loaded ankles with an adjustable stop, sheepskin heel inserts, slight knee flexion, and a contoured proximal leather band that provides further support through ischial seating (Fig. 7). This band must lie just below the ischial tuberosity. If it is too high the patient will tilt forward out of

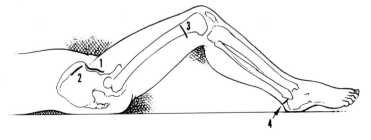

FIG. 6. Sites for percutaneous tenotomy. 1, Hip flexors; 2 and 3, bipolar tensor fasciae latae; 4, tendo achillis.

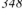

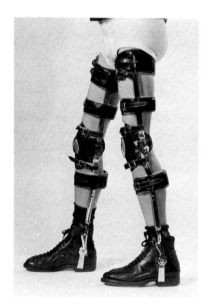

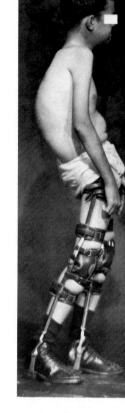

FIG. 7.   **FIG. 8.**

balance; if too low, a severe kyphosis may develop (Fig. 8). The weight of these braces is approximately 7 pounds (17).

With proper attention, brace-ambulating children seldom fall. More fractures occur from falling from a wheelchair or bed than from falls in braces. As braces require lengthening, care must be taken to bring the proximal band no higher than 2 cm below the ischial tuberosity or the braces will not permit necessary ischial seating and the patient will be unable to walk.

Preoperative knee contractures of more than 20° are corrected in serial casts to 5° or less (15). Surgical correction of knee contractures has not been found necessary, although release of the tensor fasciae incidentally corrects some knee contracture as this structure plays a role in knee flexion.

Heel cord lengthening as an isolated procedure will be unsuccessful if

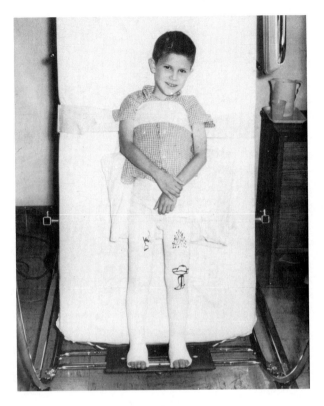

FIG. 9.

the quadriceps is weak unless long-leg bracing accompanies surgery. However, heel cord lengthening can permit better balance in patients already walking with long-leg braces. On the other hand, section of the iliotibial band can delay bracing and improve walking balance both before and after bracing (9).

Postoperative care includes the brief use of nasal oxygen and intermittent positive-pressure breathing. A Circolectric bed is used, and, on the afternoon of surgery, the patient stands in bed with his feet resting on the footboard attachment (Fig. 9). When in bed, he is positioned to stretch the hips into extension and adduction by binding the legs together at the knees and elevating the sacrum when on his back and the knees when on his abdomen (Fig. 10).

Because subcutaneous tenotomy minimizes pain and the possibility of wound dehiscence, physical therapy can be started on the afternoon of surgery. Treatment consists of standing and passive hip exercise. On the first postoperative day, the patient is walked. If in casts, the heels are fish-mouthed to avoid pressure, the bottoms pounded soft, and adhesive

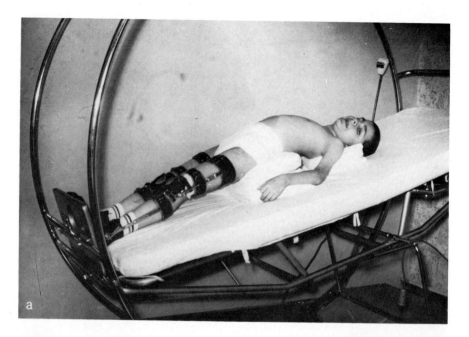

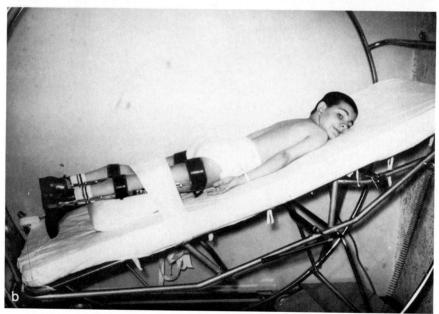

FIG. 10. Postoperative positioning on Circolectric bed. **a:** Supine. **b:** Prone.

tape is applied for friction. This is more stable than rubber walkers, and, providing firmer floor contact, it reinforces the kinesthetic supporting response.

Initially, a light aluminum walker may be necessary until the patient adjusts to his rediscovered balance. Although he finds that during walking it is still necessary to shift his torso over the supporting limb, the exaggerated postures of head and shoulder extension and the severe lumbar lordosis, which were preoperative necessities for body alignment, are no longer required. Lumbar lordosis disappears when these children sit and they walk sitting on their braces with a penguin (Alderman's) type gait (6).

Almost all day is spent in the therapy department, and during most of that time the child is standing or walking. This is continued for the better part of a week, when he is discharged to a program of home physical therapy including passive hip stretching and walking. Casts are discarded 3 weeks after surgery, and for the next 3 months, except for removal for skin care, braces are worn day and night. It is most urgent that mobility skills once regained not be lost again soon.

Although tennis shoes are best for patients out of braces because they are light and their rubber soles provide traction, high-laced surgical boots are the footwear of choice for the braced patient. However, a lightweight plastic brace is now available (13). Because it incorporates a moulded foot plate, special shoes are unnecessary for its use. Such a brace is ischial weight bearing and is molded from 5-mm stress-relieved semiopaque polypropylene. Any type of standard knee joint can be incorporated in the appliance. The final weight of the average brace is 0.68 kg (less than one-third the weight of the standard double-upright steel and leather appliance, and less than one-half that of its aluminum counterpart), but these orthoses maintain a high strength/weight ratio.

Ankle mobility in the orthosis is regulated by varying the width of the posterior strut connecting the calf piece to the foot plate. The plastic is molded with the ankle in dorsiflexion, and the strut is then trimmed until slight plantar flexion and rotation are possible.

Because the upright supporting members of the appliance are form fitted from plastic, it is less bulky than a standard brace, more comfortable and quite cosmetically acceptable. Either buckle or Velcro fittings can be used for closure, and the entire leg piece can be hidden underneath a long stocking.

Finally, all materials (including the knee pad, which can be fabricated from plastizoate and Velcro, and fittings, which can be made of aluminum) are nontoxic, radiolucent, unaffected by oils or ultraviolet light, and completely waterproof. Thus, the appliance can be washed and dried with ease, a feature contrasting severely with the difficulty of cleaning the leather used in the ordinary brace.

Because it is difficult to switch a patient from the standard double-upright brace to its plastic counterpart, it is suggested that if the plastic orthosis is to be used at all, it should be the initial brace provided.

Even after wheelchair confinement, the stability afforded by braces is appreciated by most patients as the cosmetically acceptable alignment of the lower extremities is maintained.

Because the posterior tibial muscles remain strong despite progression of weakness in other musculature, they have been transferred by Spencer (16) through the interosseous membrane and inserted through a drill hole in the third cuneiform by means of O-chromic suture tied over a bolster on the bottom of the foot. This procedure has strengthened dorsiflexion and eversion of the foot by eliminating the force of the posterior tibial, which may cause a recurrence of equinovarus deformity. The occasional case of isolated forefoot equinus can be treated with midtarsal capsulectomy and percutaneous plantar fasciotomy.

Even in patients confined to bed, the tibialis posticus and toe flexors have been graded as fair plus. This transfer, however, does not work in phase but rather on command because the tibialis posticus is a stance-phase muscle and when transferred to the dorsum it becomes a swing-phase muscle. However, relocation of its insertion removes an overactive tendency to inversion, providing an active eversion tenodesis effect (4).

Muscle tissue comprises 40% of total body weight, and over 50% of this muscle mass is lost by the end of independent ambulation, by which time patients are sometimes too weak to stand alone. Nevertheless, they are often able to walk again after correction of contractures and bracing because other factors are also influential in preventing ambulation. Joint contracture owing to disproportionate agonist-antagonist strength, and diffuse atrophy because of decreasing physical activity, obesity, emotional problems, and wheelchair immobilization imposed for the convenience of others all play a role in limiting walking potential.

Complications of lower extremity surgery may include heel decubitis ulcer, anterolateral thigh numbness (secondary to transsection of anterior branch of the lateral femoral cutaneous nerve), or any of the usual postoperative problems occurring even after short anesthesia and relatively bloodless surgery in a patient with poor respiratory toilet and generalized weakness. Fortunately, the incidence and degree of these complications have been minimal.

The usual time for surgery and bracing is between 9 and 12 years of age.[1] The patient so treated can handle his toilet needs with minimal help, and chair transfer is facilitated by locking his braces at the knees and using the legs as a long lever to tilt the patient to the standing position. The

---

[1] Almost 50% of patients stop walking by age 9. Comparison of affected brothers shows that the age at which walking ceased differed by no more than 1 year in most cases and by no more than 3 years in any instance.

average interval of extended ambulation beyond surgery is from 3 to 5 years (7). This additional period of ambulation may represent up to 20% of the life span of these children and is thus a highly significant benefit to them as maintenance of the upright posture has extended their ability to attend to all the tasks of daily living for a significant portion of their lives.

FOOT DEFORMITY

Equinocavovarus deformity (Fig. 11) was noted by Duchenne in his original description of pseudohypertrophic muscular dystrophy. As the disease progresses and weakness and contracture increase, this deformity jeopardizes alignment stability in the lower extremities and is by far the most serious foot deformity in the muscular dystrophies. Foot drop secondary to tibialis anticus weakness in facioscapulohumeral dystrophy and the steppage gait owing to weak dorsiflexion in dystrophia myotonica can both be managed with light wire-spring drop foot bracing or a floor reaction orthosis. If these appliances do not help, a standard double-upright ankle brace with a Klenzak spring dorsiflexion assist will usually correct the deformity. Such an appliance may even be necessary in the later stages of limb-girdle dystrophy. However, in classic Duchenne disease a rapidly progressive weakening of foot musculature with contracture occurs, and although this may respond temporarily to conservative measures such as passive stretch, surgical correction is ultimately necessary (10).

Overenthusiastic stretching of foot contracture should be avoided. This causes pain which prompts the patient to fight the passive force by an active effort of his own. The stretch reflex is also stimulated and this action results in strengthening of the deforming muscle or muscles. Heel cord contracture is usually more severe on one side because of the position of haunch habitually taken. Thus one foot is held in advance of the other, the partially flexed extremity developing the more severe heel cord contracture.

Equinocavovarus advances because of a selective weakening of foot musculature. The tibialis anticus is weakened early but the gastrocnemius is not. Contracture of the heel cord with its eccentric medial calcaneal insertion, augmented by unopposed tibialis posterior and toe flexor tension, forces the foot into this deformity. Rotation at the talocalcaneal joint, whose surfaces lie in an oblique anterolateral position, encourages forefoot supination (1). Once the foot is inverted beyond the tibiotalar sagittal midline, almost all dorsal and volar musculature, intrinsic and extrinsic, works to invert it further (Fig. 12).

Progressive equinocavovarus makes standing and walking uncomfortable and difficult. Pressure decubiti can develop, and the deformity eventually prevents maintenance of upright posture. Equinocavovarus is particularly disabling when combined with flexion-abduction hip contracture. In spite of correction of the hip deformity, equinocavovarus can continue.

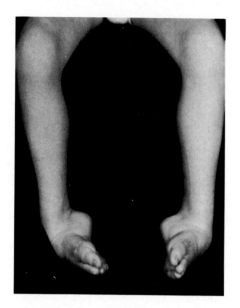

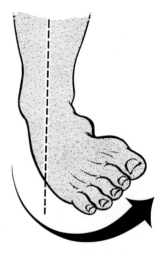

FIG. 11.   **FIG. 12.**

Attempts to forestall this condition using lateral sole and heel wedging, outer T-straps, and corrective shoe inserts [such as the University of California, Berkeley (UCB) heel-control orthoses (Fig. 13)] may temporarily be successful, but surgical correction eventually is necessary.

Bony deformity precludes the use of soft tissue release alone. Although realignment of the foot can usually be obtained through the standard techniques of triple arthrodesis or midtarsal wedge resection, these patients suffer rapid loss of strength when inactive. Operations such as these are

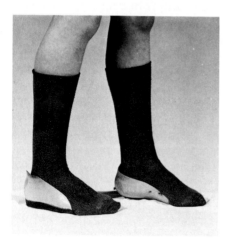

FIG. 13.

contraindicated because they require prolonged postoperative immobilization to assure bone fusion and soft tissue healing without dehiscence of multisutured surgical wounds.

However, early in the sequence of this deformity, when equinus alone is the major deforming factor and very little cavus or varus is present, isolated heel cord tenotomy can be performed. But heel cord lengthening or tenotomy removes the stabilizing force that hyperextends and locks the knee during stance so that nonbraced ambulation is usually impossible unless the quadriceps is better than fair strength.

Later, when all elements of the deformity are present, a more extensive surgical attack is necessary. Percutaneous tarsal medullostomy, combined with soft tissue release and posterior tibial tenotomy, can correct equinocavovarus, enabling the patient to stand the night of surgery and walk the next day.

SURGICAL CORRECTION OF EQUINOCAVOVARUS DEFORMITY

A 24-hr surgical skin preparation is used. Under tourniquet control a stab wound is placed over the dorsal aspect of the midtarsal area centering on the talar head. A large curette is introduced into the talar head, which is then echolated of cancellous bone. The distal calcaneus is similarly treated, when necessary, through either the same or a separate stab wound.

Percutaneous plantar fasciotomy is performed to correct cavus. The tendon of the tibialis posticus is identified distal to the medial malleolus and tenotomized percutaneously. Deformity is corrected by manipulation of the foot with collapse of the curetted bones. If single-stitch wound closure is necessary, 3–0 plain catgut is used. A well-padded long leg plaster is applied. The cast is split, its heel portion fish-mouthed, and the sole pounded soft.

The patient is encouraged to stand the evening of surgery and ambulate the next day. A walker may be necessary for a brief period until balance is rediscovered. Casts are worn for 3 weeks, followed by a return to long leg braces.

For wheelchair-confined patients who no longer stand or ambulate, advanced equinocavovarus is treated by the simple expedient of midtarsal and dorsolateral closing wedge osteotomy.

Infrequently, forefoot adductus is found as a residual or recurrent deformity (Fig. 14a). Percutaneous metatarsal osteotomy, using a thin osteotome introduced through three dorsal stab wounds, can correct this deformity permitting early postoperative ambulation in a corrective cast (Fig. 14b). In cases with residual weakness from polymyositis, the tibialis anticus is sometimes active and can be transferred to the dorsolateral aspect of the foot, thus removing a deforming inversion force and creating an active dorsiflexor in neutral or eversion.

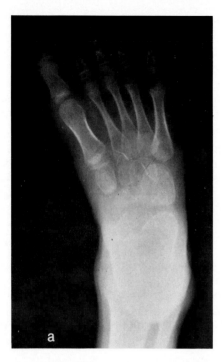 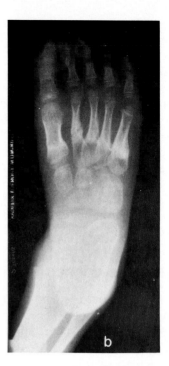

FIG. 14. Attempt to control equinocavovarus deformity with the UCB orthoses.

Correction of lower extremity instability is mandatory because even minor degrees of contracture in weight-bearing joints can interfere with balance and reduce the ability to ambulate. Relatively simple surgical procedures are available, and a judicious choice among these, followed by almost immediate postoperative ambulation, can prolong walking. As the patient's ability to stand and walk diminishes, the physician must determine whether this is the result of contracture or weakness. Experience has shown that, when indicated, the earlier surgery is done the better the result. All surgery should be bilateral, if possible, so that symmetric posture can be maintained. The subcutaneous procedures here described enable patients to maintain and significantly extend the ability to ambulate independently, thus delaying wheelchair or bed confinement.

SCOLIOSIS

Scoliosis in muscular dystrophy appears to occur with increasing age and advancing disability. Its presence depends on the type of dystrophy present; its progress is related to the severity of the primary disease. Childhood dystrophia myotonica is not complicated by spinal curvature because axial, shoulder, and pelvic musculature is weakened only late in this condition.

The onset of limb-girdle dystrophy is usually in middle or late adolescence. Weakness is most often symmetric and progression slow. Patients are ambulatory into the second or third decade, deformities occur late, and scoliosis is an uncommon finding. When it does occur, spinal growth has most often terminated and the deformity is functional rather than structural.

In Duchenne dystrophy, there is also symmetric muscular involvement and weakness, but the patient is usually younger and the vertebrae are still growing. Thus structural curvature is initiated by mechanical disequilibrium (increased gravitational stress secondary to spinal-pelvic malalignment) and appears unrelated to paralysis or asymmetry of axial muscle strength. When lower extremity contracture is relieved by tenotomy and long leg bracing, pelvic or infrapelvic tilt is obviated as a factor in the production of scoliosis. Properly braced patients walk with a stiff-legged gait, modulating the center of mass over the standing hip joint with each successive step. Because torso shift is necessary for balance, the use of rigid body support would inhibit ambulation and is contraindicated. The oscillation of body weight necessitates alternating lateral spinal bending, providing excellent symmetric spinal exercise during ambulation, thus inhibiting the production of static spinal curvature. In those patients with untreated hip, knee, and ankle contractures, several factors contribute to early spinal deformity. Most of these children stand in a hunched position, with one foot advanced for balance. This tilts the pelvis, producing a compensatory scoliotic deformity (12).

Asymmetric arm position can also cause secondary spinal deviation. Body alignment requires use of the upper extremities as stabilizing appendages (much as a tightrope walker uses a long pole for balance). Because weak deltoid muscles cannot maintain shoulder abduction, the patient hooks his thumbs over his brace tops, belt, or trouser pockets, supporting his upper extremities in shoulder extension and internal rotation, elbow flexion, and forearm pronation (Fig. 15). This posture is compensatory, necessary for balance, and should not be corrected. However, when continued, the arms tend to contract in this position, and any irregularity of upper extremity placement unbalances the torso and bends the spine. When these patients can no longer independently turn in bed, they tend also to develop a dorsal spinal curvature, convex to the side on which they lie.

Almost all patients with Duchenne dystrophy develop scoliosis rapidly after they can no longer stand and walk independently. This may be delayed, but not prevented, by prolonging ambulation as long as possible through early contracture release and bracing, and by providing a rigid (celastic or perforated orthoplast isoprene) torso support and a firm level pelvic seat when wheelchair confinement becomes inevitable, before the onset of spinal curvature. These spines are essentially flaccid and respond to the exoskeletal thoracopelvic distribution forces such a jacket provides. Spinal

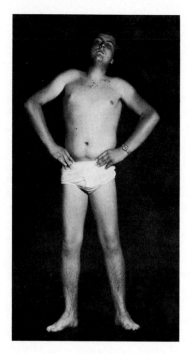

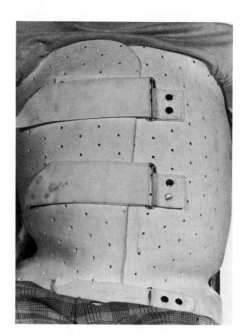

FIG. 15.   **FIG. 16.**

alignment is obtained by supporting the abdomen, elevating the ribs from a contoured pelvic foundation, and [using residual neck extension strength (5)] forcing the shoulders back and maximizing lumbar lordosis (Fig. 16). With correction of abdominal ptosis, the diaphragm is allowed increased freedom of movement and vital capacity is thereby enhanced. Such an appliance must be refitted as the child grows. The Milwaukee brace is of little use here as it is a dynamic orthosis, and patients in the later stages of muscle disease lack strength to exercise in the appliance.

Facioscapulohumeral dystrophy is rapidly progressive when onset occurs in childhood (19). It is also one of the few muscular dystrophies that may be asymmetric in distribution. Thus scoliosis is not uncommonly seen while patients are still walking, at which time spinal deformity can prevent body alignment and hinder ambulation.

Weakness in this form of dystrophy is usually less than in the other kinds of childhood myopathy, and prognosis for continued function and life expectancy is, as a general rule, more hopeful. These patients tolerate major spinal surgery well, muscle strength permits use of the Milwaukee brace, and their scolioses are generally amenable to more traditional forms of therapy.

Several illustrative cases follow.

Case 1

A 12-year-old girl was first noted to have a left midtorsal scoliosis, well compensated at age 10 (Fig. 17). She was treated conservatively with exercise for 2.5 years; at that time her curve measured 47° (Fig. 18). This was corrected to 10° in a Risser plaster jacket, and her spine fused from D-6 to D-12 (Fig. 19). She was maintained in plaster for 10 months, the first 5 of which were nonambulatory.

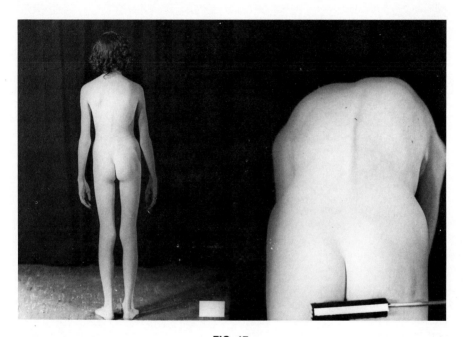

FIG. 17.

After removal of her cast she ambulated well, but some weakness of the shoulders was noted. This progressed until definite scapular winging became apparent (Fig. 20), almost 3 years after spinal fusion. Examination at that time revealed the stigmata of facioscapulohumeral dystrophy, and over the following year weakness and deformity progressed until she developed bilateral foot drop, severe lordosis, and the typical facies of this disease (Fig. 21).

She is now 30 years old, 18 years post-fusion. Her curvature has not progressed and she continues to be ambulatory. She may have had a typical juvenile idiopathic scoliosis; however, one cannot help but wonder if immobilization hastened the onset and progress of her primary muscle disease.

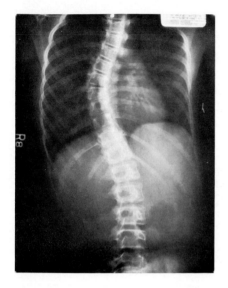

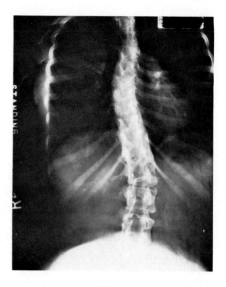

FIG. 18.   FIG. 19.

Case 2

A 13-year-old boy had far-advanced facioscapulohumeral dystrophy. A left cervical, severe, long thoracolumbar scoliosis to the right, with marked posterior rib angulation, was present (Fig. 22). A Risser-type corrective body jacket cast was applied, and it improved the patient's gait.

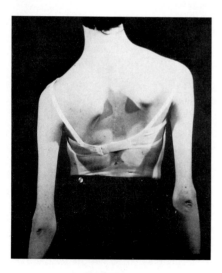

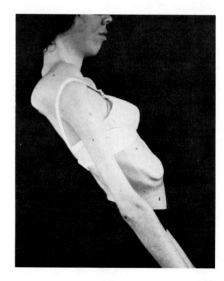

FIG. 20.   FIG. 21.

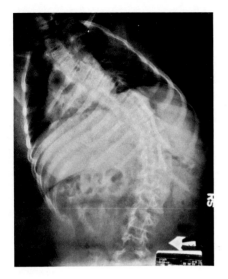

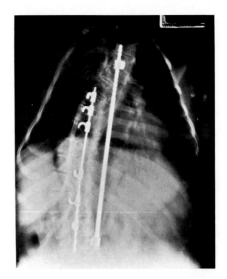

FIG. 22.   **FIG. 23.**

His curve was quite flexible in the upper portion and decreased significantly with traction. A localizer cast was fitted and a spinal fusion with Harrington rod instrumentation from D-3 to L-3 performed (Fig. 23). Shortly after surgery he was allowed up on a tilt table, and from there he progressed to parallel bars and a walker. One month later a halo was applied under local anesthesia, and this was subsequently attached to a Milwaukee brace. He was ambulated in the halo and brace. After 5 months the halo was removed and a standard Milwaukee brace chin piece substituted (Fig. 24).

In spite of severe collapsing paralytic scoliosis secondary to far-advanced myopathy, this patient tolerated surgery well, and the use of Harrington spinal instrumentation, augmented by the halo and Milwaukee brace, permitted correction of his curve with early mobilization.

In summary, the treatment of scoliosis in muscular dystrophy depends on the type and degree of myopathy present. Childhood myotonia is uncomplicated by spinal curvature. Patients with limb-girdle dystrophy, which usually begins in middle or late adolescence and progresses slowly, are often ambulatory well into the third decade and seldom show scoliosis severe enough to warrant treatment.

Duchenne dystrophics develop scoliosis only late during their ambulatory phase, and this can often be avoided by lower extremity contracture release and long leg bracing. Almost all these patients become scoliotic when they can no longer walk. This incidentally has also been noted in spastics (39% of bedridden spastics are scoliotic versus 7% of spastics still ambulatory). As patients with Duchenne dystrophy do not tolerate major spinal operations well, they are best treated by rigid torso bracing, applied after wheel-

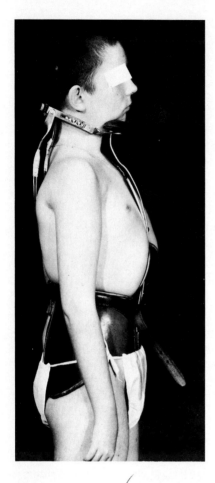

FIG. 24.

chair confinement, preferably as prophylactic therapy before the appearance of spinal curvature. The appliance must be fitted early as such patients tend to slump in the wheelchair because it takes less effort than sitting upright and, for a time at least, it is comfortable using the arms from the slumped position.

Because facioscapulohumeral dystrophy may be asymmetric in distribution, structural scoliosis is often a complication of its childhood form and can interfere with balance and walking. However, these patients are amenable to more traditional forms of treatment owing to their slow progression and relative maintenance of strength. In selected cases an aggressive program of surgery and bracing can arrest spinal deformity, thus maintaining ambulatory function.

In contrast, some patients with scoliosis secondary to infantile spinal muscular atrophy and its benign variants are candidates for spinal fusion and bracing. Generally in these cases, as in muscular dystrophy, the later the onset, the less severe the paralysis. Operative intervention in such patients is indicated when the curve is progressive and greater than 30 to 40° in spite of bracing, assuming the course of the neurological disease has stabilized. These patients require close attention to pulmonary function before, during, and after surgery. Because they have a poor pulmonary reserve, surgery causes an absolute loss of vital capacity for several weeks after operation. This is related to pain, overstretching of intercostal muscles on the concave side of the curve with relaxation of intercostals on the convex side, compression of the convex lung with overexpansion of the concave lung, and decreased reserve in the accessory muscles of respiration (H. K. Dunn, *personal communication*).

The prolonged work of postoperative breathing is exhausting to these patients, and although they can be managed with an indwelling transnasal or transtracheotomy intertracheal tube, the use of a tank respirator is better tolerated.

SUMMARY

Correction of deformity and maintenance of the upright posture have increased self-reliant skills, thus significantly enhancing the quality of life for the child with muscular dystrophy.

In addition, such techniques offer a method of prolonging independent ambulation and, in so doing, forestall confinement to a wheelchair or bed with its inevitable downhill course.

Surgery and bracing, accurately indicated and properly timed, play an important role in the total rehabilitation of the patient with muscular dystrophy.

REFERENCES

1. Archibald, K. C., and Vignos, P. J., Jr. (1959): A study of contractures in muscular dystrophy. *Arch. Phys. Med. Rehabil.*, 40:150–157.
2. Cobham, I. G., and Davis, H. S. (1964): Anesthesia for muscular dystrophy patients. *Anesth. Analg. (Cleve.)*, 43:22–29.
3. Cohen, P. J. (1972): Halogenated anesthetic and patients with elevated CPK level. *J.A.M.A.*, 220:9.
4. Eyring, E. J., Johnson, E. W., and Burnett, C. (1972): Surgery in muscular dystrophy. *J.A.M.A.*, 222:8.
5. Gibson, D. A., and Wilkins, K. E. (1975): The management of spinal deformities in Duchenne muscular dystrophy. A new concept of spinal bracing. *Clin. Orthop.*, 108:41–51.
6. Gucker, T., III (1964): The orthopedic management of progressive muscular dystrophy. *J. Am. Phys. Ther. Assoc.*, 44(4):243–246.
7. Johnson, E. W., and Kennedy, J. H. (1971): Comprehensive management of Duchenne muscular dystrophy. *Arch. Phys. Med. Rehabil.*, 110–114.
8. Miller, J. (1967): Management of muscular dystrophy. *J. Bone Joint Surg.*, 49-A(6):1205–1211.
9. Roy, L., and Gibson, D. A. (1970): Pseudohypertrophic muscular dystrophy and its surgical management: Review of 30 patients. *Can. J. Surg.*, 13:13–21.
10. Siegel, I. M. (1972): Equinocavovarus in muscular dystrophy. *Arch. Surg.*, 104:644–646.

11. Siegel, I. M. (1972): Pathomechanics of stance in Duchenne muscular dystrophy. *Arch. Phys. Med. Rehabil.,* 53:403–406.
12. Siegel, I. M. (1973): Scoliosis in muscular dystrophy. *Clin. Orthop.,* 93:235–238.
13. Siegel, I. M. (1975): Plastic-molded knee-ankle-foot orthoses in the treatment of Duchenne muscular dystrophy. *Arch. Phys. Med. Rehabil.,* 56:322.
14. Siegel, I. M., Miller, J. E., and Ray, R. D. (1968): Subcutaneous lower limb tenotomy in the treatment of pseudohypertrophic muscular dystrophy. *J. Bone Joint Surg.,* 50-A:1437–1443.
15. Spencer, G. E., Jr. (1967): Orthopaedic care of progressive muscular dystrophy. *J. Bone Joint Surg.,* 49-A(6):1201–1204.
16. Spencer, G. E., Jr. (1973): Recent advances in orthopaedics. In: *Orthopaedic Considerations in the Management of Muscular Dystrophy,* edited by J. Ahstrom, pp. 279–293. Williams & Wilkins Co., Baltimore.
17. Spencer, G. E., Jr., and Vignos, P. J., Jr. (1962): Bracing for ambulation in childhood progressive muscular dystrophy. *J. Bone Joint Surg.,* 44-A:234–242.
18. Vignos, P. J., Jr., and Archibald, K. C. (1960): Maintenance of ambulation in childhood muscular dystrophy. *J. Chronic Dis.,* 12:273–290.
19. Zundel, W. S., and Tyler, F. H. (1965): The muscular dystrophies (birth defects reprint series). *N. Engl. J. Med.,* 273:537–543.

Subject Index